Handbook of
Pediatric and Neonatal Emergencies

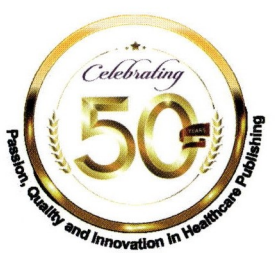

Handbook of
Pediatric and Neonatal Emergencies

Editor

S Sushamabai MD DCH FIMSA FIAP
Professor and Head
Department of Pediatrics
Pushpagiri Medical College
Pushpagiri Institute of Medical Sciences and Research Center
Thiruvalla, Kerala, India
Former Professor and Head
Department of Pediatrics
Government Medical College
Kottayam, Kerala, India
Email: drsushamabai@gmail.com

Foreword
Professor (Dr) MKC Nair

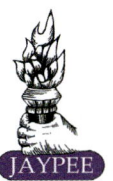

JAYPEE BROTHERS MEDICAL PUBLISHERS
The Health Sciences Publisher
New Delhi | London | Panama

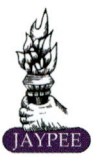
Jaypee Brothers Medical Publishers (P) Ltd.

Headquarters
Jaypee Brothers Medical Publishers (P) Ltd
4838/24, Ansari Road, Daryaganj
New Delhi 110 002, India
Phone: +91-11-43574357
Fax: +91-11-43574314
Email: jaypee@jaypeebrothers.com

Overseas Offices

J.P. Medical Ltd
83 Victoria Street, London
SW1H 0HW (UK)
Phone: +44 20 3170 8910
Fax: +44 (0)20 3008 6180
Email: info@jpmedpub.com

Jaypee-Highlights Medical Publishers Inc
City of Knowledge, Bld. 235, 2nd Floor
Clayton, Panama City, Panama
Phone: +1 507-301-0496
Fax: +1 507-301-0499
Email: cservice@jphmedical.com

Jaypee Brothers Medical Publishers (P) Ltd
Bhotahity, Kathmandu, Nepal
Phone: +977-9741283608
Email: kathmandu@jaypeebrothers.com

Website: www.jaypeebrothers.com
Website: www.jaypeedigital.com

© 2020, Jaypee Brothers Medical Publishers

The views and opinions expressed in this book are solely those of the original contributor(s)/author(s) and do not necessarily represent those of editor(s) of the book.

All rights reserved. No part of this publication may be reproduced, stored or transmitted in any form or by any means, electronic, mechanical, photocopying, recording or otherwise, without the prior permission in writing of the publishers.

All brand names and product names used in this book are trade names, service marks, trademarks or registered trademarks of their respective owners. The publisher is not associated with any product or vendor mentioned in this book.

Medical knowledge and practice change constantly. This book is designed to provide accurate, authoritative information about the subject matter in question. However, readers are advised to check the most current information available on procedures included and check information from the manufacturer of each product to be administered, to verify the recommended dose, formula, method and duration of administration, adverse effects and contraindications. It is the responsibility of the practitioner to take all appropriate safety precautions. Neither the publisher nor the author(s)/editor(s) assume any liability for any injury and/or damage to persons or property arising from or related to use of material in this book.

This book is sold on the understanding that the publisher is not engaged in providing professional medical services. If such advice or services are required, the services of a competent medical professional should be sought.

Every effort has been made where necessary to contact holders of copyright to obtain permission to reproduce copyright material. If any have been inadvertently overlooked, the publisher will be pleased to make the necessary arrangements at the first opportunity. The **CD/DVD-ROM** (if any) provided in the sealed envelope with this book is complimentary and free of cost. **Not meant for sale.**

Inquiries for bulk sales may be solicited at: jaypee@jaypeebrothers.com

Handbook of Pediatric and Neonatal Emergencies

First Edition: **2020**

ISBN: 978-93-5270-614-3

Printed at: Samrat Offset Pvt. Ltd.

Dedicated to

K Rajagopalan, my husband for the upstanding support
Raj Anand, my son for the help and encouragement
and all above
GOD Almighty for showing me the right path.

Contributors

Bibin Sajan MBBS
Resident
Department of Pediatrics
Pushpagiri Medical College
Thiruvalla, Kerala, India
Email: drbibinsajan@gmail.com

Carol Sara Cherian MD
Associate Professor
Department of Pediatrics
Pushpagiri Medical College
Thiruvalla, Kerala, India
Email: benjicarol@gmail.com

Ingale Vinod C DNB (Ped)
Senior Resident
Department of Pediatrics
Pushpagiri Medical College
Thiruvalla, Kerala, India
Email: dr. vinodingale@gmail.com

Jacob Abraham MD
Fellowship in Neonatology
Professor
Department of Pediatrics
In-charge Neonatology
Pushpagiri Medical College
Thiruvalla, Kerala, India
Email: drjacobab@hotmail.com

Manju George Elenjickal DNB (Ped)
Fellowship in Epilepsy and Neurology
Associate Professor
Department of Pediatrics
In-charge Child Development Centre
Pushpagiri Medical College
Thiruvalla, Kerala, India
Email: mysticmanju@rediffmail.com

Mathew Varghese DNB (Ped)
Senior Resident
Department of Pediatrics
Pushpagiri Medical College
Thiruvalla, Kerala, India
Email: revin_6@hotmail.com

N Krishnan Nampoothiri MD
Fellowship in Neonatology
Professor
Department of Pediatrics
Pushpagiri Medical College
Thiruvalla, Kerala, India
Former Professor and Head
Department of Pediatrics
Government Medical College
Thrissur, Kerala, India
Email: Krishnankmri54@gmail.com

P Jayasree MD DCH MRCPCH
Associate Professor
Department of Pediatrics
Pushpagiri Medical College
Thiruvalla, Kerala, India
Email: jayasreeanand6@gmail.com

S Letha MD DCH
Professor
Department of Pediatrics
Pushpagiri Medical College
Thiruvalla, Kerala, India
Former Professor and Head
Department of Pediatrics
Government Medical College
Kottayam, Kerala, India
Email: drletha@gmail.com

S Sushamabai MD DCH FIMSA FIAP
Professor and Head
Department of Pediatrics
Pushpagiri Medical College
Pushpagiri Institute of Medical Sciences
and Research Center
Thiruvalla, Kerala, India
Former Professor and Head of Pediatrics
Government Medical College
Kottayam, Kerala, India
Email: drsushamabai@gmail.com

Seany T Varghese MD
Assistant Professor
Department of Pediatrics
Pushpagiri Medical College
Thiruvalla, Kerala, India
Email: abveapen@gmail.com

Foreword

I am pleased to write the Foreword for *Handbook of Pediatric and Neonatal Emergencies*, 1st edition by S Sushamabai, because of the paucity of books solely on emergency care, especially from Kerala and also because proper management of childhood emergencies will definitely reduce the infant mortality rate. Illnesses and emergencies differ in different parts of the world as well as within a country itself, so that treatment protocols may require modification according to the situation. This book is particularly beneficial in dealing with the pediatric emergencies encountered in Asian countries.

There are 125 chapters in this book. The initial five chapters deal with the setting up of a Pediatric Intensive Care Unit and its functioning, which is helpful for the beginners in pediatrics to step into emergency care. Procedures and drug dosages are also included and the topics are presented in simple language, point projected and with systematic approach. Tables, diagrams and flowcharts are included in most chapters facilitating quick approach.

The contributors of this book are well-known faculty for their expertise, clinical acumen, astute patient care and academic excellence. S Sushamabai is one of the stalwarts in the field of pediatrics, a great academician, who has revealed a genuine interest to bring up the emergency care services for children in whichever hospitals she had worked.

I am happy to recommend this book as a bedside companion to residents in pediatrics and nurses working in pediatric emergency care department. Further, this book will be of undeniable help for the pediatricians working single-handed in peripheral health services, whether in government or private sector, since they are the group of doctors encountering the vast majority of emergencies at first.

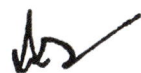

Professor (Dr) MKC Nair
MD PhD M Med Sc MBA MA FNNF FIAP FIACAM
Founder Director, Child Development Centre, Kerala, India
National President, Indian Academy of Pediatrics (IAP: 2004)
National President, National Neonatology Forum (NNF) (2011-2012)
Vice Chancellor Kerala University of Health Sciences
www.kuhs.ac.in Phone: +91 487-2207664 Fax: +91 487 2206770 e-mail: vc@kuhs.ac.in

Preface

Emergencies denote serious and unexpected situations requiring immediate intervention. In medical situations, they herald death or disability to the affected person which can be prevented by prompt and appropriate treatment.

Unlike the situation in adults, children rapidly plunge into critically ill stage because of the immaturity of organs and systems. The clinical manifestations will be subtle in them delaying the exact diagnosis and subsequently denying the right treatment. But if revived in the golden hour, the prognosis and complete recovery are far better in children, thus reducing the infant mortality rate and improving the manpower of the country. Hence, it is mandatory that the fraternity involved in child health should be updated with advances in emergency management.

This handbook deals with the childhood emergencies, especially from Asian countries. Most childhood emergencies have a typical clinical presentation, but at times may reveal the uncommon presentation of a common illness or the common presentation of an uncommon illness. I have incorporated my long years of clinical experience from wherever I have worked, which include less privileged areas to high technology centers in diagnosis and patient approach, ultimately getting good survival rate.

I sincerely hope that this book will be beneficial to every beginner in pediatrics to bring up self-skills and confidence in managing emergencies and an added help to all pediatricians working in the peripheral hospitals shouldering great responsibility.

S Sushamabai

Acknowledgments

I acknowledge the prompt and immense help of Mr VKG Nair, the Chief Librarian of the Pushpagiri Institute of Medical Sciences and Research Centre, Thiruvalla, Kerala, India, for sorting out the large number of references for this manuscript.

This textbook reflects the meritorious work of the contributors, each one having vast experience in managing pediatric emergencies. I appreciate their hard work and dedication in providing the chapters entrusted to them in time.

Ms Annamma AV and Ms Remya Krishnan deserve special thanks for taking up the huge responsibility of the computer work for this manuscript with enthusiasm and good will, sacrificing their free time.

I am thankful to Mr Sreeraj of Alumni Association, Government Medical College, Kottayam Kerala, for helping me with the emailing of important matters at the right time for the manuscript.

My husband K Rajagopalan was the real spirit and moral support behind me for preparing this text and my son Raj Anand with his amazing computer knowledge has helped me in preparing the difficult flow charts and tables for it. My grand daughters Shivani and Vedika and my daughter-in-law Dina Raj were encouraging me in bringing out this manual.

I am indebted to the innumerable number of sick children cared by me in the emergency departments of various hospitals I have worked and to their parents, for being the real eye openers stimulating me to read extensively and bring out this text.

The pediatricians working single-handed in peripheral hospitals with constraints have inspired me for the preparation of this text, which I think will be much helpful to them.

I remember with gratitude Dr V Jose Kuruvilla, my colleague for long years, but passed away in the early stage of preparation of this manuscript, who used to remind me very often the scarcity of simple books for caring the emergencies in children.

I am extremely grateful to Professor (Dr MKC Nair), Vice Chancellor, Kerala University of Health Sciences for providing a nice and generous foreword to this manuscript, in time, amidst his heavy schedules.

This is my second textbook getting published by M/s Jaypee Brothers Medical Publishers (P) Ltd., New Delhi, India. I am extremely grateful to Shri Jitendar P Vij (Group Chairman), Mr Ankit Vij (Managing Director), Ms Chetna Malhotra Vohra (Associate Director–Content Strategy) of M/s Jaypee Brothers Medical Publishers (P) Ltd, for accepting my manuscript for publication for the second time.

Contents

SECTION 1: CONCEPT OF INTENSIVE CARE

1. **Setting Up of Pediatric Intensive Care Unit** 3
   Seany T Varghese, S Sushamabai
2. **Daily Routine in PICU** 9
   Seany T Varghese, S Sushamabai
3. **PICU Rounds and Documentation** 11
   Seany T Varghese, S Sushamabai
4. **Communication in PICU** 16
   Seany T Varghese, S Sushamabai
5. **Ethics in PICU** 18
   Seany T Varghese, S Sushamabai

SECTION 2: RESUSCITATION

6. **Pediatric Basic Life Support** 23
   P Jayasree, S Sushamabai
7. **Pediatric Advanced Life Support** 31
   P Jayasree, S Sushamabai
8. **Rapid Sequence Intubation** 41
   P Jayasree, S Sushamabai
9. **Resuscitation Equipment and Drugs** 47
   P Jayasree, S Sushamabai
10. **Post-resuscitation Care** 50
    P Jayasree, S Sushamabai
11. **Anaphylaxis** 54
    S Sushamabai
12. **Oxygen Therapy** 58
    P Jayasree, S Sushamabai

SECTION 3: DETECTION OF THE ACUTELY ILL CHILD

13. **Assessment in the Emergency Room** 67
    S Sushamabai
14. **Clinical Scoring Systems** 70
    S Sushamabai

15. **Arterial Blood Gas Analysis** 74
   S Sushamabai

SECTION 4: RESPIRATORY SYSTEM

16. **Mechanical Ventilation** 83
   Carol Sara Cherian, S Sushamabai

17. **Foreign Body Obstruction of the Airway** 93
   S Sushamabai

18. **Acute Stridor** 95
   Carol Sara Cherian, S Sushamabai

19. **Acute Asthma** 100
   Carol Sara Cherian, S Sushamabai

20. **Acute Bronchiolitis** 106
   S Sushamabai

21. **Pneumonia** 111
   Carol Sara Cherian, S Sushamabai

22. **Empyema** 116
   S Sushamabai

23. **Pneumothorax and Pneumomediastinum** 120
   Carol Sara Cherian, S Sushamabai

24. **Acute Respiratory Distress Syndrome** 124
   S Sushamabai

SECTION 5: CARDIOVASCULAR SYSTEM

25. **Shock** 129
   S Sushamabai

26. **Cardiac Arrhythmias** 137
   Carol Sara Cherian, S Sushamabai

27. **Congestive Heart Failure** 143
   S Sushamabai

28. **Hypercyanotic Attacks (Tet Spells)** 147
   S Sushamabai

29. **Viral Myocarditis** 150
   S Sushamabai

30. **Rheumatic Carditis** 154
   S Sushamabai

31. **Pericardial Effusion** 158
   S Sushamabai

32. **Hypertensive Crisis** 161
S Sushamabai

SECTION 6: NERVOUS SYSTEM

33. **Raised Intracranial Pressure** 167
Manju George Elenjickal, S Sushamabai

34. **Comatose Child** 171
S Sushamabai

35. **Status Epilepticus** 176
Manju George Elenjickal, S Sushamabai

36. **Encephalitis** 182
Manju George Elenjickal, S Sushamabai

37. **Acute Bacterial Meningitis** 185
S Sushamabai

38. **Tuberculous Meningitis** 188
S Sushamabai

39. **Guillain–Barré Syndrome** 191
Manju George Elenjickal, S Sushamabai

40. **Acute Disseminated Encephalomyelitis** 194
S Sushamabai

41. **Myasthenic Paralysis** 197
Manju George Elenjickal, S Sushamabai

42. **Subdural Empyema** 201
S Sushamabai

43. **Acute Stroke in Children** 204
Manju George Elenjickal, S Sushamabai

44. **Intracranial Hemorrhage** 208
S Sushamabai

45. **Head Injury** 212
S Sushamabai

46. **Pain Management and Sedation** 216
Manju George Elenjickal, S Sushamabai

47. **Brain Death and Legal Aspects** 221
Manju George Elenjickal, S Sushamabai

SECTION 7: ENDOCRINE AND METABOLIC EMERGENCIES

48. **Diabetic Ketoacidosis** 227
S Sushamabai

49.	**Acute Adrenocortical Insufficiency** *S Sushamabai*	232
50.	**Puberty Menorrhagia** *S Sushamabai*	235
51.	**Diabetes Insipidus** *S Sushamabai*	239
52.	**Thyroid Crisis** *S Sushamabai*	242
53.	**Disorders of Electrolyte Metabolism** *S Sushamabai*	244
54.	**Hyperammonemia** *S Sushamabai*	260
55.	**Approach to Inborn Errors of Metabolism** *S Sushamabai*	265
56.	**Heat Stroke** *Manju George Elenjickal, S Sushamabai*	268
57.	**Severe Acute Malnutrition** *S Sushamabai*	272
58.	**Intravenous Fluid Therapy** *S Sushamabai*	278

SECTION 8: RENAL SYSTEM

59.	**Acute Kidney Injury** *S Sushamabai*	285
60.	**Renal Tubular Acidosis** *S Sushamabai*	291
61.	**Hematuria** *S Sushamabai*	295
62.	**Acute Pyelonephritis** *S Sushamabai*	298

SECTION 9: GASTROINTESTINAL SYSTEM

63.	**Fulminant Hepatic Failure** *Carol Sara Cherian, S Sushamabai*	305
64.	**Reye Syndrome** *S Sushamabai*	311
65.	**Acute Diarrhea and Dehydration** *Carol Sara Cherian, S Sushamabai*	314

66. **Gastrointestinal Bleeding** *Carol Sara Cherian, S Sushamabai*	321
67. **Acute Pancreatitis** *S Sushamabai*	327
68. **Ascites** *S Sushamabai*	332

SECTION 10: INFECTIOUS DISEASES

69. **Dengue Shock Syndrome** *S Sushamabai*	339
70. **Fulminant Meningococcemia** *S Sushamabai*	346
71. **Toxic Shock Syndrome** *S Sushamabai*	349
72. **Malaria** *S Sushamabai*	352
73. **Leptospirosis** *S Sushamabai*	358
74. **Rickettsial Infections** *S Sushamabai*	361
75. **Invasive Fungal Infections** *S Sushamabai*	364
76. **Hospital-acquired Infections** *S Letha, S Sushamabai*	370

SECTION 11: CONNECTIVE TISSUE DISORDERS

77. **Kawasaki Disease** *S Sushamabai*	377
78. **Macrophage Activation Syndrome** *S Sushamabai*	381

SECTION 12: HEMATOLOGY ONCOLOGY

79. **Blood and Blood Component Therapy** *S Sushamabai*	387
80. **Transfusion Reactions** *Bibin Sajan, S Sushamabai*	391
81. **Intravenous Immunoglobulin Therapy** *S Sushamabai*	395

82.	**Hemolytic Uremic Syndrome** *N Krishnan Nampoothiri, S Sushamabai*	399
83.	**Disseminated Intravascular Coagulation** *N Krishnan Nampoothiri, S Sushamabai*	402
84.	**Sickle Cell Crisis** *N Krishnan Nampoothiri, S Sushamabai*	405
85.	**Hemophilias** *S Sushamabai*	409
86.	**Oncologic Emergencies** *P Jayasree, S Sushamabai*	413
87.	**Anticoagulant and Thrombolytic Therapy** *N Krishnan Nampoothiri, S Sushamabai*	416

SECTION 13: ACCIDENTS, POISONING, AND ENVENOMATION

88.	**Drowning and Submersion Injuries** *S Letha, S Sushamabai*	423
89.	**Burn Injuries** *S Letha, S Sushamabai*	427
90.	**Inadvertent Intra-arterial Injection** *Bibin Sajan, S Sushamabai*	431
91.	**Hanging** *Manju George Elenjickal, S Sushamabai*	434
92.	**Cold Injuries** *Manju George Elenjickal, S Sushamabai*	438
93A.	**Poisoning in Children** *S Sushamabai*	442
93B.	**Other Poisonings: Symptomatology and Management** *S Sushamabai*	447
94A.	**Snake Envenomation** *S Sushamabai*	452
94B.	**Scorpion Envenomation** *S Letha, S Sushamabai*	457
94C.	**Bee and Wasp Stinging** *S Letha, S Sushamabai*	461
95.	**Rat-bite Fever** *S Sushamabai*	464

SECTION 14: NEONATOLOGY

96. **Handwashing and Sepsis Prevention** — 469
    Jacob Abraham, S Sushamabai

97. **Care of the Normal Newborn** — 471
    Jacob Abraham, S Sushamabai

98. **Danger Signs in the Newborn** — 474
    Jacob Abraham, S Sushamabai

99. **Neonatal Hypothermia** — 475
    Jacob Abraham, S Sushamabai

100. **Neonatal Resuscitation** — 478
    Ingale Vinod C, Mathew Varghese, Jacob Abraham

101. **Neonatal Ventilation** — 482
    Ingale Vinod C, Mathew Varghese, Jacob Abraham

102. **Fluid Therapy in Newborns** — 488
    Jacob Abraham, S Sushamabai

103. **Admission to the Neonatal Intensive Care Unit** — 491
    Jacob Abraham, S Sushamabai

104. **Neonatal Convulsions** — 493
    Jacob Abraham, S Sushamabai

105. **Neonatal Hypoglycemia** — 496
    Jacob Abraham, S Sushamabai

106. **Neonatal Hypocalcemia** — 498
    Jacob Abraham, S Sushamabai

107. **Neonatal Jaundice** — 500
    Jacob Abraham, S Sushamabai

108. **Neonatal Sepsis** — 505
    Jacob Abraham, S Sushamabai

109. **Apnea in Newborns** — 509
    Jacob Abraham, S Sushamabai

110. **Bleeding Neonate** — 512
    Jacob Abraham, S Sushamabai

111. **Anemia in Newborns** — 514
    Jacob Abraham, S Sushamabai

112. **Neonatal Transport** — 518
    Jacob Abraham, S Sushamabai

113. **Discharge Protocol** — 520
    Jacob Abraham, S Sushamabai

114. Audiology Screening in Neonates — 522
Jacob Abraham, S Sushamabai

115. Visual Screening in Newborns — 524
Jacob Abraham, S Sushamabai

SECTION 15: PROCEDURES

116. Lumbar Puncture — 529
S Sushamabai

117. Central Venous Access — 532
S Sushamabai

118. Peripheral Arterial Cannulation — 536
S Sushamabai

119. Intraosseous Access — 539
S Sushamabai

120. Needle Thoracocentesis — 541
S Sushamabai

121. Pericardiocentesis — 543
S Sushamabai

122. Ascitic Fluid Tap — 545
S Sushamabai

123. Suprapubic Urine Aspiration — 547
S Sushamabai

124. Liver Biopsy — 549
S Sushamabai

SECTION 16: PEDIATRIC DRUG FORMULARY

125. Pediatric Drug Formulary — 555
S Sushamabai

Index — 569

List of Abbreviations

μg	:	Microgram
ABC	:	Airway, Breathing, Circulation
ABG	:	Arterial Blood Gas
ACE	:	Angiotensin Converting Enzyme
ACHD	:	Acyanotic Congenital Heart Disease
ACT	:	Artemisinin Combination Therapy
ACTH	:	Adrenocorticotropic Hormone
ADD	:	Acute Diarrheal Disease
ADEM	:	Acute Demyelinating Encephalomyelitis
AED	:	Automated External Defibrillation
AF	:	Anterior Fontanel
AFB	:	Acid Fast Bacilli
AFP	:	Acute Flaccid Paralysis
AHA	:	American Heart Association
AKI	:	Acute Kidney Injury
ALCAPA	:	Anomalous Origin of Left Coronary Artery from Pulmonary Artery
ART	:	Anti-Retroviral Therapy
ASO	:	Antistreptolysin O
ASV	:	Anti-Snake Venom
AVPU	:	Alert, Verbal, Pain, Unresponsive
BERA	:	Brain Stem Evoked Response Audiometry
BLS	:	Basic Life Support
BMI	:	Body Mass Index
BMV	:	Bag and Mask Ventilation
BSA	:	Body Surface Area
BU	:	Blood Urea
CAH	:	Congenital Adrenal Hyperplasia
CAP	:	Community-acquired Pneumonia
CBC	:	Complete Blood Count
CBG	:	Capillary Blood Glucose
CCF	:	Congestive Cardiac Failure
CCHD	:	Congenital Cyanotic Heart Disease
CHB	:	Complete Heart Block
CHF	:	Congestive Heart Failure
CoA	:	Coarctation of Aorta
CPAP	:	Continuous Positive Airway Pressure

CPK	:	Creatinine Phospho Kinase
CPP	:	Cerebral Perfusion Pressure
CRFT	:	Capillary Refill Time
CRP	:	C-reactive Protein
CSF	:	Cerebro-spinal Fluid
CVP	:	Central Venous Pressure
CxR	:	Chest X-ray
DCT	:	Direct Coombs Test
DIC	:	Disseminated Intravascular Coagulation
DKA	:	Diabetic Ketoacidosis
DLC	:	Differential Leukocyte Count
DNS	:	Dextrose Normal Saline
DRL	:	Dextrose Ringer Lactate
EBM	:	Expressed Breast Milk
ECG	:	Electrocardiograph
ECMO	:	Extra Corporeal Membrane Oxygenation
EEG	:	Electroencephalo Graph
ESR	:	Erythrocyte Sedimentation Rate
ET/T_E	:	Expiratory Time
ETT	:	Endotracheal Tube
FiO_2	:	Fraction of Inspired Oxygen
FB	:	Foreign Body
FDP	:	Fibrin Degradation Product
Fe Na	:	Fractional Excretion of Sodium
FFP	:	Fresh Frozen Plasma
FHF	:	Fulminant Hepatic Failure
FOUR SCORE	:	Full Outline of Un Responsiveness Score
FTT	:	Failure To Thrive
GAS	:	Group A *Streptococcus*
GBS	:	Group B *Streptococcus*
GCS	:	Glasgow Coma Scale
GERD	:	Gastroesophageal Reflux Disease
HCT	:	Hematocrit
HDN	:	Hemorrhagic Disease of the Newborn
HIE	:	Hypoxic Ischemic Encephalopathy
HIV	:	Human Immunodeficiency Virus
HMD	:	Hyaline Membrane Disease
HR	:	Heart Rate
hr	:	Hourly
Hrs	:	Hours
HSV	:	Herpes Simplex Virus
HUS	:	Hemolytic Uremic Syndrome

I:E	:	Inspiration : Expiration
ICD	:	Intercostal Drainage
ICH	:	Intracranial Hemorrhage
ICP	:	Intracranial Pressure
ICS	:	Inhaled Corticosteroid
ICSOL	:	Intracranial Space Occupying Lesion
ICU	:	Intensive Care Unit
IEM	:	Inborn Errors of Metabolism
Ig	:	Immunoglobulin
IM	:	Intramuscular
INR	:	International Normalized Ratio
IO	:	Intraosseous
IT	:	Intratracheal
ITP	:	Immune Thrombocytopenic Purpura
IV	:	Intravenous
IVH	:	Intraventricular Hemorrhage
JVP	:	Jugular Venous Pressure
KD	:	Kawasaki Disease
LBW	:	Low Birth Weight
LFT	:	Liver Function Test
LGA	:	Large for Gestational Age
LP	:	Lumbar Puncture
M	:	Month/Months
M.TB	:	*Mycobacterium Tuberculosis*
MAP	:	Mean Arterial Pressure
MAS	:	Meconium Aspiration Syndrome
MCU	:	Micturating Cystourethrogram
min	:	Minutes
MODS	:	Multiorgan Dysfunction Syndrome
MP	:	Malarial Parasite
MRI	:	Magnetic Resonance Imaging
MRSA	:	Methicillin Resistant *Staphylococcus Aureus*
MUAC	:	Mid Upper Arm Circumference
Mx test	:	Mantoux test
Neb	:	Nebulization
NEC	:	Necrotising Enterocolitis
NG Tube	:	Nasogastric Tube
NIBP	:	Noninvasive Blood Pressure
NS	:	Normal Saline
O_2	:	Oxygen
OAE	:	Oto Acoustic Emission
OPA	:	Oropharyngeal Airway

ORS	:	Oral Rehydration Solution
ORT	:	Oral Rehydration Therapy
PAH	:	Pulmonary Arterial Hypertension
PALS	:	Pediatric Advanced Life Support
PCO_2	:	Partial Pressure of Carbondioxide
PCP	:	*Pneumocystis Carinii* Pneumonia
PCR	:	Polymerase Chain Reaction
PCV	:	Packed Cell Volume
PDA	:	Patent Ductus Arteriosus
PEEP	:	Positive End Expiratory Pressure
PEFR	:	Peak Expiratory Flow Rate
PEM	:	Protein Energy Malnutrition
PFO	:	Patent Foramen Ovale
PICU	:	Pediatric Intensive Care Unit
PIP	:	Peak Inspiratory Pressure
PLEDS	:	Periodic Lateralized Epileptiform Discharges
PO	:	Per Oral
PPE	:	Personal Protective Equipment
PPHN	:	Persistent Pulmonary Hypertension of Newborn
PPV	:	Positive Pressure Ventilation
PR	:	Per Rectal
PRBC	:	Packed Red Blood Cells
PRP	:	Platelet Rich Plasma
PT	:	Prothrombin Time
PTH	:	Parathyroid Hormone
PTT	:	Partial Thromboplastin Time
PVH	:	Pulmonary Venous Hypertension
RBS	:	Random Blood Sugar
RDA	:	Recommended Daily Allowance
RDS	:	Respiratory Distress Syndrome
RDT	:	Rapid Diagnostic Test
RFT	:	Renal Function Test
RHD	:	Rheumatic Heart Disease
RL	:	Ringer Lactate
RNTCP	:	Revised National Tuberculosis Control Program
Rpt	:	Repeat
RR	:	Respiratory Rate
RSI	:	Rapid Sequence Intubation
RTA	:	Renal Tubular Acidosis
SABA	:	Short Acting Beta Agonist
SAM	:	Severe Acute Malnutrition
SBP	:	Systolic Blood Pressure

SC	:	Sub cutaneous
Sch	:	Succinylcholine
SE	:	Serum Electrolytes
SGA	:	Small for Gestational Age
SIADH	:	Syndrome of Inappropriate ADH Secretion
SL	:	Sublingual
SLP	:	Serum Lipid Profile
SND	:	Sinus Node Dysfunction
SpO_2	:	Peripheral Capillary Oxygen Saturation
Sq Ft	:	Square Foot
SR	:	Sustained Release
SRUS	:	Solitary Rectal Ulcer Syndrome
SVO_2	:	Superior Venacaval Oxygen
SVT	:	Supraventricular Tachycardia
TA	:	Tricuspid Atresia
TBW	:	Total Body Water
TFT	:	Thyroid Function Test
TGA	:	Transposition of Great Arteries
Ti	:	Inspiratory Time
TOF	:	Tetralogy of Fallot
TPN	:	Total Parenteral Nutrition
TTN	:	Transient Tachypnea of Newborn
TTP	:	Thrombotic Thrombocytopenic Purpura
U	:	Unit
URT	:	Upper Respiratory Tract
USG	:	Ultra SonoGram
VAD	:	Ventricular Assist Device
VBG	:	Venous Blood Gas
VF	:	Ventricular Fibrillation
VLBW	:	Very Low Birth Weight
VSD	:	Ventricular Septal Defect
VT	:	Ventricular Tachycardia
VUR	:	Vesicoureteric Reflux
VZIG	:	Varicella Zoster Immuneglobulin
WBCT	:	Whole Blood Clotting Time
WBT	:	Whole Blood Transfusion
WHO	:	World Health Organization
WK	:	Week/Weeks
WOB	:	Work of Breathing
WPW	:	Wolf Parkinson White
Yr	:	Year

Section 1

CONCEPT OF INTENSIVE CARE

Chapter 1

Setting Up of Pediatric Intensive Care Unit

Seany T Varghese, S Sushamabai

ABSTRACT

Pediatric intensive care unit (PICU) should be separate from adult and newborn ICU. The bed number should depend upon the patient load and specialties to be cared providing 150–200 sq. ft. for each bed, should have separate isolation room, adequate equipment, electrical facilities, telephone services, and a well-placed central station to observe all patients. The staff pattern should comprise at least one intensivist, adequate number of pediatricians experienced in critical care management and mechanical ventilation round the clock, and enough residents to carry out the orders in time; experienced nurses in 1:1 ratio for unstable/ventilated patients, enough ancillary staff always available; well-equipped laboratory and radiology service close to the unit, good waste disposal system and periodic evaluation by the infection surveillance unit. Adequate equipment, periodically updated medicines and resuscitation equipment and drugs should be properly arranged. Proper register maintenance and reporting should be done by the MO in-charge.

UNIT DESIGN

Pediatric intensive care unit should be separate from neonatal and adult units dedicated solely to infants and children. Six to eight beds are ideal; should be more if the unit cares specialized surgery and trauma victims. Should be designed for future adaptability and be located near the lift, emergency department and operation theater.

Room Layout and Bed Area

- Room layout should allow actual visualization of all patients from central station.
- Patient area in open PICU should be 150–200 sq. ft.
- In a cubicle, the minimum area should be 200 sq. ft. with one wash basin.

- At least one room should have an isolation capability with an anteroom (separate area of 20 sq. ft. for handwashing, wearing mask and gown) and separate ventilation.
- The area around each bed should have enough space for performing procedures and bedside investigations.
- Easy access to head end of the patient for airway management is a must for all beds.
- Wall and ceilings should have sound absorption capability.
- Wall oxygen outlets (two), air outlet (one), suction outlets (two), and electrical outlets (10) for various equipment per bed are recommended.
- Windows should be provided in rooms to prevent the sense of isolation.
- Adequate lighting, child-friendly wall papering or painting with soothing colors and curtains are desirable.

Power Supply and Temperature Control

- Central air conditioning and central heating are preferable.
- Overhead warmers are a must if no central heating system.
- Uninterrupted power supply by backup power sources should be available.

ICU Beds

- Beds should have facility to elevate head and foot ends.
- Air/water mattresses (at least two) to prevent bedsores, should be available.
- All beds must have railing to prevent accidental fall.
- Emergency alarm button to activate code system (3) for each bed should be provided.
- There should be a cart at each bedside to keep personal belongings.

Crash Cart or Resuscitation Trolley

Resuscitation trolley should be equipped with emergency drugs and portable monitor or defibrillator; should have zones for medication preparation and cabinets for storage of medicines/materials.

Entry Doors

- Entry doors should be two in number—one for patients and another exclusively for the staff, which should be sufficiently away from the first door.
- The patient's door should be monitored by security staff.

Central Station

- Central station should have visibility to all patient areas.
- It should have ample space for necessary staff functions.

- It should be convenient enough to arrange the patients' records.
- It should provide adequate space for computer, printer, and file works for doctors and nurses.
- Three telephone lines are preferable (one dedicated to incoming calls and two for outgoing communications).
- X-ray viewer (with capacity to view several films at a time) can be placed at the central station or at a distinctive area.

Storage

- Refrigerator and essential drugs and items should be inside the PICU.
- Large patient care equipment and standby items should have a separate storeroom near the PICU; adequate area is needed for stretchers and wheelchairs.

Clean and Dirty Utility Rooms

- Clean utility room for storage of clean linen should be available.
- There must be separate dirty utility room for soiled linen and waste materials along with a separate sink.
- Provision for emptying and cleaning bedpans and urine bottles is necessary.

Waste Disposal

Waste disposal should be as per pollution control guidelines.

Communication Area

Communication area should be close to the PICU with adequate privacy.

LABORATORY SERVICES

Should have 24-hour availability with a reporting time of less than 1 hour; central along with side laboratory services are ideal.

OTHER FACILITIES

- Every PICU should have a well-prepared and updated PICU protocol for doctors and nurses.
- Doctor's duty room should be close to the PICU with intercom facility.
- PICU staff duty room with locker cabinets near the unit should be provided.
- Family waiting area for two persons (with bathroom and toilet facilities) is a must near the PICU.

EQUIPMENT (BOX 1.1)

- Equipment box should be selected on cost–benefit analysis but should be user-friendly.
- It should have proven use on pediatric patients and should be adapted for children.
- It should have warranty and biomedical service support (of the company and hospital).

> **Box 1.1:** Essential pediatric intensive care unit equipment.
>
> - Diagnostic equipment:
>   - Otoscope, ophthalmoscope, glucometer
>   - ECG, portable X-ray machine, EEG, blood gas analyzer
>   - Portable ultrasound and ECHO facilities.
> - Monitoring equipment:
>   - Oral and rectal thermometers
>   - Noninvasive multiparameter monitors
>   - Pulse oximeter
>   - Transducers
>   - Central venous pressure monitors
> - Procedural equipment:
>   - Emergency cart
>   - Butterfly needles (19–24 gauges)
>   - Micro infusion pumps
>   - Intravenous cannula (14–24 gauges)
>   - Portable suction
>   - Suction catheters (size 5–14 F)
>   - Ambu bags—neonatal (250 mL), pediatric (450 mL), adult (1000 mL)
>   - Oxygen masks—rebreather and non-rebreather (neonatal, pediatric, adult)
>   - Laryngoscope handles (pediatric, adult) with extra batteries
>   - Laryngoscope blades (straight 0–4; curved 2–3)
>   - Endotracheal tubes uncuffed (2.5–5.5), cuffed (6.0–8.0)
>   - Stylets (pediatric, adult)
>   - Laryngeal mask airway
>   - Oxygen delivery devices (nasal prongs, hood)
>   - Nasogastric tubes (6–14 F)
>   - Indwelling catheters
>   - Portable oxygen cylinders
>   - Blankets
>   - Overhead warmer/spotlight
>   - Nebulizer
>   - Oral airways (size 00–5)
>   - Nasal airways (size 12–30 F)
>   - Magill forceps (pediatric, adult)
>   - Intraosseous needles (16–18 gauges)
>   - Procedure light (portable)
>   - Ventilators (volume/pressure/PEEP support, low tidal volume capacity of 30–50 mL with nebulizer, humidifier and alarms)
>   - Noninvasive ventilator
>
> *Contd...*

Contd...

- T piece
- Tongue depressors
- Defibrillator/cardioverter
- Multilumen central catheters (4.5, 5.5, 7 F) 8 cm, 16 cm
- Sterile trays for instrument set
- Sets for cut down, lumbar puncture, thoracocentesis, bone marrow aspiration, chest tubes, and suture removal
- Miscellaneous:
  - Weighing machines
  - Bedside table
  - Overbed table
  - Intravenous pole
  - Bedside chair
  - Procedure stool
  - Torchlight with extra batteries
  - Breast pump
  - Phototherapy unit
  - Arm boards
  - Adhesive tapes
  - Cardiac arrest board/backboard
  - Splints
  - Sterile dressings
  - Stiff neck collars (small, large)
  - Television
  - Toys
  - Clocks

ORGANIZATION AND STAFFING

Doctor-in-charge

- Doctor-in-charge should be a pediatrician—trained and experienced in pediatric critical care and should implement the smooth functioning of PICU with appropriate policies and protocols in consultation with the senior faculty.
- Should maintain the PICU statistics.
- Should be the nodal person for equipment needs (Box 1.1), their updating and maintenance and should observe uninterrupted supply of PICU drugs.
- Should observe quality assurance and improvement in patient care.
- Be a member of the hospital infection control committee.
- Be prompt and responsible in reporting disease outbreaks.
- Must establish teaching and training for medical, nursing, and other staff.

Medical Staff

- Round the clock postgraduate pediatrician, good in airway skills, and having Pediatric Advanced Life Support (PALS) certification should be available.
- Residents/trainees enough in number should be available on 12-hourly rotation.

Nursing Staff

Nursing staff should be experienced in pediatric intensive care; nurse–patient ratio should be 2:1 for unstable patients; need to be 1:3 for relatively stable and unventilated patients.

Ancillary Staff

Services should be available from physiotherapist, dietician, respiratory technician, laboratory technician, radiographer, biomedical engineer, clerical staff, and social worker.

LEVELS OF PICU CARE

Level 3 Care

It has defined admission and discharge policies by a pediatric intensivist heading the unit and should have 1:1 nurse patient ratio for ventilated patients.

Level 2 Care

It is for patients requiring oxygen, nebulization, trauma monitoring, parenteral fluid therapy, and monitoring and those on follow-up care from level 3.

CONCLUSION

Pediatric intensive care unit should be well-designed with adequate and updated equipment and proper trained staff pattern.

FURTHER READING

1. Khilnani P. Indian Society of Critical Care Medicine (Pediatric Section), Indian Academy of Pediatrics (Intensive Care Chapter). Consensus guidelines for pediatric intensive care units in India. Indian Pediatr. 2002;39:43-50.

Chapter 2

Daily Routine in PICU

Seany T Varghese, S Sushamabai

ABSTRACT

Daily work in pediatric intensive care unit (PICU) if systematically carried out by all doctors and nurses, will improve the patient care and reduce the working time and medicolegal problems. Precautions for infection control, a positive preparedness to receive sick patients at any time, assessing the PICU team of the day, the status of equipment and drugs and proceeding to corrective steps in time, prioritizing the sick patients as per severity, and replacing the documents at proper places are the important points to be observed. A brief discussion of the patient's status and management should be done among the unit members (avoiding controversial points in front of caretakers). Reevaluation of the patient should not be postponed.

INTRODUCTION

Observing certain points methodically in our daily routine will be beneficial to all categories of doctors and nurses; will improve the patient care better and make it easier, and will help the one tide over medicolegal problems.

Points to Consider

- Give priority to the PICU patients for the day's work.
- Have a confident mind and determination for overcoming the problems encountered on the day, whatever be the nature.
- Be clean and modest in your attire.
- Observe precautions for infection control—change your footwear, practice proper handwashing (at least alcohol disinfection) before and after handling each patient, use sterile mask, gown, and gloves when handling highly infective patients.
- Be prepared for receiving critically ill patients at any time.
- Assess the PICU team of the day—ample in number and experienced; if not, make the appropriate arrangements.

- Evaluate the lifesaving equipment and medicines; consider urgent step for repair or replacement if at fault.
- Prioritize the patients as per disease severity, sick and unstable first and recovering patients subsequently.
- Devote ample time for each patient—do not appear to be hasty, but should not be too lengthy also.
- Decisions regarding treatment, investigations, and consultations should be taken after a brief discussion among the unit members; be careful not to discuss controversial points in front of the caretakers.
- The working diagnosis and management plan should be informed clearly to the caretakers.
- Patient's records and PICU documents should be replaced in proper places.
- Discussion of the illness of older age group children should be avoided in their presence.
- Do not postpone a reevaluation of the patient, if needed.
- Teaching, discussion, literature search, and research activities should go in pace with patient care for quality improvement.

CONCLUSION

Daily work in PICU if carried out systematically will improve patient care and time management.

FURTHER READING

1. Khilnani P. PICU – A working rounds and documentation – IAP PICU Protocols, PEDICON 2011, Jaipur.

Chapter 3

PICU Rounds and Documentation

Seany T Varghese, S Sushamabai

ABSTRACT

Routine rounds and documentation in pediatric intensive care unit (PICU) should be at least twice daily or more in critically ill patients. The resident is to present the information first which has to be verified by the senior. The format includes verification of the points in history, assessing the vitals, systemic examination by prioritization. Fluid status of the body and investigation reports need to be evaluated and orders be changed accordingly. Inform the family members regarding the condition, taking care to avoid unpleasant facts in front of older children. Order sheet and progress sheet should reveal the name, age, hospital number and time of writing on each page and in-between. Procedure notes should reveal the date, time, name of the procedure and the result obtained, medicines given, consent obtained, name of the performer and the senior consultant available. A failed procedure should be documented as such. Transfer and discharge notes should reveal the date and time, patient's details and further advice. Each documentation has to be signed with the name of the doctor along with date and time.

INTRODUCTION

Working rounds and documentation reflect the quality of care in a PICU and progress of the disease after admission.
- Assess each patient completely at least twice a day and more often if unstable.
- Master a uniform system of condensing the clinical notes; this will aid in better patient assessment, plan of action, and communication between different teams (doctors and nurses) inside the PICU.

Note: Information should be presented by the resident first.
- Get the detailed history, compiling the points obtained from the caretaker, reference letters, and others.
- Verify the patient's chart to assess the progress of the disease.
- Abridge the relevant points.

SYSTEMATIC APPROACH FOR EXAMINATION

- Appearance of the child—critical/improved?
- Verify the vital signs and note the abnormalities.
- Prioritize the systems to be evaluated; and proceed.
- Respiratory: Oxygen saturation, lung examination, arterial blood gas (ABG), chest skiagram, and ventilator settings.
- Cardiovascular: Capillary refill time, peripheral pulse volume, warmth of the extremities, IV line sites for infection, mean arterial pressure/systolic blood pressure (MAP/SBP), central venous pressure, cardiomegaly, heart sounds, murmurs, and vasopressors in use.
- *F*luids, *E*lectrolytes, *N*utrition (*FEN*): Intake (oral + parenteral including the quantity infused with medicines), output (urine as mL/kg/hr especially in last hours, stools, vomitus, aspirates), electrolyte changes, nutrition (calories, proteins, vitamins), and renal indices.
- Nervous system: Consciousness level (AVPU/GCS/FOUR score), pupils, seizures—controlled? Anticonvulsants—appropriate?
- Neurologic deficits and reflexes.
- CT/MRI, electroencephalography reports, cerebrospinal fluid studies.
- Gastrointestinal tract and abdomen: Oral ulcers, thrush, abdominal distension (girth) tenderness, mass, bowel sounds, perineum (edema, hernia, skin changes), and perianal excoriation or ulcers.
- Infectious diseases: Body temperature, status of the initial septic focus, hospital-acquired illness, white blood counts, culture reports, day of antibiotics, and review for antibiotic change as per sensitivity.
- Hematology: Anemia, bleeding from puncture sites, skin or mucosal bleeds, platelet count, and coagulation status.
- Limbs: Perfusion, color, swellings, tenderness or compartmental syndrome, and pulsations of the arteries.
- Invasive lines, catheters: Consider the need for central lines, Foley's catheter or peripheral lines.
- Hepatic: Fetor hepaticus, flapping tremor, palmar erythema, liver span (increasing /rapidly decreasing).
- Laboratory results: Review all.
- Prescription charts: Review drugs and dosages, assess nurse's chart for proper timing of drug administration.
- Plan or alter the therapy based on these assessments.
- Discuss clearly the plan among the unit members.
- Specialist's opinion if needed should be obtained.
- Communicate to the family members clearly about the probable diagnosis, treatment adopted, expected course of the illness, and probable outcome.

DOCUMENTATION

Writing good notes is an art; complete and accurate documentation ensures continuity of care and will be a defense to the doctor in an hour of crisis.

POINTS TO REMEMBER

- Be truthful, never add to or delete an old controversial chart or note.
- Make a new corrected entry for deleted orders.
- Document what you tell to the family.

GENERAL GUIDELINES

- Note heading, date, and time.
- Be legible, no erasers—strike through mistakes and rewrite.
- Sign and write name with designation—for multipage notes sign, rewrite date and time.
- Following documentations should be clear and concise:
  - Admission notes
  - Progress report
  - Prescription
  - Procedure details
  - Transfer notes
  - Discharge summaries.

ADMISSION NOTES

- Be concise, clear, and complete; diagrammatic representation is better.
- For documenting physical examination, diagrams are better explanatory.
- Evaluate the investigations ordered and the results.
- Proceed to assessment; write diagnosis if sure only; otherwise, consider possible differential diagnosis.
- Plan the investigations and time of starting medicines.

PROGRESS NOTES

- Title, date, and time.
- Follow the SOAP format (**S**ubjective—what the patient says, **O**bjective—examination findings, **A**ssessment, **P**lan); vital signs are mandatory.
- Signature, name, and designation.

PRESCRIPTIONS

- Each sheet should reveal patient's name, age, hospital number, provisional diagnosis, and weight of the child.
- Enter the date and time.
- Write the orders legibly.
- Drug strength should be in standard units (as mg/g, not as mL/tab).
- Dosing intervals should be in hours (q 8 hr or q 12 hr).
- To correct an order, strike through and rewrite.
- To discontinue (DC) an order, write a dated and timed DC order.
- Verbal or phone orders have to be signed within 24 hours.
- Discuss with the nurse the orders which are written not during routine rounds time.

A time tested prescription writing in priority order is shown below:
- *Monitoring*: T, P, R, BP, I/O chart, daily weight, etc. according to the provisional diagnosis.
- *Lifesaving medicines* as oxygen, nebulization, etc.
- *Specific drug* for specific etiology, e.g. antibiotics.
- *Supportive therapy* like intravenous fluids.
- *Symptomatic therapy* like paracetamol, saline nasal drops, etc. which provide subjective well-being, but will not alter the outcome of the illness.

PROCEDURE NOTES

Procedure notes always should be written with date and time:
- Name of the procedure, indications, whether written consent obtained, site, date and time, duration, sedation, analgesia given, actual procedure including equipment used, condition after the procedure, performer, and senior expert present.
- If unsuccessful, it has to be noted.

TRANSFER NOTES

Transfer can be made from PICU to ward or to another hospital as follows:
- Transfer to ward—enter the progress notes, rewrite orders, indicate pending laboratory reports, and inform the parents regarding ward shift.
- When transferred to another hospital, document the reason for transfer in the hospital record. Brief summary revealing the diagnosis, investigation reports, medicines given, course in the hospital, reason for transfer and the mode of transport, and condition at the time of transfer—all should be documented in the reference letter.

- The reason for transfer to another hospital should be informed to the parents.
- The emergency services in the receiving hospital should be informed if possible.
- A medical team (doctor and nurse) capable of handling the emergency care of critically ill children should accompany.

DISCHARGE SUMMARY

- Remember—others judge the quality of your care from the discharge summary.
- Brief clinical summary, investigations, diagnosis, hospital course, procedures, complications, condition at discharge, advice, follow-up date, pending investigation reports, and further points to be considered at follow-up, are to be documented.

CONCLUSION

Pediatric intensive care unit routine rounds should be systematic and documentation should be clear, both of which will reflect the quality of care given in PICU.

FURTHER READING

1. Khilnani P. PICU – A working rounds and documentation – IAP PICU protocols, PEDICON 2011, Jaipur.

Chapter 4

Communication in PICU

Seany T Varghese, S Sushamabai

ABSTRACT

Timely and appropriate communication is a must in pediatric intensive care unit (PICU) to provide confidence among the caretakers about the diagnosis and management provided. The room for communication is to be near the PICU and wait area. A fixed time after the morning rounds will be ideal for the main communication. The senior most faculty available should give the counseling at least once, others have to listen and act as spokespersons at other times. The parents and near relatives can participate and clarify doubts. The provisional diagnosis, complications anticipated, and treatment provided should be detailed. Transfer to a higher center if opted, discuss the merits. Before doing costly or invasive investigations, the need and the untoward problems expected, have to be explained and written consent is to be obtained.

INTRODUCTION

Counseling is very important in patient care. In spite of expert medical management, parents and patients may go unsatisfied if proper counseling is not done.

Consider the following points:
- Ideally a senior staff member should discuss the details every day. Junior doctors and nurses should attend the session to ensure consistency. Further progress details of the child can be informed by the residents acting as spokespersons of the senior doctor (after discussion).
- A separate room near the PICU and wait area is the ideal one for communication. A fixed time period after the morning rounds will enable some close relatives also to be present for the session.
- The patient's parents, near relatives, and a senior respected person if available (who will be more receptive and be able to communicate more to the parents and help them make decisions) can be allowed.

- Explain in simple language the nature of the illness (includes the diagnosis and pathogenesis), overall laboratory data, treatment plan, usual outcome, and specific risk factors for the patient.
- The relatives should be given opportunity to clarify their doubts.
- Try to communicate in accordance with the level of the parent's educational status.
- A correct balance between optimism and pessimism should be maintained while explaining the progress. Excessive pessimism may lead to denial of care, marked depression, and anxiety in parents. On the other hand, undue optimism may produce blame on the doctor if the outcome is adverse.
- Undue reactions of rage may be encountered at times out of guilt and despair. Efforts to maintain patience and project a caring attitude both in speaking to parents and handling the patient should be mastered by all the health staff. The senior consultant should set a model for such behavior. The junior doctors and other health staff (usually overworked and tired) should be periodically reminded by the seniors not to become impatient and to cultivate patience and empathy by self-training.
- A brief documentation of the communication with date and time is a must in the doctor's progress notes and nurse's report.
- Before doing costly laboratory investigations, invasive procedures, and life-sustaining organ support, the need, benefit for the patient, and the risks encountered (if done/not done) should be explained in detail and written consent with date and time should be obtained.

CONCLUSION

Good communication in PICU can provide better patient confidence and should be mastered by all doctors and nurses.

FURTHER READING

1. Parvathy VK, Mammen DS. How to communicate? In: Sushamabai S, editor. Clinical evaluation of newborns, infants and children. 2nd Ed. New Delhi: Jaypee brothers Medical Publishers (P) Ltd; 2009.

Chapter 5

Ethics in PICU

Seany T Varghese, S Sushamabai

ABSTRACT

Ethical issues in treating sick children include balancing the benefits, burdens, and harms of therapy in the face of uncertainty. Providing benefit only, never harming, permitting autonomy for decisions and justice are the major principles of medical ethics. Informed consent up to the age of 18 years should be obtained from parents only. For withholding and withdrawing life support, correct advice should be provided to the parents.

INTRODUCTION

Critically ill children in PICU may recover fully, die or survive with disability. Major principles of medical ethics are:

Beneficence

Provide care that benefits to the patients, e.g. parents of children may face tragic choices about support of a sick child whose survival with disability could endanger the economic or psychological integrity of the rest of the family.

Nonmaleficence

Avoid harming patients.

Autonomy

Individuals should decide their own best interests, i.e. medical decision should be in accordance with the patients and/or family's perspective (which may at times be according to their religious benefits also).

Justice

Provide service without bias from factors irrelevant to the medical situation.

TRANSITIONING THE GOALS OF CARE

Informed Consent

Children have no legal rights to make decisions for themselves before 18 years of age. Usually parents serve as the valid surrogates for their children. Parents or other surrogates must have adequate decision making capacity. Presently, doctors have less freedom to treat patients according to their own feelings and benefits.

Withholding and Withdrawing Life Support

A correct decision and communication should be made by the doctor when continued existence of the patient does not serve any purpose and burdens outweigh the benefits. To decide about withdrawing treatment, adequate assessment, clinical trial to detect poor prognosis, and the least likelihood of a successful outcome are to be confirmed.

Documentation

Dated (with time) documentation from the parents/surrogates should be obtained for any decision taken.

CONCLUSION

Ethics in pediatric intensive care unit (PICU) should be strictly followed in managing sick children.

FURTHER READING

1. American Academy of Pediatrics, Committee on Bioethics. Ethics and the care of critically ill infants and children. Pediatrics. 1996;98:149.

Section 2

RESUSCITATION

Chapter 6

Pediatric Basic Life Support

P Jayasree, S Sushamabai

ABSTRACT

Basic life support (BLS) is the cardiopulmonary resuscitation (CPR) procedure, given to a person found to be unconscious, by a lay person. Presently, it is advised in CAB (chest compressions, airway, breathing) sequence. Assess for breathing in 10 seconds; if no breathing/ineffective breathing, start chest compression—ventilation in 30:2 ratio, open the airway and send someone to get the emergency system. After 2 minutes of CPR, if the victim is not responding and has no pulse, get automated external defibrillator (AED), provide shock and continuing CPR, transport the victim to the nearest medical facility.

GUIDELINES FOR LAY RESCUERS

Start the steps of CPR when the victim is found unconscious. The recommended sequence of CPR has previously been known by the initials "ABC": Airway, Breathing/ventilation, and Chest compressions (or Circulation). The *2010 AHA Guidelines for CPR and ECC* recommend a CAB sequence (chest compressions, airway, breathing /ventilations).

GUIDELINES FOR HEALTHCARE PROVIDERS AND OTHERS TRAINED IN 2-RESCUER CPR

The sequence of basic life support (BLS) for healthcare providers is similar to that for lay people with some variation as indicated below (Flowcharts 6.1, 6.2 and Fig. 6.1):

Shockable rhythms—principles: Ventricular fibrillation (VF) and pulseless ventricular tachycardia (VT) need immediate CPR and defibrillation.
- Children with sudden witnessed collapse (during an athletic event) are likely to have VF or pulseless VT.
- Manual defibrillator is preferred for infants, the first energy dose being 2 J/kg. If second dose is required, provide double dose—4 J/kg.

Flowchart 6.1: Pediatric BLS—Steps in Cardiopulmonary Resuscitation (CPR)—2010 American Heart Association (AHA) guidelines.

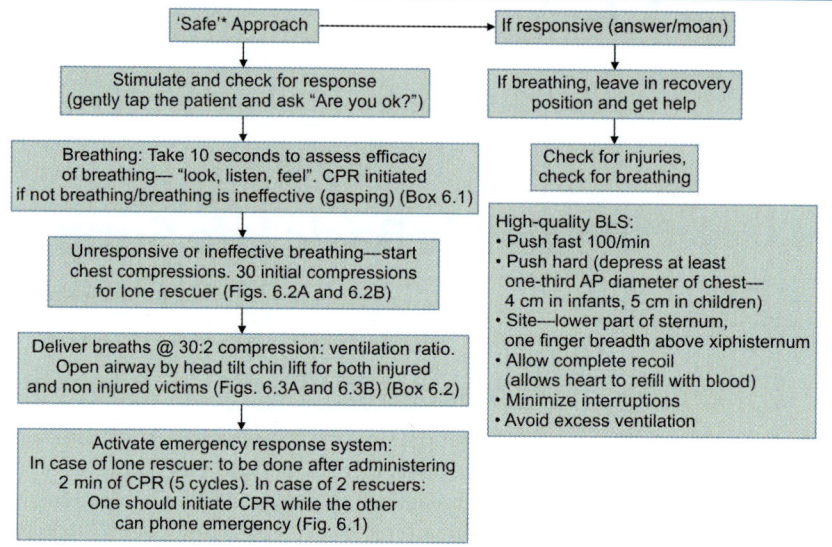

*Fire, explosives, electricity short circuit, suffocation
(AP, anteroposterior; BLS, basic life support; CPR, cardiopulmonary resuscitation)

Flowchart 6.2: Pediatric BLS—Approach to unresponsive child—2010 American Heart Association (AHA) guidelines.

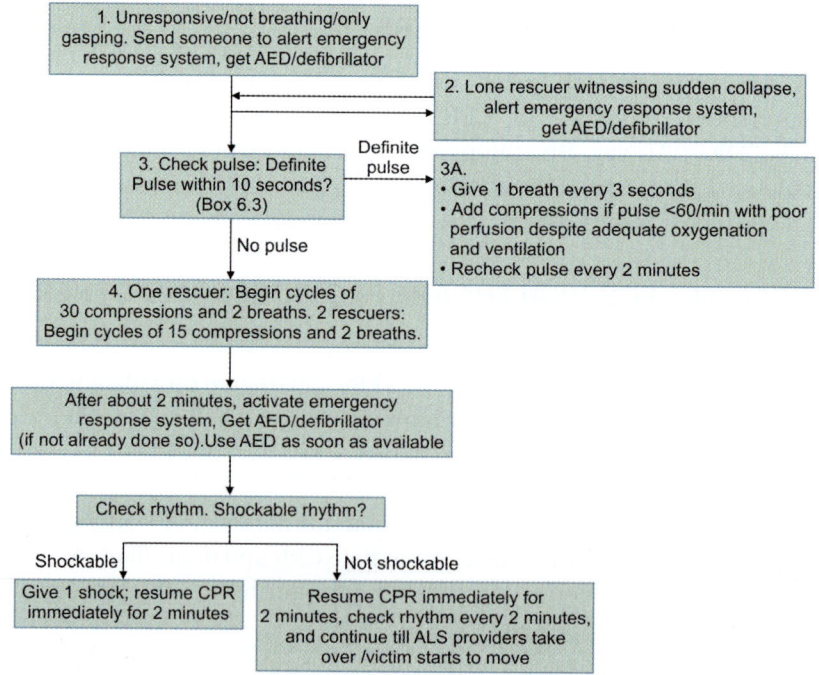

(AED, automated external defibrillator; ALS, advanced life support; CPR, cardiopulmonary resuscitation)

Chapter 6: Pediatric Basic Life Support

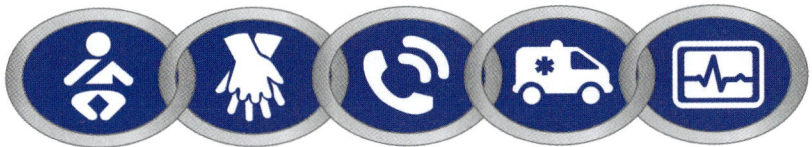

Fig. 6.1: Pediatric chain of survival.

> **Box 6.1:** Useful tips "SAFE APPROACH"—2010 American Heart Association (AHA) guidelines.
>
> **S**hout for help
> **A**pproach with caution*
> **F**ree from danger (for rescuer and patient)
> **E**valuate ABC
> **The size of the child influences four areas of resuscitation technique:**
> - Head position
> - Rescue breaths
> - Pulse assessment
> - Chest compressions
>
> **Head position:**
> - Infants: neutral
> - Small child-sniffing
> - Bigger child-gargling
>
> **Breaths:**
>   Infant: mouth over mouth and nose
>   Child: mouth to mouth
>
> **Pulse assessment:**
>   Infant: at the brachial or femoral artery
>   Child: at the carotid or femoral artery
>
> **Chest compressions:**
>   Infants: 2 rescuers-use both hands to encircle the chest and compress with the thumbs; lone rescuer: use the 2-finger chest compression.
>   Child: one or both hands positioned a finger's breadth above xiphisternum.
>   Opening airway: After 30 compressions (15 compressions if 2 rescuers), open the airway with a head tilt–chin lift and give 2 breaths. If spinal injury is suspected, use a jaw thrust without head tilt to open the airway. Proceed to head tilt–chin lift maneuver if the jaw thrust does not open the airway.
>
> *Caution against fire, explosives, electricity short circuit, suffocation.

> **Box 6.2:** Useful tips for breaths—2010 American Heart Association (AHA) guidelines.
>
> - Breathe into the patient over 1–1.5 seconds to cause a chest rise similar to normal breath.
> - To give breaths to an infant, use a mouth-to-mouth-and-nose technique; to give breaths to a child, use a mouth-to-mouth technique (pinch the nose closed while doing this)
> - In an infant, if you have difficulty in making an effective seal over the mouth and nose, try either mouth-to-mouth or mouth-to-nose ventilation
> - If chest does not rise, presume that airway is not open, so reposition the head between each attempt and consider "jaw thrust". Remove any foreign matter easily seen.
> - If 5 attempts to make chest rise are ineffective, treat for presumed foreign body obstruction (*"choking child"*).

Box 6.3: Useful tips for circulation—2010 American Heart Association (AHA) guidelines.

Take 10 seconds to assess the adequacy of circulation:
- All ages—look for signs of life like breathing, moving, and swallowing.
- If there are signs of circulation, then treat as respiratory arrest.
- If unsure of pulse or pulse <60/min or no signs of life, start chest compressions.

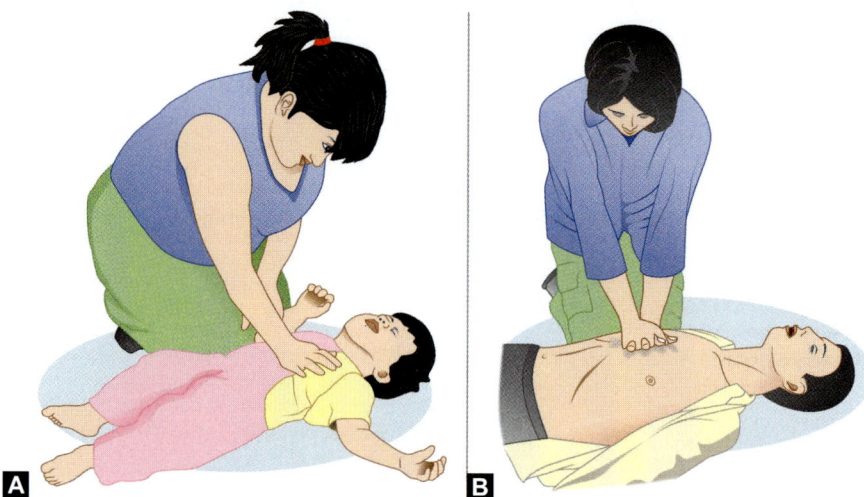

Figs. 6.2A and B: Methods of chest compression in children using one hand/both hands.

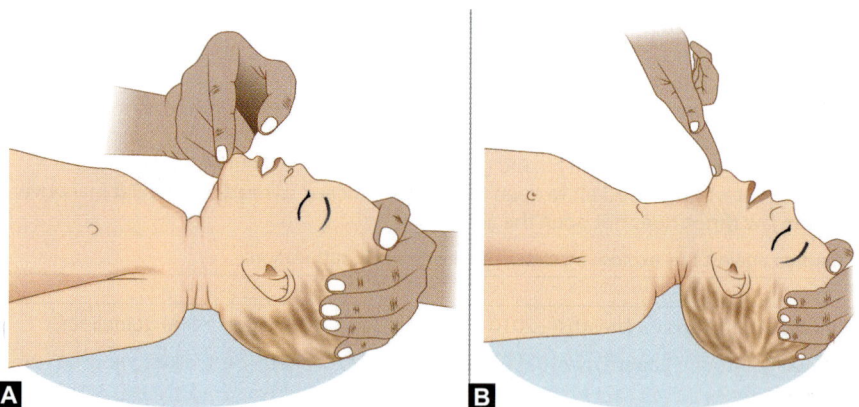

Figs. 6.3A and B: Neutral head position (ideal for infants) and sniff position (ideal for children) while administering breaths.

- If no manual defibrillator, an AED equipped with a pediatric attenuator is preferred for infants and for children less than 8 years.
- If neither is available, an AED without a dose attenuator may be used.

- Automated external defibrillators with high energy doses have been successfully used in infants with minimal myocardial damage and good neurological outcomes.

CHOKING CHILD

Method of Back Blows: Conscious Child (Flowchart 6.3)

- *Infant:* Position the infant safely along your arm or your knee, face downward, head at lower level than bottom. Place one hand under

Flowchart 6.3: Pediatric BLS—Approach to choking child—2010 American Heart Association (AHA) guidelines.

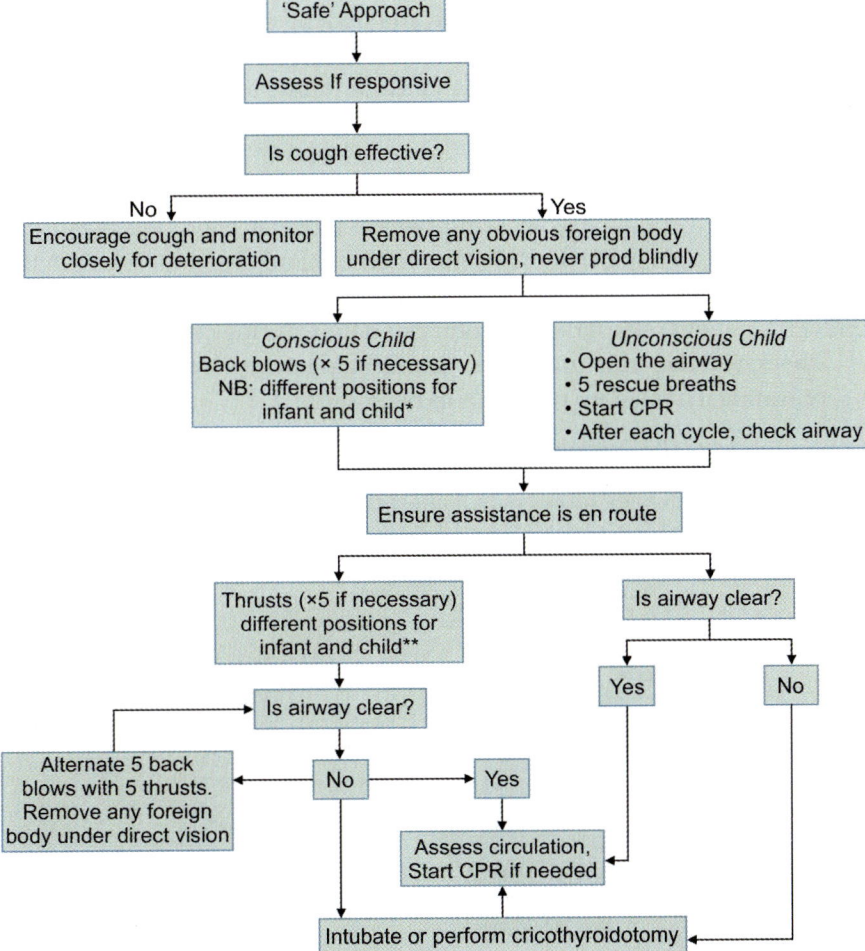

*Position of the infant as shown in Figure 6.4A
**Indicates position of the child as shown in Figure 6.4B
(CPR, cardiopulmonary resuscitation)

infant's chin to support the head and airway. Using the heel of the other hand apply a sharp blow between the scapulae (Fig. 6.4A).
- *Child:* Lean the patient forward over your extended arm so that the head is lower than chest. Tell the child what you are going to do before giving a sharp blow between the scapulae with heel of your hand (Fig. 6.4B).
- Check whether this maneuver has dislodged the foreign body before repeating it further up to 5 times as necessary.

If back blows are unsuccessful and airway remains obstructed, ensure that assistance is on the way before proceeding to thrusts.

Method of Thrusts

Infant: Perform chest thrusts. Support the patient's head and turn the face upward. Place two fingers on the infant's chest as for chest compressions. Press slowly and deliberately on the chest to mimic its movement as when the infant coughs (Fig. 6.4A).

Child: Perform abdominal thrusts. Tell the patient what you are going to do. Kneel behind a small child or stand behind a bigger child. Place your fist just above the umbilicus; then place your other hand over your fist. Stabilize yourself against the patient's back before pulling your fist upward and inward under the patient's diaphragm to mimic its action during cough (Fig. 6.4B).
- Check whether this maneuver has dislodged the foreign body before repeating it further up to 5 times as necessary.

Continuation of the Procedure

Infant: Alternate 5 back blows with 5 chest thrusts.
Child: Alternate 5 back blows with 5 abdominal thrusts.

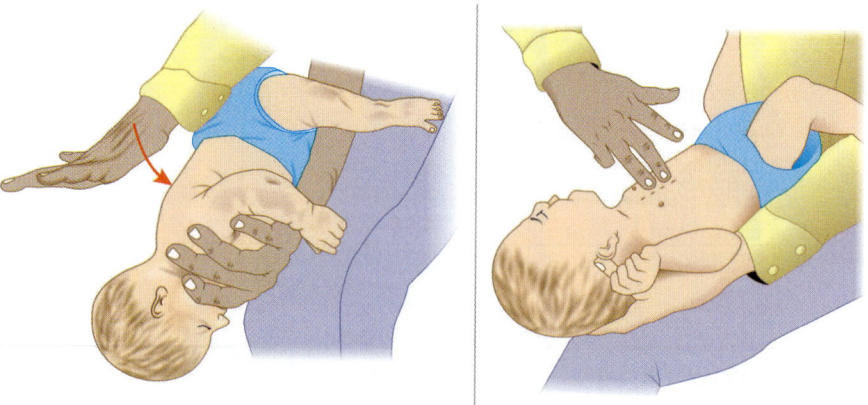

Fig. 6.4A: Method of back blows and chest thrusts in infants.

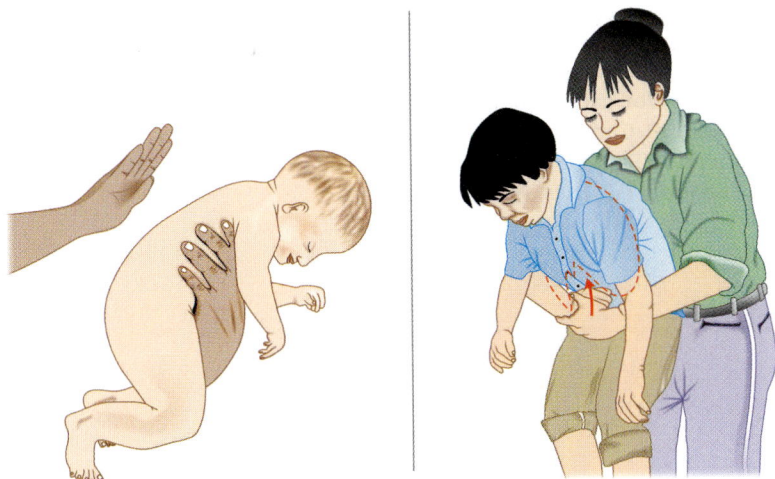

Fig. 6.4B: Method of back blows and abdominal thrusts in children.

Unconscious Child (Flowchart 6.3)

If the patient has lost consciousness following choking, initiate BLS:
- Inspect the airway
- Open the airway—head tilt-chin lift
- Assess breathing
- Attempt rescue breaths: Try to deliver five rescue breaths, if necessary, reposition the head between each breath.
- If unsuccessful with rescue breaths, continue BLS by delivering chest compressions at the rate of 100/minute (compression:breaths ratio 15:2 if 2 rescuers, 30:2 for lone rescuer)
- After each cycle of compressions, look in the mouth to see if the compressions have been effective in removing the obstruction.
- Ensure assistance.
- Advanced life support interventions include:
  - Direct visualization of the foreign body with laryngoscope and removal with Magill's forceps or suction
  - Ventilation with bag and mask to displace object to one of the bronchi
  - Attempt intubation and ventilation.
  - Emergency needle cricothyroidotomy while preparing for bronchoscopy
  - Emergency tracheotomy only in children above 12 years.

CONCLUSION

Basic life support is the life-saving emergency resuscitation provided by any person, to a victim found unconscious at any place.

FURTHER READING

1. Berg MD, Schexnayder SM, Chameides L, et al. American Heart Association guidelines for cardiopulmonary resuscitation and emergency cardiovascular care, part 13, Circulation. 2010;122(Suppl 3):S862-S75.
2. Hartman ME, Cheifetz IM. Pediatric Emergencies and Resuscitation. In Nelson Textbook of Pediatrics, 19/e; 2011.

Chapter 7

Pediatric Advanced Life Support

P Jayasree, S Sushamabai

ABSTRACT

Advanced life support (ALS) should be provided to the patient not responding to basic life support (BLS). Change to bag and mask ventilation or endotracheal intubation and mechanical ventilation so as to provide adequate oxygenation; obtain IV/IO access; parallel investigations, chest X-ray (CXR), and electrocardiography (ECG) to assess shockable or nonshockable cardiac rhythm. Give indicated drugs or DC shock as per cardiac electrical activity. Maintain perfusion with fluid and electrolytes and rectify correctable causes of cardiac arrest.

STEPS IN ADVANCED LIFE SUPPORT

- When/if no recovery with BLS, continue cardiopulmonary resuscitation (CPR), and proceed to ALS.
- Advanced life support follows ABC principle:
  - *A, B—airway and breathing:*
    - Adequate correction of ventilation and oxygenation with bag and mask using high flow oxygen.
    - Apply oropharyngeal airway (OPA) until endotracheal tube is placed successfully.
  - *C—circulation:*
    - Establish cardiac monitoring.
    - Pause compressions to check for rhythm and feel pulse.
    - Determine whether defibrillation is necessary [i.e. ventricular fibrillation (VF)/pulseless ventricular tachycardia (VT)].
    - Sixty percent of pediatric arrests are asystolic (nonshockable), secondary to hypoxia and acidosis.
    - Obtain vascular access for giving drugs—intravenous (IV) or intraosseous (IO).

- *Evaluate for reversible causes of arrest (6H's and 4T's):*
  - *6H's:* Hypoxia is the leading cause;[1] others are hypovolemia, hypothermia, hypoglycemia, H ions (acidosis), hyper/hypokalemia/hypocalcemia (metabolic).
  - *4T's:* Tension pneumothorax, tamponade, toxins, thromboembolism.[2]
- *Drugs:* While resuscitation is being done, depute one staff to record all the drugs administered.

GENERAL GUIDELINES

- Continue CPR 15:2.
- Intubate as soon as possible, give 8–10 breaths/minute.
- Secure vascular access (IV/IO).
- Send blood samples for glucose, urea, electrolytes, creatinine, complete blood count (CBC), culture, grouping and cross-matching, and coagulation parameters—prothrombin time (PT) or activated partial thromboplastin time (APTT), and arterial blood gas (ABG).
- Obtain finger prick glucose.
- Chest skiagram
- Proceed to detailed history and physical examination for correctable causes.
- Deliver CPR in 2 minute cycles. A new rescuer should take over the delivery of compressions each cycle or earlier as necessary to ensure consistently effective compressions. Treat reversible causes.
- Give adrenaline every 3–5 minutes. Reassess rhythm and pulse after every cycle and respond.
- Return of pulse—proceed to post-cardiac arrest care.

AIRWAY

- *Oropharyngeal airway:* Should be introduced if the patient is not conscious and gag reflex is absent. Size—distance from the corner of the patient's mouth to ear lobe.[3]
- *Nasopharyngeal airway:* Useful in those who have gag reflex.
- *Laryngeal mask airway (LMA):* Is advised if oxygenation cannot be maintained with bag and mask ventilation (BMV) and endotracheal intubation is not established but should be introduced by an experienced doctor.

Method of Insertion of OPA

- Using a head tilt-chin lift, a modified jaw thrust, or by grasping the tongue and jaw by placing your thumb in the patient's mouth, move the tongue forward and position the OPA (Figs. 7.1A to E).[3] Now slowly insert it.

Chapter 7: Pediatric Advanced Life Support   33

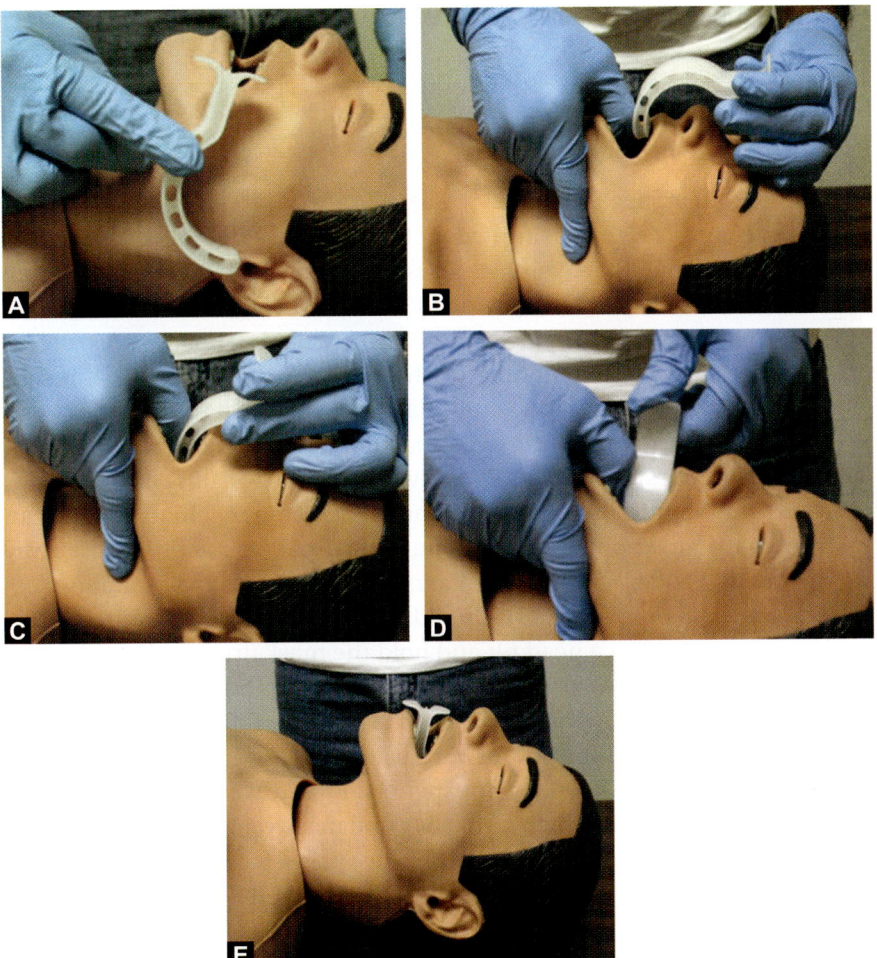

Figs. 7.1A to E: (A) Assessing the required size of oropharyngeal airway; (B) Method of insertion of oropharyngeal airway; (C) Advancing oropharyngeal airway; (D) Rotating oropharyngeal airway 180°; (E) Oropharyngeal airway position after insertion.

- As the OPA is being inserted, slight resistance will be felt, but continue insertion simultaneously rotating the OPA 180° and advance it until the flange is resting on or just above the patient's teeth.[4]
- Oropharyngeal airway is removed by simply pulling it out of the patient's mouth (without rotating).[4]
- In children below 8 years of age, OPA is inserted from either corner of mouth and rotating the device 90° as it is inserted or by using a tongue depressor to hold the tongue while the OPA is inserted anatomically with patient's airway.[3]
- Airway should be placed into patient's mouth always, before starting bag and mask ventilation (BMV).

- If the patient gags while placing the airway, remove it, but start direct BMV.
- Maintain Hb status and cardiac output.

Bag and Mask Ventilation

- Insert oropharyngeal airway.
- Use the correct size of self-inflating bag (Fig. 7.2) and mask. In general, bag delivers half of its volume. Thus, a 500 mL bag will deliver 250 mL which is suitable for children up to 15–20 kg. The right-sized mask is one which covers the tip of chin, the nose and mouth, but not the eyes. Before using, ensure the functioning of the device by checking whether air pressure is felt if the mask is firmly placed against the hand and squeezed.
- While squeezing the bag, the force and tidal volume should be just enough to make the chest rise visibly. Excessive ventilation will impede the venous return and reduce the cardiac, cerebral, and coronary blood flow.[5] It can also cause air trapping and barotrauma in patients with small airway obstruction and also stomach inflation, regurgitation, and aspiration.[5]
- The hand holding the mask should perform two tasks simultaneously [C-E grip—perform a head tilt and hold the mask firmly against the face while lifting the jaw. For this, use the thumb and index finger to make a "C", pressing the edges of the mask to the face.[6] Perform and maintain the "head tilt' and hold the jaw forward using the last three fingers forming an "E" (Fig. 7.3A). Ideally two experienced and well-trained providers should work together while giving bag and mask ventilation.
- One provider should hold the mask firmly against face of the patient using two hands creating a leak proof seal while lifting the patient's jaw at the same time. The other squeezes the bag slowly and gently taking 1 second per ventilation (Fig. 7.3B).

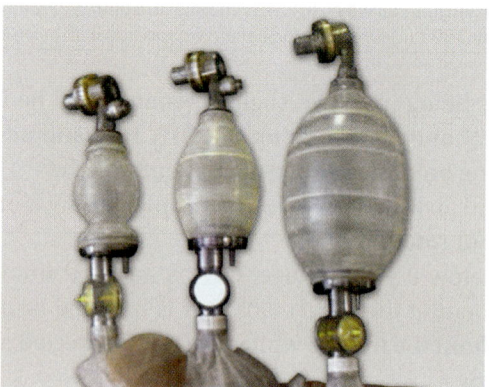

Fig. 7.2: Bags of sizes 250 mL (newborns), 500 mL (children up to 20 kg), 1,500 mL (children >20 kg).

Chapter 7: Pediatric Advanced Life Support

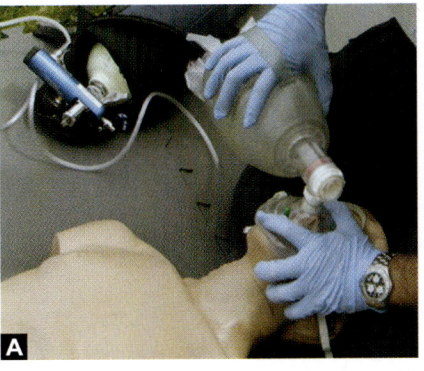 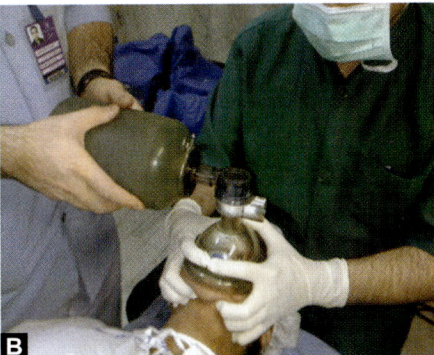

Figs. 7.3A and B: (A) One provider giving bag and mask (E-C grip); (B) Two providers giving bag and mask.

- The seal and volume problems do not arise once the bag is connected to an advanced airway inserted to the patient (endotracheal tube, laryngeal mask airway).[6]
- Once the patient has advanced airway in place, two rescuers no longer provide CPR in cycles (alternating compressions with ventilations in the ratio 15:2).[7]
  - Provide chest compressions at a rate of 100/minute.[8]
  - The provider delivering ventilations gives it at a rate of one ventilation every 6–8 seconds (8–10/minute).
  - Providers switch roles every 2 minutes to avoid compressor fatigue which affects the effectiveness of chest compressions, minimize the interruptions in chest compressions and avoid excess ventilation.[6]

MANAGEMENT OF PULSELESS CARDIAC ARREST[9]

The algorithm for management of pulseless cardiac arrest is described in Flowchart 7.1 and Figures 7.4A to D.

Flowchart 7.1: Management algorithm of pulseless cardiac arrest.[9]

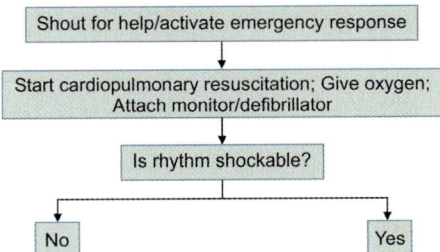

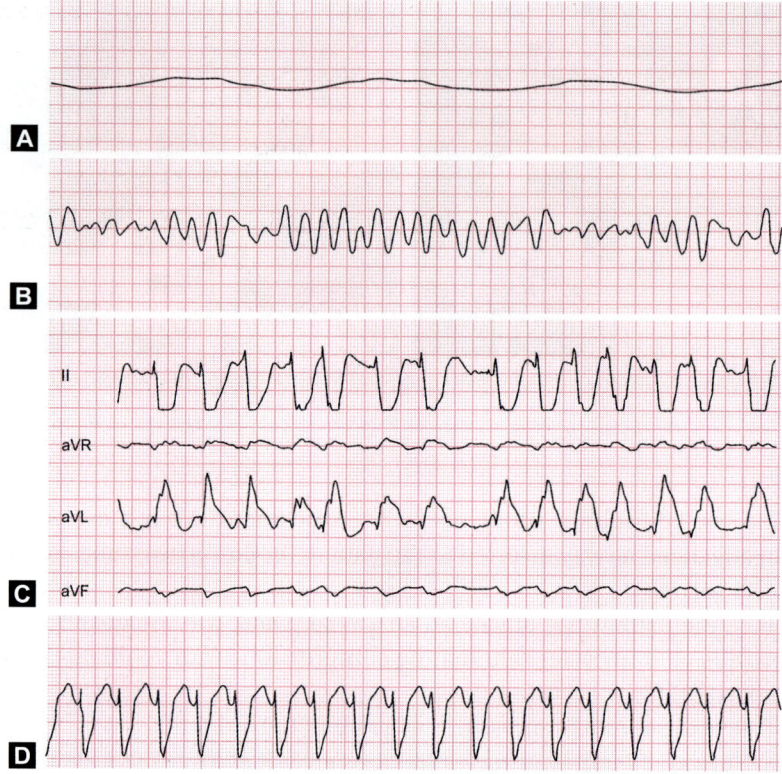

Figs. 7.4A to D: (A) Asystole; (B) Ventricular fibrillation (VF); (C) Pulseless electrical activity (PEA); (D) Ventricular tachycardia (VT).[10]

MANAGEMENT OF ASYSTOLE OR PULSELESS ELECTRICAL ACTIVITY (NONSHOCKABLE RHYTHM)

The algorithm for management of asystole or pulseless electrical activity is described in Flowchart 7.2.

MANAGEMENT OF VT AND PULSELESS VENTRICULAR TACHYCARDIA (SHOCKABLE RHYTHM) (FLOWCHART 7.3)

- *Aim*: To defibrillate as quickly and as safely as possible.
- Continue CPR while preparing for defibrillation.
- Do not delay shocks; intubation and venous access being important can be done between shocks.
- Confirm a shockable rhythm by ECG tracings before proceeding.
- Oxygen:
  - Provide 100% O_2 to maintain SpO_2 >94%
  - Avoid hyperoxia by reducing FiO_2.

Chapter 7: Pediatric Advanced Life Support

Flowchart 7.2: Management of asystole or pulseless electrical activity (nonshockable rhythm).[11]

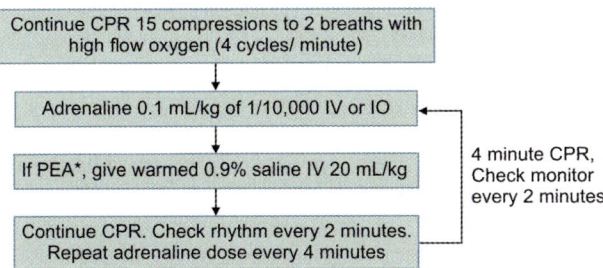

(CPR, cardiopulmonary resuscitation; *PEA, pulseless electrical activity)

Flowchart 7.3: Management of ventricular tachycardia and pulseless ventricular tachycardia.

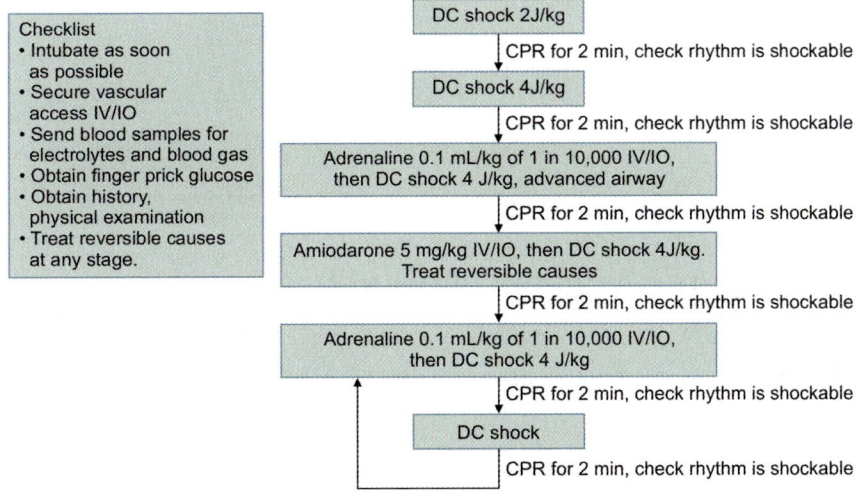

(CPR, cardiopulmonary resuscitation; DC, direct current; IV, intravenous; IO, intraosseous)

PEDIATRIC BRADYCARDIA (WITH A PULSE AND POOR PERFUSION)[12-14]

The pediatric bradycardia algorithm is described in Flowchart 7.4.

Drug Dosages

- *Epinephrine IV/IO:*[15] Dose 0.01 mg/kg (0.1 mL/kg 1:10,000 concentration).[12] Repeat every 3–5 minutes. If IV/IO not available, but endotracheal tube (ET) in place, may be given ET, dose being 0.1 mg/kg (0.1 mL/kg of 1:1,000).[15]
- *Atropine IV/IO dose:* 0.02 mg/kg. Minimum dose 0.1 mg and maximum single dose 0.5 mg.[15]

Flowchart 7.4: Pediatric bradycardia algorithm (With a pulse and poor perfusion).[12]

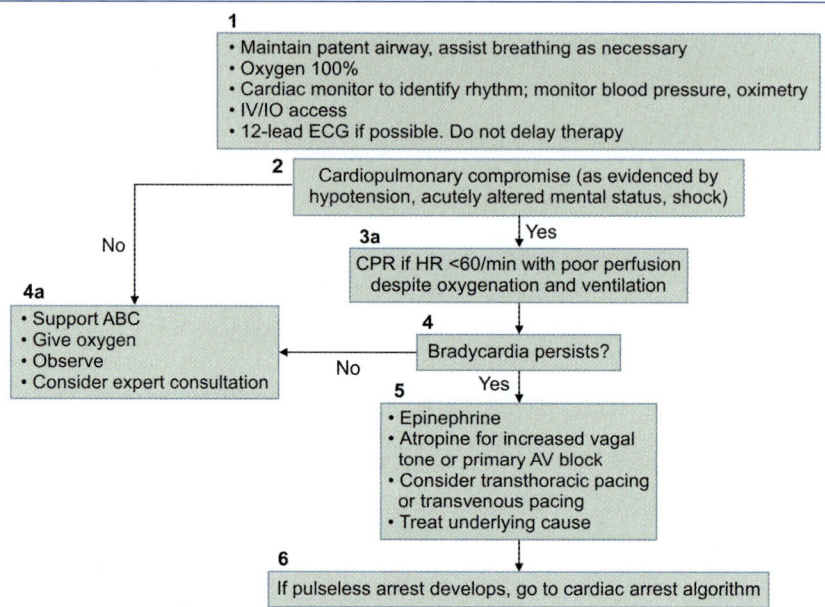

(AV, atrioventricular; ABC, airway, breathing, circulation; CPR, cardiopulmonary resuscitation; HR, heart rate; IO, intraosseous; IV, intravenous)

PEDIATRIC TACHYCARDIA (WITH A PULSE AND POOR PERFUSION)[2]

The pediatric tachycardia algorithm is described in Flowchart 7.5.

Drug Dosages

- *Synchronized cardioversion:* Begin with 0.5–1 J/kg; if not effective, increase to 2 J/kg. Sedate if needed, but do not delay cardioversion.[14]
- *Adenosine IV/IO dose:* First dose 0.1 mg/kg rapid bolus (maximum 6 mg); second dose 0.2 mg/kg rapid bolus (maximum 12 mg), each dose should be followed by saline push and ECG recording.[14]
- *Amiodarone IV/IO dose:* 5 mg/kg over 20–60 minutes *or* procainamide IV/IO dose—15 mg/kg over 30–60 minutes; do not routinely administer amiodarone and procainamide together.[17]

Flowchart 7.5: Pediatric tachycardia algorithm.[2,14,16,17]

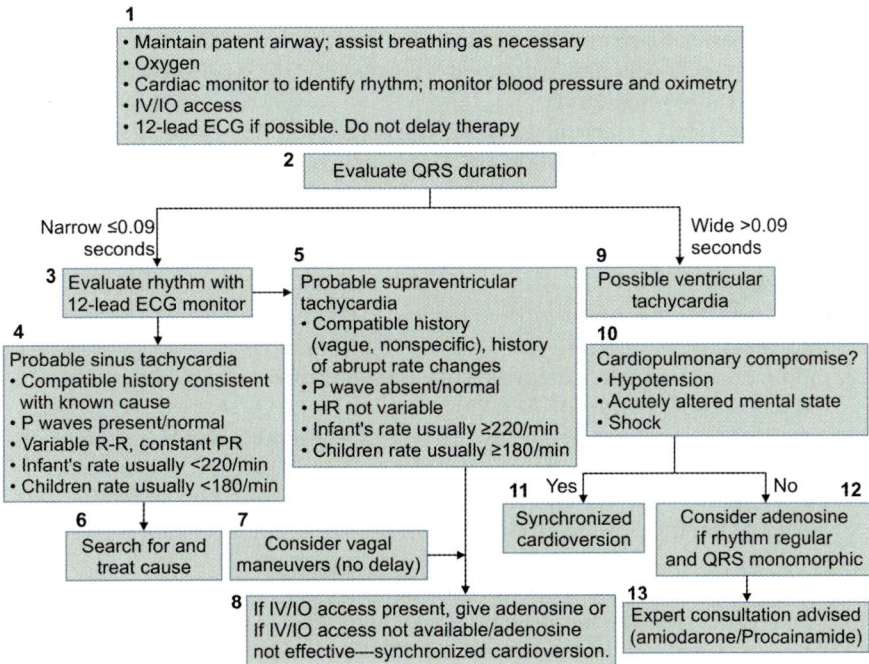

(HR, heart rate; IO, intraosseous; IV, intravenous; ECG, electrocardiography)

CONCLUSION

When BLS fails in CPR, proceed to ALS to establish ventilation and perfusion in a well-equipped emergency setup by an expert team.

REFERENCES

1. http://www.ypeda.com/attachments/article/150/2016_PALS_Manual_Final_Online.pdf (Internet from 24-Dec-2017).
2. Burmester M. Appendix A: Resuscitation Algorithms. In: Daubeney PEF, Rigby ML, Niwa K, Gatzoulis MA (Eds). Pediatric Heart Disease: A Practical Guide. US: Blackwell Publishing Ltd; 2012. pp. 282-6.
3. http://iausnursing.blogfa.com/post-22.aspx (Internet 01-Sep-2014).

4. http://centigra../wp-content/uploads/2013/06/Oral-Pharyngeal-Airway.pdf (Internet from 19-Mar-2015).
5. http://www.sothep.com/files/CPR%202010.pdf (6- Jan-2015).
6. http://cpr-acls-pals.com/wp-cntent/uploads/2012/01ACLS-pre-course-study-pdf (Internet 03-Aug-2014).
7. American Heart Association. (2005). American Heart Association guidelines for cardiopulmonary resuscitation and emergency cardiac care.
8. http://www.csems.org/download/Protocols%202014.pdf (Internet 10-May-2014)
9. Basic Clinical Anesthesia, 2015.
10. http://www.greencoeducation.com/gcepals05supplement.pdf (Internet 10-May-2014).
11. http://www.gerties.org/userfiles/Standard TreatmentGuide.pdf (Internet 11-Jun-2014).
12. http://drkermanshahi.kums.ac.ir/kums_content/media/digitallibrary/2014/11/book11/11.pdf (Internet 07-APR-2017).
13. http://www.scmca.org/Protocols/MasterProtocolCombined.pdf (Internet 01-Feb-2015).
14. https://archive.org/stream/feri clinical advisor 2014/feri clinical advisor 2014 djvu. txt (Internet 28-Aug-2016).
15. http://www.eugene-or.gov/portal/server.pt/gateway/PTARGS_0_2_175840_0_0_18/Section%20A%20 Intermediate.pdf (Internet 15-Oct-2011).
16. "Emergency Care". Pediatric Board Study Guide.2015.
17. http://ncecc.net/wp-content/uploads/2012/03/ALS-protocols-May-15-2012pdf (Internet 10-Nov-2012).

Chapter 8

Rapid Sequence Intubation

P Jayasree, S Sushamabai

ABSTRACT

Rapid sequence intubation (RSI) is the quick intubation of the airway by an experienced team in an emergency, without producing aspiration, cardiac compromise or neurologic problems. Patient assessment, adequate preparation, preoxygenation, premedication, sedation, cricoid pressure, neuromuscular blockade, airway placing, endotracheal tube placement and confirmation, and post-intubation care are the steps involved.

INTRODUCTION

Rapid sequence intubation is a coordinated procedure to secure the airway quickly using sedatives and neuromuscular blocking agents so as to reduce the risk of aspiration and undesirable cardiovascular and neurologic responses.

INDICATIONS FOR RSI

- All patients with risk of pulmonary aspiration
- Rapidly progressing neuromuscular paralysis
- Respiratory arrest with full stomach
- Unresponsive child
- Coma with raised abdominal pressure
- Head injury with full stomach or last meal unknown.

POINTS TO REMEMBER

- Rapid sequence intubation should be done only by proficient doctors in airway management using sedatives and neuromuscular blocking agents.
- A secondary plan must be there to manage the airway in the event that intubation cannot be achieved.
- Do not paralyze the "difficult airway" patient at the time of intubation; instead sedate, intubate, and then paralyze—"awake intubation".

CONTRAINDICATIONS

- Patients with short neck, anatomical anomalies of spine, micrognathia, cleft palate, etc.
- Laryngotracheal problems—anatomical, infection, edema, and tumors
- History of cervical radiation therapy
- Patients who cannot be orally intubated.

RSI PROCEDURE

- *Step 1: Rapid assessment*
    - *History:* **AMPLE** (**A**llergies, **M**edications, **P**ast medical history, **L**ast meal, **E**vent history).
    - *Assessment:* Vitals, neck anatomy, micrognathia, cleft palate, injuries, and other diseases.
- *Step 2: Preparation—***SOAPMM** (**S**uction, **O**xygen, **A**irway, **P**eople, **M**onitors, and **M**edicines [Table 8.1]).
- *Step 3: Preoxygenation—*give bag and mask ventilation with 100% oxygen for 3–5 minutes to wash out nitrogen so that 3–4 minutes of apnea without arterial desaturation is possible.
- *Step 4: Premedication—*this is to reduce the adverse effects of laryngoscopy, sedatives and paralytic drugs, e.g. bronchospasm, raised intracranial, ocular and gastric pressures, increased sympathetic discharge, and bradycardia.

Table 8.1: Rapid sequence intubation preparation—SOAPMM (check everything and keep ready at the bedside).

1	Suction Oxygen	Large bore Yankauer catheter attached to wall suction Central supply ideal
2	Airway	(i) Two functioning laryngoscopes, the blades appropriately sized and shaped. (ii) Two endotracheal tubes—one appropriately sized and one smaller size (ETT size—internal diameter (a) uncuffed: 3.5 mm up to 1 year age, 4 mm from 1 year to 2 years, 4 + age/4 >2 years. (b) cuffed ETT: 3 mm up to 1 year age, 3.5 mm from 1 year to 2 years, 3.5 + age/4 >2 years)
3	People	Professionals needed during and post-procedure phase: Doctors, nurses, respiratory therapist, etc.
4	Monitors	Pulse oximetry, heart rate, blood pressure and continuous ECG monitoring
5	Medications	At least one patent IV line, specific RSI medications (Table 8.2), their dose and frequency determined, drawn up and labeled

(ECG, electrocardiography; ETT, endotracheal tube; RSI, rapid sequence intubation)

Table 8.2: Medications in rapid sequence intubation.

A. Premedication:

No.	Drug	Indication	Mechanism	Dose (IV)
1	Lidocaine	Raised ICP, head injury, hyperreactive airway disease (HRAD)	Decreases intracranial response to intubation, decreases bronchospasm in HRAD	1–1.5 mg/kg
2	Atropine	Children <8 years—with first dose of Sch >8 years—with second dose of Sch	Reduces bradycardia response to Sch and intubation	0.02 mg/kg; minimum dose 0.1 mg

B. Sedatives:

No.	Drug	Dose (IV)	Onset of action	Duration of action	Advantages	Adverse effects
1	Midazolam	0.1–0.3 mg/kg	30–60 seconds	15–30 minutes	Reversible, Amnesic, Anticonvulsant	Apnea, no analgesia
2	Thiopental	2–5 mg/kg	<30 seconds	5–10 minutes	↓ICP, ↓cerebral O_2 consumption	Hypotension, laryngospasm
3	Ketamine	1–2 mg/kg	45–60 seconds	10–20 minutes	↑BP, bronchodilator	↑secretions, laryngospasm, hypertension, hypotension in CCF
4	Etomidate	0.3 mg/kg	15–45 seconds	3–12 minutes	Safe for ↑ICP	Myoclonic jerks
5	Fentanyl	1–5 µg/kg	30–60 seconds	20–30 minutes	Minimal side effects compared to other opiates	Chest wall rigidity, should not be used with MAO inhibitors
6	Propofol	1.5–3 mg/kg	<30 seconds	5–10 minutes		Hypotension, bradycardia, apnea

C. Paralytic agents:

No.	Drug	Dose (IV) for intubation	Onset	Duration	Adverse effects
1.	Succinylcholine	1–2 mg/kg	45–60 seconds	6–12 minutes	Fasciculations, hyperkalemia, bradycardia, malignant hyperthermia, bronchospasm
2.	Vecuronium	0.1–0.2 mg/kg	90–120 seconds	60–75 minutes	Tachycardia, bradycardia, hypotension
3.	Rocuronium	0.6–1.2 mg/kg	50–75 seconds	30–60 minutes	Tachycardia, hypotension, bronchospasm

(ICP, intracranial pressure; MAO, monoamine oxidase; Sch, succinylcholine)

Table 8.3: Choice of sedatives for rapid sequence intubation.

Normotensive	Hypotensive/hypovolemic	Head injury/status epilepticus	Status asthmaticus
Midazolam or etomidate or thiopental or propofol	Etomidate or ketamine or midazolam (avoid in severe hypotension)	Normotensive: thiopental or propofol or etomidate Hypotensive: Etomidate or low-dose thiopental	Ketamine or midazolam

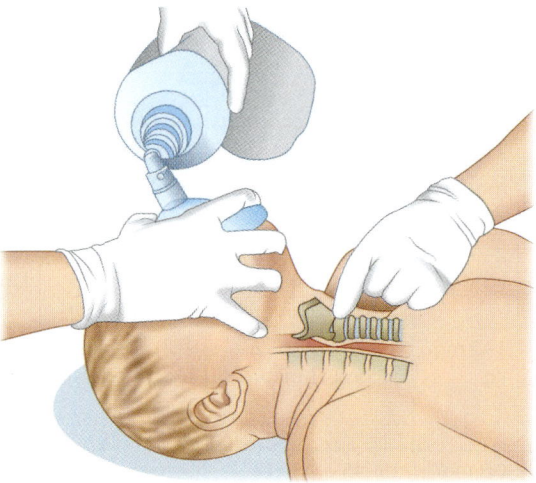

Fig. 8.1: Cricoid pressure.

- Intravenous atropine in all children less than 8 years of age with the first dose of succinylcholine (Sch) and with second dose of Sch in children more than 8 years. Intravenous lidocaine for head injury, raised intracranial pressure, and reactive airway disease (Table 8.2).
- *Step 5: Sedation*—use one of the following:
  - IV midazolam/thiopental/ketamine/etomidate
  - Choice of sedation shown in Table 8.3.
- *Step 6 (a): Protection of airway by Sellick maneuver (Fig. 8.1)*—apply cricoid pressure just sufficient to compress the esophagus as the patient becomes unconscious to prevent regurgitation of gastric contents and aspiration. Maintain the pressure till successful intubation and verification.
- *Step 6 (b): Paralysis*—use one from Table 8.2.
  - IV succinylcholine/rocuronium/vecuronium
  - Succinylcholine can cause bradycardia with first dose in infants and with subsequent doses in older children. Premedicate with atropine.

- Succinylcholine can cause hyperkalemia in patients with muscle injury and burns.
 - Avoid Sch in neuromuscular disease, ocular trauma, and family history of malignant hyperthermia.
 - Succinylcholine induces fasciculations in children more than 5 years of age and hence administer vecuronium or rocuromium prior to Sch.
- *Step 7: Positioning of the airway*
 - *Less than 2 years of age:* Large occiput leads to head and neck flexion and airway obstruction; hence elevate the shoulders with a towel roll.
 - *More than 2 years of age:* Place towel roll under the head, gently hyperextend the head at the atlantoaxial joint for optimal alignment of tracheal, pharyngeal, and oral axes.
- *Step 8: ETT placement*
 - Confirm muscular paralysis by gently grasping the jaw for flaccidity.
 - With the laryngoscope in the left hand, gently open the mouth with right hand, insert the laryngoscope into the right of the patient's mouth and sweep the tongue to the left.
 - While proceeding, if the glottis aperture is not easily visible, an assistant can perform the BURP maneuver (Backward, Upward, Rightward Pressure) on larynx to improve the view of the glottis.
 - Through the visible glottis, gently insert the ETT with the right hand until the cuff is 2–3 cm past the vocal cords and then remove the stylet, inflate the cuff.
- *Step 9: Confirm endotracheal tube placement*
 - Do not release Sellick maneuver until confirmation of correct ETT placement is made by the following methods:
   - Visualizing ETT passing through the vocal cords
   - Auscultation of breath sounds heard over both lungs equally, especially the axillae
   - Symmetrical chest rise with ventilation
   - Fogging of ETT during ventilation
   - Pulse oximetry (due to prior hyperoxygenation, SpO_2 may not decline even without effective ventilation for as long as 3 minutes)
   - End tidal CO_2
   - Absence of gastric inflation sounds over stomach
   - Chest skiagram.
- *Step 10: Post-intubation care*
 - Secure the ETT (taped or tied)
 - Gastric decompression
 - Monitor vitals
 - Administer a longer acting sedative as the patient may awaken before the muscle relaxant wears off.

Flowchart 8.1: Algorithm rapid sequence intubation.

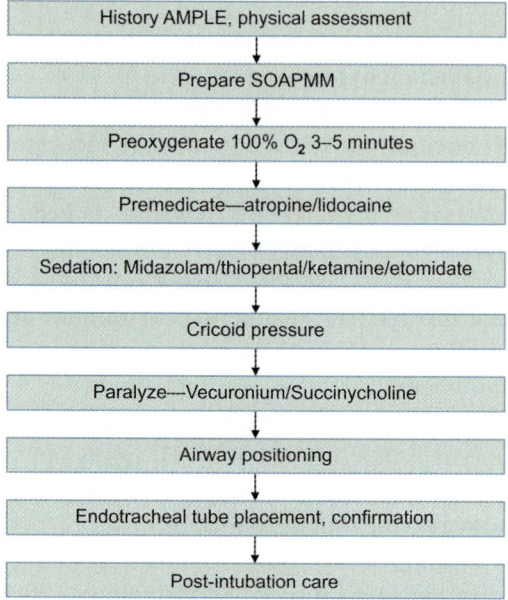

The algorithm of rapid sequence intubation is described in Flowchart 8.1.

CONCLUSION

Rapid sequence intubation is an emergency endotracheal intubation by an expert team and is often required in a pediatric intensive care unit.

FURTHER READING

1. http://centegra.org/wp-content/uploads/2011/01/Oral-Pharyngeal-Airway.pdf. Accessed on 25th December 2012.
2. Journal of the American Heart Association. (2010). 2010 American Heart Association Guidelines for Cardiopulmonary Resuscitation and Emergency Cardiovascular Care Science. Available from http://cardiologiadepanama.org/uploads/2010-aha-guidelines.pdf. [Accessed on September 2018]
3. Kelly I. Basic life support. In: Emergencies in Pediatrics and Neonatology. Crisp S and Stuart J (Eds). Great Ormond Street, Oxford: Oxford University Press; 2010. pp. 52-60, 64-75.
4. Tress EE, Kochanek PM, Saladino RA, et al. Cardiac arrest in children. J Emerg Trauma Shock. 2010;3(3):267-72.
5. www.scottishintensivecare.org.uk/education/RSI%20brochure.pdf. Accessed on 27th December 2012

Chapter 9

Resuscitation Equipment and Drugs

P Jayasree, S Sushamabai

ABSTRACT

In all patient care areas (emergency rooms, PICU, NICU, general wards, procedure rooms), resuscitation may be warranted at any time. Hence a resuscitation area should be maintained in all these areas. The area should be easily approachable, having a resuscitation cart in which emergency equipment and drugs are systematically arranged and updated daily. A nurse and medical officer are to be in charge for this arrangement but all staff need to have sufficient knowledge about the area and the arrangements available.

INTRODUCTION

For successful resuscitation, necessary equipment and drugs should be available in time. The resuscitation area should have the equipment and drugs arranged in a resuscitation cart, regularly checked and updated, and kept in an accessible location known to all concerned staff.

DRUGS (IV, IM, PR PREPARATIONS)

- Adenosine
- Adrenaline (1 in 1,000, 1 in 10,000)
- Amiodarone
- Antibiotics (Broad-spectrum)
- Anticonvulsants (diazepam, midazolam, lorazepam, fosphenytoin, phenobarbitone, sodium valproate)
- Atropine sulfate (0.1 mg/mL)
- Calcium gluconate (10%)
- Corticosteroids (hydrocortisone, methyl prednisolone, dexamethasone)
- Dextrose (10%, 25%)
- Diphenhydramine
- Dopamine, Dobutamine

- Etomidate
- Fentanyl
- Ketamine
- Lidocaine
- Naloxone
- Pancuronium
- Potassium chloride (10%)
- Propofol
- Ranitidine
- Rocuronium
- Salbutamol nebulization
- Sodium bicarbonate (7.5%)
- Succinylcholine
- Vecuronium
- Intravenous fluids: Normal saline, 5% dextrose, Ringer lactate, 0.45% saline, 3% saline, 5% dextrose in 0.45% saline, and 10% dextrose.

EQUIPMENT

- Bags: Valve, mask (250 mL, 450 mL, and 1,000 mL)
- Endotracheal tubes (uncuffed 2.5 mm to 5.5 mm; cuffed 3 mm to 8 mm)
- Glucometer
- Laryngoscope handles (pediatric, adult); with extra batteries, bulbs
- Laryngoscope blades (straight 0 to 4, curved 2 to 3)
- Magill forceps (pediatric, adult)
- Nasal airways (size 12 to 30 Fr)
- Nasogastric tubes (size 6 to14 Fr)
- Nebulizer
- Noninvasive multipara monitor
- Oral airways (size 00 to 5)
- Oxygen masks (rebreathing and non-rebreathing with reservoir)
- Oxygen source (central, cylinders with flow meters)
- Pulse oximeter
- Stylets (pediatric, adult)
- Suction device
- Suction catheters (size 5 to 14 Fr).

FLUID MANAGEMENT

- Adhesive tape
- Arm boards
- Butterfly needles: 19 to 25 gauges
- Central vein catheters (size—infant, child)

- Infusion pumps/syringes
- Intraosseous needles
- Intravenous cannula (14 to 24 gauges)
- Intravenous tubing, micro drip sets.

MISCELLANEOUS

- Cardiac arrest board/backboard
- Defibrillator
- Preprinted drugs with doses
- Sphygmomanometer (with infant, child, adult, and thigh cuffs)
- Splints, sterile dressings
- Stiff neck collars (small, large).

CONCLUSION

Resuscitation equipment and drugs are to be systematically arranged and maintained updated in all patient care areas and should be readily accessible to all medical staff when in need.

Chapter 10

Post-resuscitation Care

P Jayasree, S Sushamabai

ABSTRACT

Systematic post-resuscitation care will definitely improve the outcome in a pediatric intensive care unit. The steps involved are review of history and physical examination to know the etiology of cardiopulmonary arrest, and to implement subsequent measures to prevent recurrence, continuing stabilization of the vital organs, and to implement measures to improve long-term outcome. Reexamine each system, review the investigations and make corrections, reset the ventilator arrangements, continue monitoring of the heart for postmyocardial infarction, maintain high normal BP, anticipate and treat for nonconvulsive seizures, and maintain normothermia, but if facilities are available, induce hypothermia for the needy patient. Maintain adequate perfusion by keeping urine output 1–4 mL/kg/hr. Start early enteral feeds, avoid hyper and hypoglycemia. Consider packed RBC tranfusion if Hb is less than 7 g/dL; detect and correct coagulopathy.

OBJECTIVES

- Optimize and stabilize cardiopulmonary function and vital organ perfusion (brain, kidneys).
- Identify the causes of cardiopulmonary arrest and treat them to prevent recurrence.
- Safe transport of the patient to appropriate critical care unit if needed.
- Institute measures to improve long-term neurological outcome.

APPROACH

Documentation

- Events leading to cardiopulmonary arrest if possible.
- Events encountered during cardiopulmonary resuscitation (CPR).
- Type and dose of drugs given.
- Time required for return of spontaneous circulation (ROSC) (good outcome declines with the length of resuscitation process).

System-wise Approach

Respiratory System

- Monitoring and support of the airway.
- Oxygenation: After ROSC, maintain blood oxygen saturation (SpO_2) 94–98%; prevent hyperoxia.
- Use appropriate ventilator setting adjustment.
- Assess arterial blood gas (ABG) and plasma lactate half an hour later and correct the problem.
- Chest skiagram for endotracheal tube (ETT) positioning, lung (pneumothorax, aspiration pneumonia) or heart problems (pneumomediastinum, pneumopericardium, cardiomegaly).
- Monitor for post-arrest acute respiratory distress syndrome; set ventilation adjustments for lung protection.
- Adequate sedation and analgesia for responsive intubated patients.
- 30° head end elevation nursing (if not in shock); keep neck in midline.
- If patient's condition deteriorates, consider *DOPE*; detect the problem and make appropriate correction. (DOPE: D, for displacement of tube; O, for obstruction of tube; P, for pneumothorax; E, for equipment failure).

Cardiovascular System

- Secure two IV lines, remove IO line; central venous access is preferred for inotrope administration, arterial access is ideal for blood pressure monitoring.
- Assess hemodynamic status periodically by extremity warmth, capillary refill time, heart rate, BP, oxygen saturation (pulse oximetry), and urine output.
- Treat hypotension aggressively by bolus normal saline, inotropes, and vasopressors.
- Post-arrest myocardial dysfunction can precipitate cardiac arrest again for 48 hours; continuous ECG monitoring and bedside echocardiograms are needed to assess cardiac status; ideal inotrope is epinephrine.
- Continue with maintenance fluids after deficit therapy.

Nervous System

- Maintain high-normal BP for adequate cerebral perfusion.
- Anticipate and treat convulsive and nonconvulsive seizures; consider continuous bedside EEG monitoring and prophylactic anticonvulsant therapy; correct metabolic derangements of glucose, sodium, calcium and magnesium.

Temperature Homeostasis

- Hypo- and hyperthermia can occur after cardiac arrest.
- Hyperthermia worsens neurologic outcome; prevent shivering by sedation; control fever with paracetamol; detect and treat infections.
- Induce hypothermia up to 32–34°C body temperature for 12–24 hours following resuscitation if facilities are adequate.

Renal System

- Monitor urine output, if less than 1 mL/kg/hr—consider fluid boluses (prerenal failure) or dialysis (renal failure).
- Polyuria: Urine output more than 4 mL/kg/hr may indicate glycosuria, osmotic diuresis (mannitol) or neurogenic diabetes insipidus; consider corrective measures.
- Avoid nephrotoxic drugs; adjust the dose of medicines having renal excretion.

Gastrointestinal System

- Monitor gastric aspirate—quantity and color.
- Provide stress ulcer prophylaxis by H_2 blockers or proton pump inhibitors.
- Start early enteral feeds.
- Watch for abdominal compartmental syndrome (reduced urine output, acidosis, increasing ventilator requirements); intra-abdominal pressure more than 20 cm H_2O requires decompression if associated with any two of the above features.
- Ischemic hepatitis revealed by transient elevation of liver enzymes is self-regressing.

Hematologic System

- Anemia (due to bleeding or repeated blood collection) should be corrected by packed cells to maintain Hb more than 7 g%.
- Bleeding can be due to platelet and coagulation defects or infection; should be corrected by whole blood or component therapy and empirical antibiotics pending culture reports.

Metabolic Problems

- Hyper- and hypoglycemia can occur; monitor blood glucose periodically; maintain euglycemia (120–180 mg/dL).
- Monitor sodium, potassium, calcium, and magnesium as indicated and correct the derangement.

Counseling the Family

The critical situation of the patient should be periodically communicated to the family in an empathetic way; risk factors for poor outcome should be properly informed.

CONCLUSION

Post-resuscitation care to assess the cause of cardiopulmonary arrest and continuing organ support is highly important.

Chapter 11

Anaphylaxis

S Sushamabai

ABSTRACT

Anaphylaxis is acute life-threatening allergic event usually IgE-mediated. The chapter deals with the etiology, clinical presentation, differential diagnosis, and management. Mild episodes can be treated in emergency room with intramuscular (IM) adrenaline and oral antihistamines and prednisolone. Children with severe episodes require pediatric intensive care unit (PICU) care. Those with predominant respiratory distress should be treated with O_2, adrenaline and salbutamol nebulization, IV hydrocortisone, and IV fluids in addition to inj. adrenaline, ranitidine, and other antihistamines. Patients with shock should be kept foot end elevated with O_2, IV fluids, IV hydrocortisone, and dopamine along with antihistamines. Since recurrence can occur, patients should be observed for 24 hours. Proper advice should be given for prevention at discharge.

INTRODUCTION

Anaphylaxis is sudden life-threatening allergic reaction produced by potent biologically active mediators from mast cells and basophils. Anaphylactoid reaction has similar clinical presentation requiring similar treatment but is not IgE-mediated and does not recur.

ETIOLOGY

- Drugs: Including vaccines and intravenous fluids
- Foods: Especially nuts, milk, egg, and seafoods
- Insect bites: Wasp and bee
- Materials: Latex.

MANIFESTATIONS

- Skin: Itching, urticaria, and flushing
- Respiratory: Dyspnea, stridor (laryngeal edema), and wheezing (bronchospasm)

- Cardiovascular: Hypotension, collapse, arrhythmia, and tachycardia
- Gastrointestinal: Nausea, vomiting, colicky abdominal pain, and diarrhea
- Central nervous system: Unconsciousness (hypoxia, shock), convulsions.

Note: Infants present with irritability, profuse sweating, drooling, hoarseness of voice, stridor, vomiting, flushing, and sudden unresponsiveness; older children express feeling of warmth, weakness, apprehension, and impending doom.

ONSET

- Immediate—within 30 minutes
- Delayed—30 minutes to 8 hours
- Late—8 hours to 24 hours
- Biphasic—recurrence within 24 hours (mostly within 4 hours).

DIFFERENTIAL DIAGNOSIS

- Respiratory: Foreign body aspiration, acute severe asthma, and vocal cord dysfunction.
- Cardiovascular: Cardiogenic shock, arrhythmias, and myocardial infarction.
- Central nervous system: Vasovagal episodes and seizures.

INVESTIGATIONS

- Serum selective IgE antibodies, plasma histamine, and plasma β tryptase—all are of diagnostic support but not helpful for immediate management.
- Consider relevant investigations to exclude the differential diagnosis and to detect organ damage.

PATIENT APPROACH

Quick history, parallel assessment, stabilization, and therapy as per severity.

Categorization and Treatment (Flowchart 11.1)

Mild Episode

Features are urticaria, sneezing, vomiting, and colic.
- Manage in emergency room.
- Withdraw the trigger.

Section 2: Resuscitation

Flowchart 11.1: Algorithm for anaphylaxis treatment.

```
                        Stabilize ABC
                         Categorize
                              │
         ┌────────────────────┼────────────────────┐
         ▼                                         ▼
┌─────────────────────┐                  ┌──────────────────┐
│ Mild –ER observation│                  │ Severe PICU admit│
│ Withdraw trigger    │                  └──────────────────┘
│ IM adrenaline       │                           │
│ DPH/PNR/CTR (0)     │                ┌──────────┴──────────┐
│ Ranitidine (0)      │                ▼                     ▼
│ ± Prednisolone (0)  │      ┌──────────────────┐   ┌──────────────────┐
└─────────────────────┘      │ Stridor ± wheeze │   │ Shock            │
         │                   │ IV/IM adrenaline │   │ 30° elevation    │
         ▼                   │ Oxygen 100%      │   │   foot end       │
┌─────────────────┐          │ Neb. adrenaline  │   │ IV/IM adrenaline │
│ Assess vitals   │→ Unstable│ Neb. salbutamol  │   │ 100% oxygen      │
│   × 24 h        │          │ IV Hydrocortisone│   │ Two IV access    │
└─────────────────┘          │ IV DPH /PNR      │   │ IV DPH+ ranitidine│
         │                   │ IV ranitidine    │   │ IV HC/MP         │
         │    Severe category│ IV fluids        │   │ IV NS/RL         │
         │    ◄──────────────│ Assess vitals    │   │ IV colloids +MF  │
         ▼         Taper drugs└──────────────────┘  │ IV dopamine      │
     Stable ◄──────                │                │ Monitor          │
         │              ┌──────────┼──────────┐     └──────────────────┘
         ▼              ▼          ▼          ▼              │
    Discharge        Stable  Respiratory              ┌──────┴──────┐
         │                    distress                ▼             ▼
         ▼                       │                 Stable       Unstable
 Cetirizine ±              Bag and mask               │             │
 prednisolone × 3d         ventilation            Taper drugs     APLS
 Prevention, education         │                      │
                               ▼                      ▼
                        Cricothyroidotomy         Discharge
                               │                  48 to 72 h
                               ▼
                       Mechanical ventilation
```

(CTR, cetirizine, DPH, diphenhydramine; ER, emergency room; HC, hydrocortisone; MF, maintenance fluid; MP, methyl prednisolone; O, oral; PNR, pheniramine)

- Administer adrenaline IM 0.01 mg/kg (maximum 0.3 mg, >12 years 0.5 mg); Repeat q15 minutes up to 3 doses if needed (has rapid onset of action).
- H_1 antihistamine (any one): Diphenhydramine 1.25 mg/kg/dose q 6 hr (PO, IM, IV) or pheniramine 0.1 mg/kg/dose q 6 hr or cetirizine 0.25 mg/kg q 24 hr (has slower onset of action).
- Prednisolone 1 mg/kg/dose q 12 hr (prevents recurrence).
- Assess vitals; change to severe category if no improvement or deterioration.
- If stable for 24 hours, discharge.
- Advice cetirizine + prednisolone for 3 days.
- Inform and educate on preventive therapy.

Severe Episode

Features are acute stridor, respiratory distress, and collapse.
Admit in PICU—classify and treat as:
- *With stridor or wheeze:*
    - Adrenaline IM/IV × 3 doses 15 minutes interval
    - Oxygen (100%) by non-rebreathing mask till blood oxygen saturation (SpO_2) is stable more than or equal to 94%

- Nebulized adrenaline (2.5 mg/5 mL) with oxygen × 3 doses 20 minutes apart.
- Nebulized salbutamol 0.5 mL to 1 mL + saline 3 mL with oxygen × 3 doses 20 minutes apart till PS is less than or equal to 4
- IV hydrocortisone 1–5 mg/kg/dose q 6 hr or methylprednisolone 1–2 mg/kg/dose q 6 hr for 24–48 hours
- IV ranitidine 1–2 mg/kg/dose q 8–12 hr slowly (max 50 mg) × 24–48 hours
- IV normal saline 30 mL/kg in 1 hour followed by maintenance fluid therapy
- Monitor vitals every 30 minutes.
- If compromised respiration—position the patient to open the airway, start bag and mask ventilation, and proceed for cricothyroidotomy or intubation and mechanical ventilation.

- *With shock—30° elevation of foot end of cot:*
  - IV/IM adrenaline (lateral thigh) × 3 doses every 15 minutes.
  - Supplementary oxygen 100% by non-rebreathing mask.
  - Secure two intravenous accesses.
  - IV H_1 and H_2 receptor antagonists q 8 to 6 hr.
  - IV hydrocortisone or methyl prednisolone q 6 hr.
  - IV normal saline or Ringer lactate up to 30 mL/kg in 1 hour followed by colloids 10 mL/kg in 20 minutes followed by slow infusion in 2–4 hours.
  - Switch over to maintenance fluids; if no improvement after 40 mL/kg bolus fluid, give IV adrenaline 0.01 mg/kg followed by IV dopamine infusion 5–10 µg/kg/minute.
  - Proceed to advanced pediatric life support (APLS) if still unstable.
  - Recovery can occur at any stage; start gradual tapering of drugs and consider discharge if stable for 24 hours.
  - Discharge advices as in mild episode.

CONCLUSION

Anaphylaxis is an allergic event which can present as acute life-threatening episode and should be detected and treated at the earliest to save life.

FURTHER READING

1. Tse Y, Rylance G. Emergency management of anaphylaxis in children and young people: new guidance from the resuscitation Council (UK). Arch Dis Child Educ Pract Ed. 2009;94:97-101.

Chapter 12

Oxygen Therapy

P Jayasree, S Sushamabai

ABSTRACT

Oxygen therapy is often needed in pediatric intensive care unit to prevent death due to hypoxia from trivial to serious illnesses. Low flow systems are blow by, nasal cannula, oxygen mask and partial rebreathing mask and provide 30–60% oxygen. High flow systems are non-rebreathing mask, O_2 hood or head box, oxygen tent, ambu bag, anesthesia bag, and endotracheal tube and deliver 50-100% O_2. Monitoring of O_2 therapy is by clinical parameters, pulse oximetry, and arterial blood glucose analysis. Adverse effects of O_2 therapy are retinal damage in preterm babies and by excess free radicals causing alveolar capillary damage.

INTRODUCTION

Oxygen (O_2) therapy is the method to increase the concentration of inspired O_2 to treat or prevent tissue or cellular hypoxia. Atmospheric air contains 21% O_2. Hypoxemia and hypoxia denote reduced O_2 concentrations in blood and tissues, respectively.

POINTS TO REMEMBER

- Though oxygen is a component of the atmospheric air, for therapy the concentration should be appropriately calculated and untoward effects should be properly assessed.
- Assess the patency of airway before therapy.
- Only humidified O_2 should be administered.

INDICATIONS

- Situations with hypoxemia (SpO_2<90% or paO_2<60 mm Hg)—anemia and respiratory compromise.
- Diseases with hypoxia in which O_2 saturation is normal, e.g. shock and cardiac failure; by increasing the O_2 content of the blood, O_2 delivery to the tissues is maximized.
- Home therapy as palliative care in chronic lung disease.

OXYGEN DELIVERY SYSTEMS

- Low-flow systems
- High-flow systems.

Low-flow Systems

O_2 mixes with room air during inspiration in these systems.
- *Blow by*—is blowing oxygen past a child's face. Not a reliable method.[1] Can be used to provide oxygen to infants who get agitated by other methods of delivery. Provides less than 30% O_2, needs 6–10 L/min O_2 flow with tubing very close to child's nostrils.
- *Nasal prongs (Fig. 12.1):* Simple device, allows easy feeding and chest physiotherapy. Two soft prongs inserted into the anterior nares deliver oxygen to the nasopharynx where it mixes with air and acts as reservoir.[1] Flow rate 1–4 L/min, the concentration of oxygen received by the lungs being 25–40%. In newborns and infants, limit the flow rate up to 2 L/min as it can cause inadvertent positive end-expiratory pressure (PEEP).
- *Simple oxygen mask (Hudson mask) (Fig. 12.2):* Simple and cheap, provides 24–55% O_2 at a flow rate of 4–10 L/min; useful for short periods as for procedures and patient transport. Exhaled gas escapes through the side holes in the mask. During inspiration, air enters the mask through these side ports and mixes with O_2 from the tube connected to the mask. A flow more than 5 L/min is recommended to prevent rebreathing CO_2 accumulation.[1]
- *Partial rebreathing mask:* Simple mask with an attached reservoir and one-way valve at the exhalation ports which permits air expulsion, but prevents air entrapment:
- No valve between mask and reservoir bag.

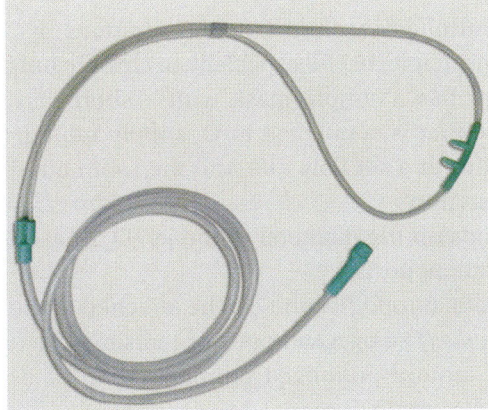

Fig. 12.1: Nasal prongs.

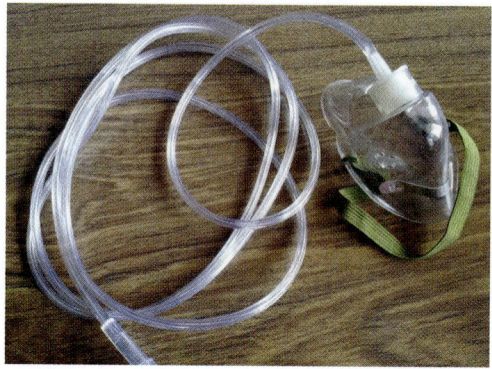

Fig. 12.2: Hudson mask.

- Air is drawn during inspiration from fresh O_2 inflow as well as the reservoir which contains the initial one-third of O_2-rich exhaled gas.[1]
- Requires O_2 flow of 10–15 L/min to provide 60–80% O_2 concentration.
- Recommended for children with high O_2 requirement.

High-flow Systems

- *Non-rebreathing masks:* Supply the highest concentration of oxygen to a spontaneously breathing patient (FiO_2 0.6–1)
  - Includes mask with reservoir and two systems of one-way valves—between the bag and mask and also over the exhalation ports.[2]
  - With flow rates of 15 L/min, patient gets 100% O_2 during inspiration from the dual supply of O_2 from the reservoir bag and from the fresh O_2 source.
  - Exhaled gas escapes via one-way valve to the atmosphere.
  - Gas inlet safety valve allows room air to enter if the O_2 source is accidentally disconnected.[2]
- *Venturi masks:*
  - Deliver controlled inspired O_2 concentrations of 25–60% based on Bernoulli principle; useful especially in chronic lung disease.
  - The system has a simple mask with a short corrugated hose and a jet orifice that is connected to O_2 supply tubing; O_2 flows through the jet orifice at a set flow rate and the room air enters through the entrainment ports.
  - FiO_2 depends on the diameter of the jet, O_2 flow rate, and the size of the entrainment ports.[2]
  - Supplemental humidification can be attached to the hose.
- *Enclosure systems:* The oxygen hoods or tents may be used for infants or children who require prolonged administration of oxygen but cannot tolerate a nasal cannula or mask.[1]

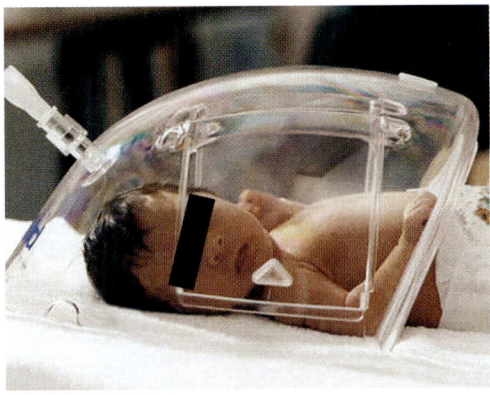

Fig. 12.3: Baby inside oxygen hood.

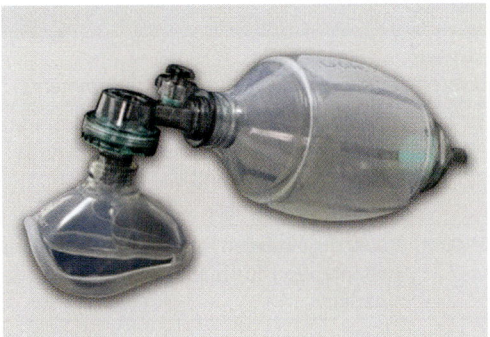

Fig. 12.4: Ambu bag.

- O_2 *hoods/head boxes (Fig. 12.3):*
    - Transparent plastic boxes that encompass the infant's head.
    - Oxygen enters the hood through a gas inlet; exhaled gas exits through the opening at the neck.[1]
    - Up to 95% O_2 can be supplied with oxygen flow rates of more than 10–15 L/min.[1]
    - Babies are accessible for monitoring and care.
- O_2 *tents:*
    - Clear, plastic shells that surround the child's head and upper body.
    - Provide up to 50% O_2 using high oxygen flow rates, but mixing with room air occurs whenever the tent is opened.[1]
    - Limits access to the child by family and clinical staff.[1]
- *Ventilation bags:* Provide O_2 through a mask or an artificial airway (such as an endotracheal tube).[1] They are of two types:
    - *Self-inflating bags (Ambu bags) (Fig. 12.4):*
        - Reinflate with a recoil mechanism.
        - Diluted O_2 is delivered to the patient with an O_2 source since room air is entrained inside the bag.[1]

- Higher O_2 can be delivered to the patient if a reservoir is attached to the bag.
- *Flow-inflating (anesthesia) bags:*
  - Require a gas source to remain inflated.
  - 100% oxygen can be delivered by adjusting the flow of O_2 and outlet control valve.[1]
- *Endotracheal tubes:*
  - Useful to administer through nasopharynx in continuous positive airway pressure (CPAP) and in mechanical ventilation.
  - Not used for oxygen therapy alone.

Table 12.1 summarizes salient points of O_2 therapy.

Table 12.1: Salient points of O_2 therapy.

System	% oxygen delivered	Indications	Comments
Blow by	<30%	Spontaneously breathing infants who require low doses of oxygen and do not tolerate a mask	Monitor pulse oximetry for hypoxemia
Nasal cannula/prongs	25–40%	Low dose oxygen to spontaneously breathing patients	Can cause nasal mucosal damage
Simple mask	35–50%	Low dose oxygen to spontaneously breathing patients	Assess correct mask fit
Partial rebreather mask	50–60%	Used to conserve oxygen	
Nonrebreather mask	Up to 95%	High-dose oxygen to spontaneously breathing patients	Tight mask fit required to deliver higher concentrations of oxygen
Venturi mask	25–60%	Delivers controlled inspired O_2	Ideal for prolonged O_2 therapy in chronic lung disease
Hood	80–90%	Infants less than 1 year of age	Noisy for patient; *Candida* infection on prolonged periods of use
Tent	<50%	Children who require 30% oxygen or less	Mist may obscure view of the patient; noisy for patient
Self-inflating ventilation bag	95–100% with reservoir	To provide assisted ventilation and oxygen	Must use with a reservoir to provide higher oxygen concentration
Flow-inflating ventilation bag	100%	To provide assisted ventilation and oxygen	Requires experience to use reliably

MONITORING OF OXYGEN THERAPY

Clinical

Improvement in patient's sensorium, cyanosis, restlessness, heart rate, respiratory rate, and chest retraction.

Pulse Oximetry

- Monitors the percentage of O_2-saturated hemoglobin.
- Value less than or equal to 92% indicates hypoxemia.
- O_2 saturation of 95% is ideal.
- Not reliable if the patient is in shock or has carbon monoxide poisoning.

Arterial Blood Gas Analysis

- Helps to measure the oxygen pressure obtained by blood gas analysis.
- PaO_2 value less than 60 mm Hg and more than 100 mm Hg indicates hypoxia and hyperoxia, respectively; both are dangerous.
- Procedure is traumatizing; limb ischemia can follow very rarely.

ADVERSE EFFECTS OF OXYGEN THERAPY—IF EXCESS ADMINISTERED

- Retinal damage in premature babies less than 32 weeks gestation.
- Excess free radical release causing alveolar capillary damage and alveolar edema at all ages.

These adverse effects can be prevented by proper monitoring. O_2 if used in less than 50% concentration, toxic effects can be eliminated even in prolonged therapy as in preterm babies and for home therapy in chronic hypoxic diseases.

CONCLUSION

Oxygen is a life-saving drug for patients with hypoxia, but in excess can cause serious organ damage and hence its therapy is to be strictly monitored.

REFERENCES

1. http://www.neumologica.org/POSTGRAD0%/202008/Articulos%20 virtuals% 20 oxigenoterapla/oxygen%20delivery%20systems%20for%20infants%20and%20 children. (Internet from 21-Sep-2011)
2. Ranjit S. Acute respiratory failure and oxygen therapy. Indian J Pediatr. 2001;68(3):249-55.

Section 3

DETECTION OF THE ACUTELY ILL CHILD

Chapter 13

Assessment in the Emergency Room

S Sushamabai

ABSTRACT

Rapid and systematic assessment of the child in the emergency room detects life-threatening problems in time and their prompt correction. The assessment steps are primary, secondary, and tertiary. Primary assessment should be within minutes by parallel history and quick physical examination based on assessment pentagon along with stabilization. Secondary assessment is to be completed within hours by detailed history and physical examination. Tertiary assessment is evaluating relevant investigations and the duration is variable.

INTRODUCTION

Rapid and systematic assessment of the child enables one to:
- Identify the immediate threats to life
- Provide timely correction.

The assessment steps are primary, secondary, and tertiary.

PRIMARY ASSESSMENT

- Assess within minutes by parallel history and physical examination.
- The steps are—ask, look, feel, assess, and then act as per the situation.

Different assessment scales are available worldwide. The Pediatric Advanced Life Support (PALS curriculum format of ABCDE approach to the patient as in *Figure 13.1* is one easily adaptable;
(**A**—airway, **B**—breathing, **C**—circulation, **D**—disability, **E**—exposure).
A: Airway—assess the patency by:
- Observing the movements of chest and abdomen
- Listening for breath sounds, stridor, and snoring
- Feeling for air movement at mouth and nose.

Proceed to clearance of airway immediately if obstructed.

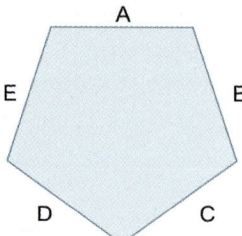

Fig. 13.1: Assessment pentagon.

B: Breathing—assess by:
- Respiratory rate—count for 30 seconds by inspection of chest movements.
- Bradypnea and apnea herald immediate intervention.
- Tachypnea or fast breathing is to be considered if the respiratory rate (RR) is more than 60/min for less than 60 days age; more than or equal to 50/min for more than or equal to 60 days to 1 year; more than or equal to 40/min for more than 1 year to 5 years; and more than or equal to 30/min for more than 5 years age.
- Severe tachypnea: Less than 1 year more than 70/min; More than 1 year more than 50/min.
- Observe for increased work of breathing as revealed by—chest retraction, suprasternal indrawing, and head nodding with respiration.
- Auscultate the lungs for added breath sounds which include—grunting, stridor, crackles, and wheeze.
- Record pulse oximetry which if less than 94% indicates hypoxemia.

C: Circulation—assess by:
- Look and feel of the skin—for color, mottling, and warmth; pale/cyanosed and cold extremities and mottled skin indicate compromised cardiac output.
- Heart rate (HR) and rhythm—auscultate for 5 seconds and multiply by 12. At any age, HR less than 60/min is bradycardia and more than 180/min is tachycardia, both require further evaluation. Heart rate if more than three times the age-wise normal RR is tachycardia.
- Delayed capillary refill time (CRFT): Elevate the upper limb 15° above the precordial level, gently press the finger tip for 3 seconds, assess the time for blanching to disappear. CRFT more than or equal to 3 seconds indicates peripheral circulatory failure.
- Blood pressure evaluation—consider hypotension if systolic blood pressure is less than or equal to 60 mm Hg for neonate, less than or equal to 70 mm Hg for 1 month to 1 year age, less than or equal to 70 + (2 × age in year) for 1–10 years age, and less than or equal to 90 mm Hg for all more than 10 years age.

D: Disability—refers to neurologic dysfunction for the level of consciousness and cortical function; assess by:
- Pupillary size and response to light
- AVPU scale (A—alert, V—response to call, P—response to pain, U—unresponsive to all).

E: Exposure—assess by:
- Undressing the child completely to detect injuries, burns, bleeding, bite marks, and fractures.
- Recording the body temperature to detect hypothermia and fever.

SECONDARY ASSESSMENT
- Start as early as possible after the primary assessment and stabilization.
- Assess by focused history and physical examination.
- Should be completed within few hours to arrive at a clinical diagnosis.

TERTIARY ASSESSMENT
- Proceed to appropriate investigations relevant to the clinical diagnosis.
- Duration depends on the type of emergency.

CONCLUSION
Systematic assessment of the patient in the emergency room as primary, secondary, and tertiary steps will enable for timely, effective stabilization and to reduce death and morbidity.

Chapter 14

Clinical Scoring Systems

S Sushamabai

ABSTRACT

Scoring systems applying clinical signs with or without investigations are helpful to understand the critical stage of the patient and for counseling the parents. Two widely applied scoring systems are the Acute Illness Observation Scale (AIOS) and the Pediatric Risk of Mortality 3rd Version (PRISM III). In AIOS (applicable to babies >3 months age only), six clinical parameters are used, score 6 predicting good survival and score 30 revealing 10-fold increase in chance of serious illness. In PRISM III, 17 physiologic variables subdivided into 26 ranges are assessed—score more than 10 predicting higher mortality and long pediatric intensive care unit (PICU) stay.

INTRODUCTION

Scoring systems are helpful in assessing the severity of illness in PICU so that information regarding the critical stage and the probable outcome can be communicated more objectively. Two scoring systems—*AIOS*[1-5] and *PRISM III*[6] used for this purpose are described below:

Acute illness observation scale (AIOS).

Six observation items and their scales that have reliably and validly identified serious illness in febrile children are given below. Total score is 6 × 5 = 30. The scale is not applicable in babies < 3 m age.

	Observation item	Normal		Moderate impairment		Severe impairment	
1.	Quality of cry	Strong with normal tone or content and not crying	☐ ☐	Whimpering/ sobbing	☐	Weak / moaning/ high pitched	☐ ☐
2.	Reaction to parent stimulation (effect on consoling)	Cries briefly, then stops/content and not crying	☐ ☐	Cries off and on	☐	Continual cry/ Hardly responds	☐ ☐

Contd...

Contd...

	Observation item	Normal		Moderate impairment		Severe impairment	
3.	State variation	If awake, then stays awake or if asleep and stimulated, wakes up quickly	☐ ☐	Eyes close briefly, then awakens or awakens with prolonged stimulation.	☐ ☐	Will not rouse or Falls to sleep	☐ ☐
4.	Color	Pink	☐	Pale hands and feet or Acrocyanosis	☐ ☐	Pale/blue or Ashen (gray) or mottled	☐ ☐ ☐
5.	Hydration	Skin normal, eyes, mouth moist	☐	Skin, eyes normal mouth slightly dry	☐ ☐	Skin doughy or tented & eyes may be sunken & dry eyes and mouth	☐ ☐
6.	Response to social overtures	Smiles or alerts (2 months or less)	☐ ☐	Brief smile or alerts briefly (2 months or less)	☐ ☐	No smile, face anxious or Dull expressionless No alerting (2 months or less)	☐ ☐ ☐

Scoring: Normal – 1; Moderate impairment – 3; Severe impairment – 5
The best possible score – 6 x 1 = 6; worst score – 6 x 5 = 30
Chance of serious illness
1–2% if total score ≤ 10; 10-fold increase if total score > 10.

PEDIATRIC RISK OF MORTALITY (3RD VERSION)

It is based on 17 physiologic variables, subdivided into 26 ranges. Mortality and duration of PICU stay are found to increase as the PRISM III score exceeds 10 in sick children.[7] The parameters and scores are given below:

Cardiovascular/neurologic vital signs.

Systolic blood pressure (mm Hg)
Measurement ....

	Score = 3	Score = 7
Neonate	40–55	<40
Infant	45–65	<45
Child	55–75	<55
Adolescent	65–85	<65

Heart rate (beats/min)
Measurement........................

	Score = 3	Score = 4
Neonate	215–225	>225
Infant	215–225	>225
Child	185–205	>205
Adolescent	145–155	>155

Contd...

Contd...

Temperature
Measurement ....
        Score = 3
All ages   <33° C (91.4° F) or
        >40.0° C (104.0° F)

Pupillary reflexes
Measurement............................
        Score = 7   Score =11
All ages   One fixed   Both fixed
                              One reactive

Mental status
Measurement.......................
        Score = 5
All ages   Stupor/Coma (GCS < 8)

Acid–base or blood gases.

Acidosis   Total CO_2 mmol/L or pH
Measurement.....................
        Score = 2   Score = 6
All ages   pH 7.0–7.28   pH <7.0
        or T CO_2 5–16.9   or T CO_2 <5

Total CO_2 (mmol/L)
Measurement................
        Score = 4
All ages   >34.0

pH
Measurement.....................
        Score = 2   Score = 3
All ages   7.48–7.55   >7.55

PaO_2 (mm Hg)
Measurement.....................
        Score = 3   Score = 6
All ages   42.0–49.9   <42.0

PCO_2 (mm Hg)
Measurement ....
        Score = 1
All ages   50.0–75.0

Score = 3
>75.0

Chemistry tests.

Glucose
Measurement......................
        Score = 2
All ages   > 200 mg/dL or
        > 11.0 mmol/L

Potassium (mmol/L)
Measurement ....
        Score = 3
All ages   > 6.9

Creatinine
Measurement......................
        Score = 2
Neonate   > 0.85 mg/dL or 75 μmol/L
Infant   > 0.90 mg/dL or 80 μmol/L
Child   > 0.90 mg/dL or 80 μmol/L
Adolescent   > 1.30 mg/dL or 115 μmol/L

Blood urea nitrogen (BUN)
Measurement ....
        Score = 3
Neonate   > 11.9 mg/dL or
        > 4.3 mmol/L
All other ages   > 14.9 mg/dL or
        > 5.4 mmol/L

Hematology tests.

White blood cell count (cells/mm³)

Measurement ....

	Score = 4
All ages	< 3,000

Platelet count (cells/mm³)

Measurement ....

	Score = 2
All ages	100,000–200,000

Prothrombin time (PT) or Partial thromboplastin time (PTT) (sec)

Measurement ....

	Score = 3
Neonate	PT > 22.0 or PTT > 85.0
All other ages	PT > 22.0 or PTT > 57.0

	Score = 4	Score = 5
	50,000–99,999	< 50,000

Total Prism III score ....

CONCLUSION

For sick children in PICU applying clinical scoring systems is highly helpful to prognosticate the disease status, anticipating organ supportive therapy and counseling the family.

REFERENCES

1. McCarthy PL, Sharpe MR, Speizel SZ, et al. Observation scales to identify serious illness in febrile children. Pediatrics. 1982;70:802.
2. https://www.nice.org.uk/guidance/CG160/documents/feverish-illness-in-children-update-appendix-h-evidence. (Internet from 02-Jul-2017).
3. Jaskiewicz JA, McCarthy CA. Evaluation and management of the febrile infants 60 days of age or younger. Pediatr Ann. 1993;22(8):477-80, 482-3.
4. http://indianpediatrics.net/jan2002/jan-12-22htm. (Internet from03-Oct–2008).
5. Bulloch B. Fever without focus in the older infant. In: Moyer VA, Elliott EJ, Gilbert R, Klassen T, Logan S, Mellis C, Henderson-Smart DJ, Williams K (Eds). Evidence-based Paediatrics. BMJ; 2007.
6. Pollack MM, Patel KM, Ruttimann UE. PRISM III: An updated pediatric risk of mortality score. Crit Care Med. 1996;24:743-52.
7. Nishad AK, Carol SC, Sushamabai S, et al. Role of PRISM III score in predicting the outcome of children in pediatric intensive care unit. Pushpagiri Medical Journal. 2015;7:18-25.

Chapter **15**

Arterial Blood Gas Analysis

S Sushamabai

ABSTRACT

Arterial blood gas (ABG) is the most important investigation to detect rapidly the derangements in the body physiological status. The parameters assessed are pH, pCO_2, pO_2, HCO_3, base excess, and anion gap. The blood sample for assessment should be collected and transported to laboratory as per standard directions. The abnormalities encountered are metabolic acidosis, respiratory acidosis, metabolic alkalosis, and respiratory alkalosis as simple or mixed error. The treatment is to control the basic illness, ventilatory support for hypoxia and hypercarbia, intravenous (IV) sodium bicarbonate or tris (hydroxymethyl) aminomethane (THAM) for metabolic acidosis, normal saline for metabolic alkalosis, proper ventilation and oxygen for respiratory acidosis and rebreathing into a bag for respiratory alkalosis. Isolated ABG abnormalities without clinical signs need not be corrected. Finally calculate the anion gap and correct the electrolyte derangement.

INTRODUCTION

Arterial blood gas provides information regarding the acid-base status, oxygenation, ventilation, electrolytes, and hemoglobin status of the body. Basic knowledge of ABG analysis is mandatory for treating critically ill children since derangements of these parameters is fatal and should be corrected as emergency.

INDICATIONS FOR ABG ANALYSIS

- Acute severe respiratory distress
- Critically ill child
- Chronic persistent respiratory distress
- Acute cardiac disorders
- Renal failure—acute or chronic
- Suspected inborn errors of metabolism.

PARAMETERS TO BE INTERPRETED

- pH: Denotes the H⁺ concentration otherwise the acid status of the body.
- pCO_2: Denotes the arterial CO_2 level or the ventilation status.
- pO_2: Indicates the oxygen tension in the blood or the oxygenation status.
- HCO_3: Represents the base status.
- Base excess: Measures the renal metabolic component of base status.

A simplified version of ABG interpretation in 10 steps is described next.

Note: ABG interpretation should be always based on history and physical examination.

- *Step 1: Collection of blood sample*
  Arterial blood is ideal. Venous blood is adequate for acid–base interpretation alone when frequent evaluation is needed as in diabetic ketoacidosis or renal disease. Use heparinized syringe (0.05–0.1 mL heparin/1 mL blood). Excess heparin increases H⁺ concentration. Transport the sample to the laboratory (chilled in ice) without delay. The report should be ready within minutes.

- *Step 2: Recollect the basic normal values:*

  pH: 7.40 ± 0.04 pCO_2: 40 ± 4 mm Hg
  HCO_3: $24 + 4$ mEq/ PaO_2: 80–100 mm Hg
  Hb: 11–12 g/dL Base excess: +/-2

- *Step 3: Assess the pH—whether normal, acidosis or alkalosis*
  - $N = 7.40 \pm 0.4$
  - Less than 7.35: Acidosis
  - More than 7.45: Alkalosis.

- *Step 4: Find out whether the abnormality is respiratory or metabolic.*

	Acidosis	Alkalosis
Respiratory	CO_2 ↑	CO_2 ↓
Metabolic	HCO_3 ↓ or Base excess ↓	HCO_3 ↑ or Base excess ↑

- *Step 5: Assess the compensation whether appropriate or not.*

Disorder	Expected compensation
Metabolic acidosis	$pCO_2 = 1.5 \times (HCO_3) + 8 \pm 2$ (Winter's formula)
Metabolic alkalosis	pCO_2 increase by 7 mm Hg for each 10 mEq/L increase in the serum (HCO_3) or $pCO_2 = 0.7 \times (HCO_3) + 21 \pm 1.5$
Respiratory acidosis	
Acute (<24 hr respiratory distress)	HCO_3 increases by 1 for each 10 mm Hg increase in pCO_2
Chronic (>2 days respiratory distress)	HCO_3 increases by 3.5 for each 10 mm Hg increase in pCO_2
Respiratory alkalosis	
Acute	HCO_3 falls by 2 for each 10 mm Hg decrease in pCO_2
Chronic	HCO_3 falls by 4 for each 10 mm Hg decrease in pCO_2

Comparable values for venous blood gas.

	Arterial blood gas	Venous blood gas
pH	7.4	7.37
pCO_2	40 mm Hg	45 mm Hg
pO_2	97 mm Hg	40 mm Hg

- *Step 6: Confirm your findings with the base excess and pH*
  - Low pH with negative base excess: Acidosis
  - High pH with positive base excess: Alkalosis
  - If the base excess disagrees with the pH, it is compensating for a respiratory abnormality.
- *Step 7: Assess whether the disorder is simple or mixed*
  - Simple acid–base disorder: pCO_2 and HCO_3 change in the same direction
  - Mixed disorder: pCO_2 and HCO_3 change to the opposite directions
  - Common mixed disorders are: acute severe asthma, shock, cardiopulmonary arrest, respiratory distress syndrome (RDS) in the newborn, salicylate poisoning, and diuretic therapy (Flowchart 15.1).
- *Step 8: Assess the oxygen status, give correction immediately*
  - Keep the oxygen supplementation appropriate to maintain PaO_2 between 80 mm Hg and 90 mm Hg to avoid oxygen toxicity.
  - Irrespective of the oxygen status, if the child is critically ill with cardiorespiratory problem, provide 100% oxygen.
- *Step 9: Assess the Hb status to account for hypoxia*
  Consider packed red blood cell transfusion if Hb is less than 7 g/dL.
- *Step 10: Assess the anion gap*
  - Plasma anion gap is useful for evaluating patients with metabolic acidosis.
  - It divides the patients into 2 diagnostic groups—normal or increased anion gap.
  - Anion gap = Na − (Cl + HCO_3); normal value is 4 to 11.
  - Increased anion gap indicates an increase in unmeasured anions.

The common causes of normal and increased anion gap metabolic acidosis.

Normal anion gap metabolic acidosis	Increased anion gap metabolic acidosis
Diarrhea	Methanol poisoning
Renal tubular acidosis	Uremia
	Diabetic ketoacidosis
	Infections
	Lactic acidosis
	Ethylene glycol poisoning
	Starvation ketosis
	Salicylate poisoning
	Inborn errors of metabolism (organic acidemias)

Flowchart 15.1: Interpretation of acid-base disturbances.

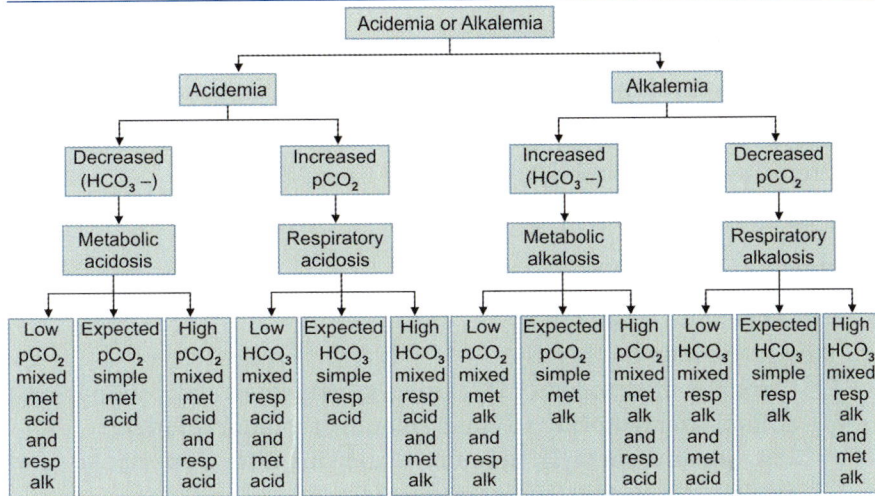

(met acid, metabolic acidosis; resp acid, respiratory acidosis; met alk, metabolic alkalosis; resp alk, respiratory alkalosis)

Table 15.1: Estimation of H⁺ from pH.

pH	Estimated (H^+)
7.0	98
7.10	78
7.20	63
7.30	50
7.40	40
7.50	32
7.60	26
7.70	20

Laboratory error: To be verified if the ABG values do not agree with the clinical situation.

Evaluate whether the three given values are mutually compatible according to Henderson–Hasselbalch equation in which,

$$H = 24 \times pCO_2/HCO_3 \text{ (pH is presented as } H^+ \text{ ion concentration)}$$

For example: If HCO_3 is 20 mEq/L, pH 7.40, pCO_2 33, calculate the value closer to pH using the above formula:

$$H = 24 \times 33/20 = 40$$
$$\text{pH: estimated } (H^+) \text{ (refer to Table 15.1)}$$

THERAPY IN BLOOD GAS DERANGEMENT

Metabolic Acidosis

Clinical Features (May be masked by the underlying illness)

- *Acute:* Deep breathing showing air hunger (Kussmaul breathing), drowsiness, resistant shock, and cardiac irregularity.
- *Chronic:* Lethargy, failure to thrive, and unexplainable dehydration.

Treatment

- Treat the underlying illness
- If pH is less than 7:
  - IV sodium bicarbonate (7.5%) 1 mEq/kg as bolus or add to the patient's IV fluid after removing an equal amount of sodium chloride.
  - Tris (hydroxymethyl) aminomethane in mixed metabolic and respiratory acidosis: 2 mEq/kg/dose (1 mEq = 3.3 mL)
  - Hemodialysis in renal insufficiency.

Respiratory Acidosis

Causes

- *Respiratory:* Asthma, pneumonia, acute respiratory distress syndrome, and fatigue
- *Central nervous system:* Drug-induced (narcotics), encephalitis, head trauma, and respiratory paralysis.

Clinical Features

Mainly due to etiology: Headache, confusion, asterixis, coma, and seizures.

Treatment

- Treat the underlying cause.
- Mechanical ventilation if pCO_2 is more than 75 mm Hg in acute conditions
- Avoid bicarbonate therapy.

Metabolic Alkalosis

Causes

- Chloride loss: Emesis, NG tube aspiration, diarrhea, endocrine disorders, and diuretic therapy
- Excess base therapy
- Severe hypokalemia.

Clinical Features

- Features of the underlying illness
- Apathy, stupor
- Tetany due to hypocalcemia
- Hypotonia and abdominal distention due to hypokalemia.

Treatment

- Treat the underlying cause
- Stop excess base therapy
- Change the diuretic
- Potassium supplementation
- IV normal saline if HCO_3 is more than 32 mEq/L

Respiratory Alkalosis

Causes

Tachypnea due to asthma, bronchiolitis, pneumonia, and hyperventilation.

Clinical Features

- Only in severe and acute stage
- Paresthesia and numbness.

Treatment

- Treat the underlying cause.
- Rebreathing into bag in hyperventilation.

CONCLUSION

Arterial blood gas analysis is a must in all sick children. Collection and transport of the blood sample should be careful; interpretation and corrective therapy should be done correlating with the clinical condition.

Section 4

RESPIRATORY SYSTEM

Chapter **16**

Mechanical Ventilation

Carol Sara Cherian, S Sushamabai

ABSTRACT

Mechanical ventilation is respiration maintained by an equipment connected to the patient's airway. The indications are respiratory and nonrespiratory, which ultimately lead to derangement in blood gas pattern. Anticipate mechanical ventilation in any patient, at any time in the pediatric intensive care unit (PICU). Hence the expert staff and updated equipment and properly functioning ventilators should be always ready in the PICU. Ventilate the patient at the earliest indication. First intubate the patient, assess the endotracheal (ET) tube functioning by bagging and adjust the ventilator settings according to the disease process and the weight of the child. Set the initial FiO_2 at 0.6 to at 100% O_2 and reduce the FiO_2 to less than 0.5 to maintain SpO_2 at 95%, ensure humidification and set the alarms. Administer midazolam and morphine for sedation and analgesia. One trained staff should be solely devoted to care the patient. Parameters for weaning and extubation are control of the precipitating illness, SpO_2 = 95% with FiO_2 less than 0.4, stable cardiovascular status, intact cough and gag reflexes, and low level of ventilator settings.

INTRODUCTION

Mechanical ventilation is the movement of air in and out of the lungs by a ventilator connected directly to the patient's airway. The device may also be a resuscitation bag.

NORMAL VERSUS MECHANICAL VENTILATION

In normal ventilation, negative intrathoracic pressure created during chest expansion results in inspiration. Expiration follows passively by the elastic recoiling of the lungs. In mechanical ventilation most commonly positive pressure is applied to the upper airway to drive in air into the lungs raising the airway pressure (and its adverse effects). Negative pressure ventilators which simulate physiologic ventilation (are more scientific) are not well-established because they are technically complex.

INDICATIONS FOR MECHANICAL VENTILATION

- Respiratory failure revealing blood gas derangement as PaO_2 less than 60 Torr while breathing 60% O_2, $PaCO_2$ more than 60 Torr, and pH less than 7.25.
- Clinical situations as:
    - Apnea, cardiac arrest, Glasgow Coma Scale less than 8, and unable to protect the airway
    - Refractory status epilepticus and fluid refractory shock
    - Respiratory paralysis (Guillain-Barré syndrome, envenomation, poisoning, and paralytic poliomyelitis)
    - Acute life-threatening asthma and severe bronchiolitis
    - Alveolar diseases (severe pneumonia, ARDS)
    - Post-cardiac surgery and pulmonary edema
    - Head and spinal cord injuries
    - Chest trauma—flail chest and pneumothorax.

TERMINOLOGIES USED

- *Tidal volume (V_T):* The volume of air that flows in and out of the chest during quiet breathing. Normal value is 6–12 mL/kg. Restricting V_T to the lower limit, i.e. lung protective ventilation reduces ventilation-induced lung injury *(VILI)*.
- *Frequency/ventilation rate (V_F/V_R):* Respiratory rate set in the ventilator depending on the indication for mechanical ventilation and the physiologic norm of the patient's age. Normal range is 15–30/minute.
- *Peak inspiratory pressure (PIP):* Highest pressure that can be met during inspiration. Normal value is 15–20 cm H_2O. Should be kept to the lowest possible to prevent barotraumas.
- *Positive end-expiratory pressure (PEEP):* Pressure regulated in the expiratory valve of the ventilator so as to prevent end-expiratory alveolar collapse. PEEP improves oxygenation by opening diseased alveoli and increases functional residual capacity (FRC). Normal value is 4–10 cm H_2O (physiological PEEP). Can be increased up to 15 cm in noncompliant lung as in acute respiratory distress syndrome (ARDS). PEEP can be increased by reducing the expiratory time. Value more than 15 cm H_2O can cause barotraumas.
- *IE ratio (I:E):* Ratio between inspiratory and expiratory time. Normal value I:E = 1:1.5 to 1:2. Can be altered by adjusting the inspiratory time *(Ti)*. Normal Ti = 0.5 – 1.5 seconds. Oxygenation can be improved by increasing Ti.
- *Fractional inspired oxygen (FiO_2):* Fraction of inspired oxygen. 100% O_2 is represented as I. Room air O_2 is 21% (0.21).

- *Mean airway pressure (MAP):* Average positive pressure generated in the lung over time can be displayed on the ventilator. Determines the oxygenation and the possibility for barotrauma. Determined by PIP, PEEP, Ti, VR, and flow rate.

PHASES OF MECHANICAL VENTILATION

Consider four factors along with the patient's clinical condition:
1. *Mode (initiation and control of respiration)*
2. *Inspiratory phase characteristics (duration of inspiration and volume/pressure delivered)*
3. *Termination of respiration (cycle)*
4. *Expiratory phase characteristics (application of PEEP).*

Goal is to assist patient's respiratory effort. In the absence of patient's effort, respiratory muscle deconditioning may occur making weaning difficult.

Mode

In control mode, breath is initiated entirely by the ventilator. It can be:
- *Controlled mechanical ventilation (CMV):* Ventilator determines and carries out *all parts of respiration; applied in* completely apneic patients (Fig. 16.1).
- *Intermittent mandatory ventilation (IMV):* Ventilator initiates *respiration* at a set frequency. Patient can breathe spontaneously in between. Asynchrony can occur between the patient and ventilator, requiring sedation and pharmacologic paralysis.

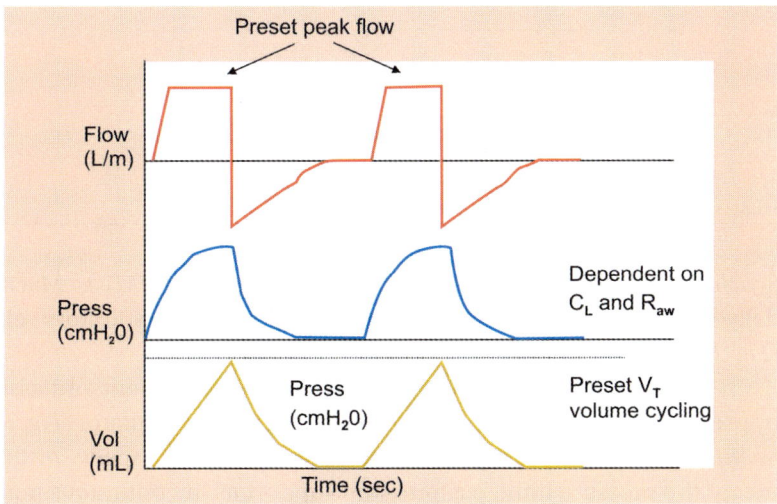

Fig. 16.1: Controlled mechanical (mandatory) ventilation (CMV).

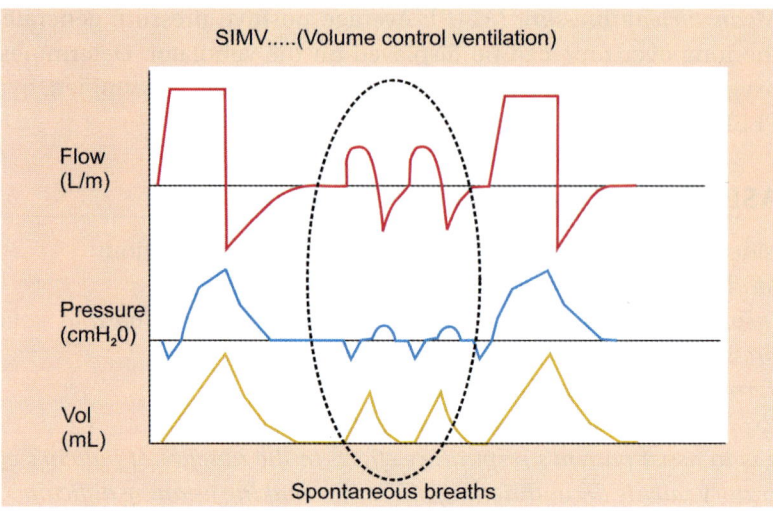

Fig. 16.2: Synchronized intermittent mandatory ventilation (SIMV).

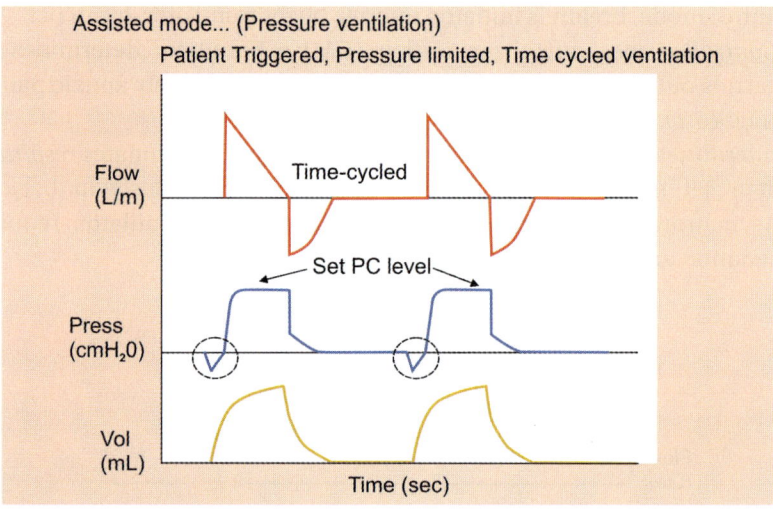

Fig. 16.3: Assist-control mode (AC mode).

- *Synchronized intermittent mandatory ventilation (SIMV):* Machine-delivered breaths are triggered by the patient's inspiratory efforts *(Fig. 16.2)* so that ventilator–patient asynchrony is less.
- *Assist-control (AC) mode:* Breath is triggered by the patient and assisted by preselected inspiratory pressure or volume by the ventilator *(Fig. 16.3).*
- *Spontaneous mode:* The patient has control over all aspects of breath except the pressure limit, e.g. pressure support as in continuous positive airway pressure (CPAP) *(Fig. 16.4).*

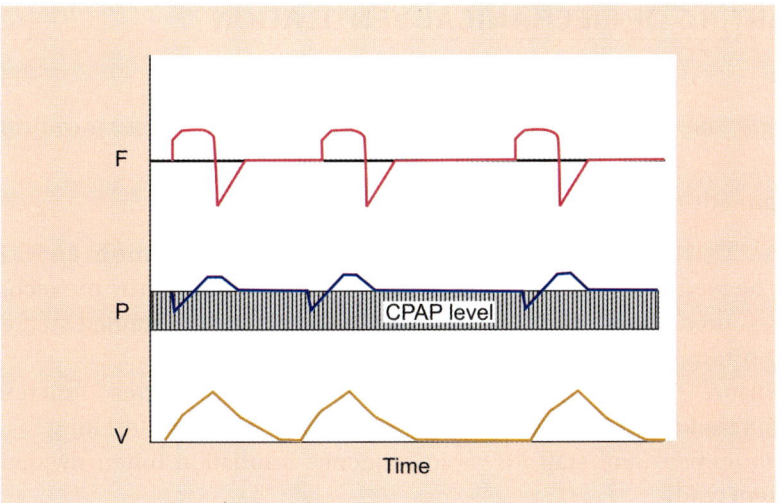

Fig. 16.4: Continuous positive airway pressure.

- *Control variable:* Can be tidal volume [volume-controlled ventilation *(VCV)*] or pressure delivered by the machine [pressure-controlled ventilation *(PCV)*]. PCV is preferred in children and also in asthma as it results in delivery of more tidal volume for the same inflation pressure. Pressure-regulated volume control *(PRVC)* combines the advantages of VCV and PCV.

Inspiratory Phase Characteristics

These should be adjusted to suit the patient's respiratory mechanics. In PCV, Ti is directly set in (seconds) the ventilator. In VCV, Ti is adjusted by controlling the inspiratory flow. Ti need is longer in diseases with low FRC such as ARDS and pulmonary edema.

Termination of Inspiration (Cycle)

It can be time cycled or volume cycled. For time cycled, breath inspiration is terminated after the preselected Ti. In volume cycled, breath inspiration ends after a preselected volume is delivered.

Expiratory Phase Characteristics

These consider the application of optimal PEEP.

STARTING OF MECHANICAL VENTILATION

Goal

To maintain oxygenation and ventilation till the disease process is controlled.

Preparation and Monitoring

- Anticipate mechanical ventilation to be started at any time in an ICU.
- The Medical Officer and the nurse in-charge should verify the technical resources, equipment efficacy, and the availability of trained staff every morning.
- Ensure O_2 and air sources, suction, monitors, alarms, function of humidifier, and "system self check" with the circuit and test lung.
- Equipment and staff for rapid sequence intubation (often needed) be kept ready.
- Intubate the patient; assess endotracheal (ET) tube functioning and continue bagging.
- Set the ventilator parameters according to the disease as SIMV/AC control mode/PCV/VCV/PRVC as variables and PS/VS. Connect the patient to the ventilator.
- Consider PCV in infants less than 8 kg because of the small tidal volume. Set the PIP to have adequate chest rise, good oxygenation, and hemodynamic stability. VCV—set V_T 6–8 mL/kg. Make adjustment as per response.
- PCV—set PIP 10–20 cm H_2O above the PEEP. Assess clinically and by SpO_2.
- Select Ti and IE ratio.
- Set the initial FiO_2 0.6 to 1 for SpO_2 100%. Reduce to less than 0.5 as the oxygenation improves to maintain SpO_2 at 95%.
- Set PEEP at 5 cm H_2O. Can be increased up to 15 cm in decreased compliance to maintain SpO_2 90% at FiO_2 0.5–0.6.
- Ensure humidifier function.
- Set the alarms—high pressure at 8–10 cm H_2O above the set PIP and low pressure 5–10 cm H_2O below the set PIP.

Table 16.1 reveals the ventilator settings in different respiratory disorders.

- Proper sedation and analgesics to prevent patient distress—use a combination of midazolam (1–2 µg/kg/min) + morphine (30–60 µg/kg/min) or others as per disease condition (Chapter 8).

Subsequent monitoring (Refer post-resuscitation care—Chapter 10).

Clinical: Frequently (at least hourly)

Table 16.1: Disease-based ventilator parameters.

Problem	V_F /min	V_T mL/kg	PIP (cm H_2O)	PEEP (cm H_2O)	I:E	Ti	Any others
Normal lung	15–30	7–10	15–20	4–10	1:2	0.8–1	
Bronchial asthma	8–12	10–12	30–40	0–4	1:2–4		
Bronchopneumonia	25–40	6–7	15–25	4–8	1:1.5–2	0.4–0.5	
ARDS	25–40	6 mL for LBW	<30	Optimal for SpO_2 90%	1:1 to 1:3		

(ARDS, acute respiratory distress syndrome; PEEP, positive end-expiratory pressure; I:E, inspiratory to expiratory time; PIP, peak inspiratory pressure; Ti, inspiratory time; V_F, ventilatory frequency; V_T, tidal volume)

Remember: One trained staff nurse should constantly care the patient.
- Frequency of ventilation or asynchrony.
- Vitals, capillary refill time, and equal air entry in chest.
- Neurological status.
- Abdominal distension, bowel sounds, gastric aspiration, and urine output.

Ventilator Assessment

- Ventilation rate and spontaneous breathing.
- Pulse oximetry and continuous monitoring of vitals (non invasive).

Radiological

Chest skiagram once daily till improvement and whenever any deterioration. Confirm the position of the ET (at the level of the 2nd rib) and nasogastric tube; assess for hyperinflation, air leak, atelectasis, pneumonia, and cardiac size.

Laboratory Investigations

Arterial blood gas within 1 hour of intubation and then at least 12 hourly, after major setting changes or if any change in condition.

Goal: pH 7.35–7.45; pO_2 60–90; pCO_2 35–45.

Other laboratory tests: Complete blood count, renal function test, electrolytes as indicated, and culture of ETT secretions.

CARE OF THE CHILD ON VENTILATOR

- Prevent aspiration: Head-end elevation 30–45°.
- Frequent (2 hourly) position change.

- 4 hourly ET suction or more frequently if more secretions.
- Frequent suctioning of oral and deep pharyngeal secretions to prevent aspiration.
- Apply 2% chlorhexidine thrice daily orally.
- Deflate the cuffed tube intermittently.
- Promote drainage of the ventilator condensate.
- Continue sedation and analgesics till signs of recovery.
- Maintain general hygiene.
- Protect pressure areas and eyes.
- Start nasogastric feeds with age appropriate protein, calories, micronutrients and adequate fluids at the earliest; avoid if ileus.
- Bowel and bladder care by enema/laxative and indwelling catheter.
- Maintain strict asepsis.
- A pleasant environment in the PICU with musical background, frequent caretaker visits, touch and tender loving care to speed up the recovery.
- Parent counseling at least twice daily by senior doctors and in between as per situation (by duty staff) regarding the patient's progress is very important.

VENTILATOR PROBLEMS ENCOUNTERED

Rapid Deterioration—Suspect and Rectify

- Change in heart rate, respiratory rate, hypotension, cyanosis, pallor, poor perfusion (delayed CRFT), increased work of breathing (WOB), struggling patient, poor lung aeration, and alarm activation.
- Close monitoring helps detection before alarm activation:
    - Rule out DOPE [**D**-displaced tube, **O**-obstructed tube, **P**- pneumothorax, pneumopericardium, **E**-equipment failure (disconnection)].
    - Disconnect the patient from the ventilator, initiate bag and mask with 100% oxygen; do gastric decompression.
    - Equipment failure: Check for leaks, disconnection; check ventilator function with a test lung, rectify the problem, and reconnect.
- Bag and mask ventilation if still unstable:
    - Check tube patency: Provide vigorous suction.
    - Cannot pass suction catheter? Deflate the cuff and continue suction.
    - No improvement: Laryngoscopy to visualize ETT position; reintroduce the tube if displacement is observed.
    - Endotracheal tube in position: No block but no improvement—suspect air leak or worsening of lung disease.
    - Manually ventilate with a PEEP device; order chest X-ray (CXR) urgently, treat as per pathology.

- *Airway disease (asthma, bronchiolitis)*: Suspect auto PEEP. Confirm by CXR revealing hyperinflation. Disconnect the ventilator for 20–30 seconds, brief manual squeeze, reset ventilator connections and parameters so as to improve expiration. Sedate properly.
- No problems in DOPE, patient still unstable—look for patient ventilator dyssynchrony. Assess by ventilator rate and spontaneous rate along with PIP, SpO_2 and exhaled volume. Reset the ventilator parameters.

Gradual Deterioration

Causes are:
- Partial tube occlusion
- Sepsis, pneumonia (VAP), and lung collapse
- Biochemical disturbances
- Myocardial dysfunction
- Ventilator-induced lung injury
- Poor humidification.

Assess and do appropriate correction.

WEANING AND EXTUBATION

- Indicate the process of discontinuing the ventilator support.
- Rapid discontinuation is possible in the majority especially in upper airway obstruction.
- Longer period is required in conditions like Guillain–Barré syndrome and muscle diseases.
- Traditional methods involve gradual reduction on the ventilator support over days, e.g.:
  - IMV to SIMV with PS and gradual reduction
  - Noninvasive CPAP 5–8 cm H_2O.
- Extubation, if prolonged for more than 7 days, failure rate is more.

Parameters to be Satisfied

- Recovery from the primary indication for mechanical ventilation, e.g. status epilepticus.
- Glasgow Coma Scale more than 11, stable cardiovascular status, no/minimal tachypnea or tachycardia, no more increased WOB, stable $SpO_2 = 95\%$ on FiO_2 less than 0.4.
- Intact central respiratory effort and airway protective reflexes (cough, gag).
- Low level of ventilator support—SIMV 5/min, PS—5 cm H_2O, PEEP 5–7 cm H_2O, PIP less than 20 cm H_2O, and no gross dyselectrolytemia or acidosis.

Spontaneous Breathing Trial

- Should be assessed before extubation.
- Assess all parameters as above are satisfied.
- Start CPAP on less than or equal to 5 cm H_2O or low-level ventilator support.
- Observe for cardiovascular or respiratory compromise (tachypnea, tachycardia, increased WOB, prolonged CRFT).
- If stable, continue for 30 minutes; if unstable, terminate spontaneous breathing trial (SBT).
- Repeat SBT in failed cases should only be after 24 hours stabilization and support.
- Older method is T-piece trial.

Procedure for Extubation

- IV dexamethasone 0.5 mg/kg q 6 hr; start 24 hrs prior to planned extubation, continue 4–6 doses.
- Keep nil oral for 4 hours, NG aspiration just prior to extubation.
- Suction of oral cavity, ETT, and nostrils.
- Withdraw the tube during positive pressure inflation of ambu bag.
- Nurse the child head elevated; administer warm and humidified oxygen as required.
- Give adrenaline nebulization or Heliox if post-extubation stridor occurs.
- Assess ABG 20 minutes after extubation.

CONCLUSION

Mechanical ventilation is an expert invasive process for patient survival often required in PICU and the staff and equipment in PICU should always be well prepared for it.

FURTHER READING

1. Venkatraman ST. Mechanical ventilation and respiratory care. In: Fuhrman BP, Zimmerman J (Eds). Pediatric Critical Care, 3rd edition. Philadelphia PA: Mosby Elsevier; 2006. pp. 683-719.

Chapter 17

Foreign Body Obstruction of the Airway

S Sushamabai

ABSTRACT

Foreign body (FB) of the airways is not uncommon in children especially in the 1–3-year age group. The child can present as sudden choking, acute respiratory distress, recurrent or persistent wheeze or with chronic cough and wheeze. This chapter deals with the clinical presentation, patient approach, investigations, and emergency and late management. Chest skiagram is helpful to detect partial or complete obstruction of the airway. Immediate stabilization, salbutamol nebulization, and oxygenation should be given. Specific therapy is prompt endoscopic removal of FB with rigid bronchoscope.

INTRODUCTION

Foreign body obstruction of the airway can end up in sudden death, acute respiratory distress, persistent wheezing or chronic and recurrent respiratory illness in children. Common age is between 1 year and 3 years because of the mouthing habit to explore the objects they come across.

COMMON MATERIALS ASPIRATED

- *Small babies:* Liquid food items, rarely objects may be given to them by older siblings so that parents will be totally unaware of the situation.
- *Infants and toddlers:* Peanuts, food items, seeds, vegetable pieces, leaves, fruits, toys or their parts, chewing gums, fish bones, and medicines as tablets or capsules.

CLINICAL PRESENTATION

- Suspect foreign body aspiration in a lone child found unresponsive. If a large foreign body is obstructing the larynx, the child will be unable to cry, cough or breathe.
- Consider FB aspiration in the differential diagnosis of cardiac arrest, postictal phase, and acute laryngeal edema due to anaphylaxis or fume inhalation.
- Child witnessed to have sudden choking, gagging, paroxysmal cough, stridor, hoarseness of voice, and inability to speak.

- Child brought with history of FB aspiration but symptoms subsiding after some time. The diagnosis may be overlooked in this asymptomatic period of FB getting lodged.
- Any child with prolonged wheezy episode, recurrent cough, wheeze, and respiratory infection not responding to conventional treatment.

PATIENT APPROACH

- *Lone unresponsive child*: Immediate stabilization (refer APLS—choking child). Proceed to expel the FB by back blow and chest trusts in infants (<1 year) or Heimlich maneuver above 1 year age.
- *Open the airway*: Remove the FB if visible, do not perform blind sweep.
- Give *positive pressure breaths* with bag and mask.
- If ventilation fails and foreign body cannot be expelled out; attempt intubation and try to push FB into right or left main bronchus.
- Continue cardiopulmonary resuscitation if patient goes into arrest.

Child Witnessed or Suspected to have FB Obstruction

- Assess the severity of obstruction: Cyanosis, marked chest indrawing, inability to speak, weak cry, and poor or no air entry—all indicate severe obstruction.
- Stabilize immediately; obtain expert help for airway management.

INVESTIGATIONS

- Chest radiographs including abdomen—expiratory posteroanterior and lateral views. Obstructive emphysema with persistent inflation of the lung on the affected side and mediastinal shift to the opposite side indicate partial obstruction of bronchial lumen. Collapse is a late finding.
- CT chest in selected cases with recurrent symptoms suspicious of FB obstruction.

SPECIFIC TREATMENT

- Prompt endoscopic removal of FB with rigid instruments.
- Preoperative investigations and fluid and electrolyte stabilization should be observed.
- Salbutamol nebulization for bronchospasm.

CONCLUSION

Foreign body obstruction of the airway is more common in young children and should be diagnosed and managed promptly.

Chapter 18

Acute Stridor

Carol Sara Cherian, S Sushamabai

ABSTRACT

Acute stridor is a medical emergency in children due to different etiology. The common conditions are acute laryngotracheobronchitis (ALTB), acute epiglottitis, acute infectious laryngitis, acute bacterial tracheitis, retropharyngeal abscess, foreign body aspiration, angioedema, and spasmodic croup. The differentiating clinical features are described. Downe's score clinical scoring for severity assessment using stridor, cough, accessory muscle activity, cyanosis, and inspiratory sound is described. Score up to 6 can be managed in ER with adrenaline nebulization and dexamethasone. Those with score more than 7 should be treated in the pediatric intensive care unit with intensive supportive therapy, repeated doses of adrenaline nebulization and dexamethasone, and intubation if severe obstruction.

Specific therapy for the associated condition should be provided.

INTRODUCTION

Stridor is abnormal respiratory sound, predominantly inspiratory, resulting from critical narrowing of the upper airway (UAW). Acute stridor is a serious and potentially life-threatening affliction leading to respiratory compromise requiring immediate and expert management. The underlying illness can be acute or acute exacerbation of a preexisting chronic illness.

COMMON CAUSES AND SALIENT FEATURES

Acute Laryngotracheobronchitis

Caused by many viral agents especially influenza A virus and mycoplasma. Common age group—3 months to 5 years. Features are low-grade fever, barking cough, hoarseness of voice, and early onset of inspiratory stridor; may rarely progress to severe UAW obstruction.

Acute Epiglottitis

Pathogens—(mainly bacterial) *Haemophilus influenzae b, Streptococcus pyogenes, Streptococcus pneumoniae,* and *Staphylococcus aureus.* Common age group is 1 year to 7 years. Features—high fever, sore throat, and rapid progression to respiratory obstruction. Stridor is a late sign.

Acute Infectious Laryngitis

Mainly viral and bacterial infection by *Corynebacterium diphtheriae* can occur in unimmunized children. Low-grade fever, rhinitis, cough, hoarseness and loss of voice, and early stridor are the symptoms. In diphtheria, prominent cervical lymphadenitis (bull neck), dysphagia, and membranous tonsillitis are characteristics and can progress to rapid airway obstruction.

Spasmodic Croup

Possible allergy to viral agents. Age group 1 year to 3 years. Evening coryza, hoarseness of voice, barking cough progressing to stridor at night are characteristic; repeated episodes at subsequent nights are usual.

Acute Bacterial Tracheitis

It is a life-threatening infection. Agents are *S. aureus, Moraxella catarrhalis, H. influenzae,* and anaerobic bacteria. Mean age 5 years to 7 years. Present with high fever, brassy cough, toxicity, and stridor rapidly progressing to respiratory distress.

Retropharyngeal Abscess (RPA)

Polymicrobial infection by *group A Streptococcus*, anaerobic bacteria, *S. aureus, H. influenzae b, Klebsiella,* and *Mycobacterium avium intracellulare.* Common age group is less than 4 years. Clinical features include fever, dysphagia, drooling, neck stiffness, torticollis, stridor, and bulging of posterior pharyngeal wall on throat examination.

Foreign Body Aspiration

Common age group 1 to 3 years. Acute onset of violent paroxysms of cough, choking, and gagging are the common features. Stridor and progressive respiratory distress, if impaction occurs in larynx or trachea.

Angioedema

History of allergy, associated itching, urticaria, and angioedema are the other features.

Table 18.1: Downe's score (DS) for upper airway obstruction.

Physical finding	Score		
	0	1	2
Stridor	None	Inspiratory	Inspiratory and expiratory
Cough	None	Hoarse	Barky
Retraction and nasal flaring	None	Flaring, suprasternal retractions	Flaring, suprasternal and subcostal retractions
Cyanosis	None	In room air	In 40% O_2
Inspiratory breath sounds	Normal	Harsh and wheezy	Delayed

Score < 3, Home management; 4–7, high dependency unit care; >7, PICU admission, consider intubation if not responding to medicines.

PATIENT APPROACH

- Diagnosis and severity of respiratory distress is by clinical assessment.
- Quick history, physical examination, and ABC stabilization if the child is having severe respiratory distress (Refer—choking child for foreign body aspiration).
- Severity assessment can be done by clinical scoring such as—Downes score *(Table 18.1)* or Westley score.

TREATMENT OF AIRWAY OBSTRUCTION

Downes Score Less than 4

- Allow the child to assume comfortable position (parent's lap).
- Minimize upsetting examination or procedures.
- Oxygen therapy to keep blood oxygen saturation (SpO_2) more than 93% (face mask and non-rebreathing mask).
- Nebulized epinephrine (1: 1000) 0.5 mL/kg (max. 5 mL) with 3 mL saline in 20 minutes.
- Dexamethasone 0.6 mg/kg single dose PO/IM.
- Assess every 30 minutes for 4 hours.
- Assess the lower airway for infection or bronchospasm; treat accordingly.
- Discharge criteria—no stridor at rest, normal sensorium, and SpO_2 >93% at room air.

Downes Score More than or Equal to 4 or Increasing Stridor

- Nebulized epinephrine three doses 20 minutes interval followed by one dose every 1–2 hour as indicated. Watch for tachycardia. Taper frequency as the child improves.

- Dexamethasone 0.6 mg/kg IM followed by 0.2 mg/kg IM q 12 hr for 48 hours.
- Nebulized budesonide 2 mg in 4 mL saline (irrespective of weight) single dose.
- IV fluids—correction of dehydration followed by maintenance therapy.
- Consider intubation (expert anesthetist is needed) if the child is in impending respiratory arrest, drowsy or cyanosed.

SPECIFIC THERAPY FOR UNDERLYING ETIOLOGY

- Foreign body removal
- Retropharyngeal abscess—antibiotics and incision drainage
- Epiglottitis—antibiotics
- Bacterial tracheitis—antibiotics
- Empirical antibiotics—ceftriaxone + cloxacillin/clindamycin (+anaerobic coverage in RPA)
- Specific therapy in diphtheria.

INVESTIGATIONS

- Should be done after stabilization; not a must for diagnosis.
- Chest skiagram to exclude lower respiratory illness.
- X-ray neck anteroposterior—steeple sign in ALTB.
- X-ray neck lateral—thumb sign in acute epiglottitis and widening of retropharyngeal space in RPA.
- Complete blood count, blood culture—diagnostic help in bacterial infections.
- Throat swab culture and pus culture in RPA.
- Arterial blood gas analysis to decide about intubation.

MONITORING

Vitals, Downes score, sensorium, and SpO_2.

PROGNOSIS

- Excellent if early diagnosis and appropriate treatment initiated.
- Excellent for ALTB, laryngitis and spasmodic croup.

The algorithm for approach to a child with acute stridor has been described in Flowchart 18.1.

Flowchart 18.1: Algorithm for approach to a child with acute stridor.

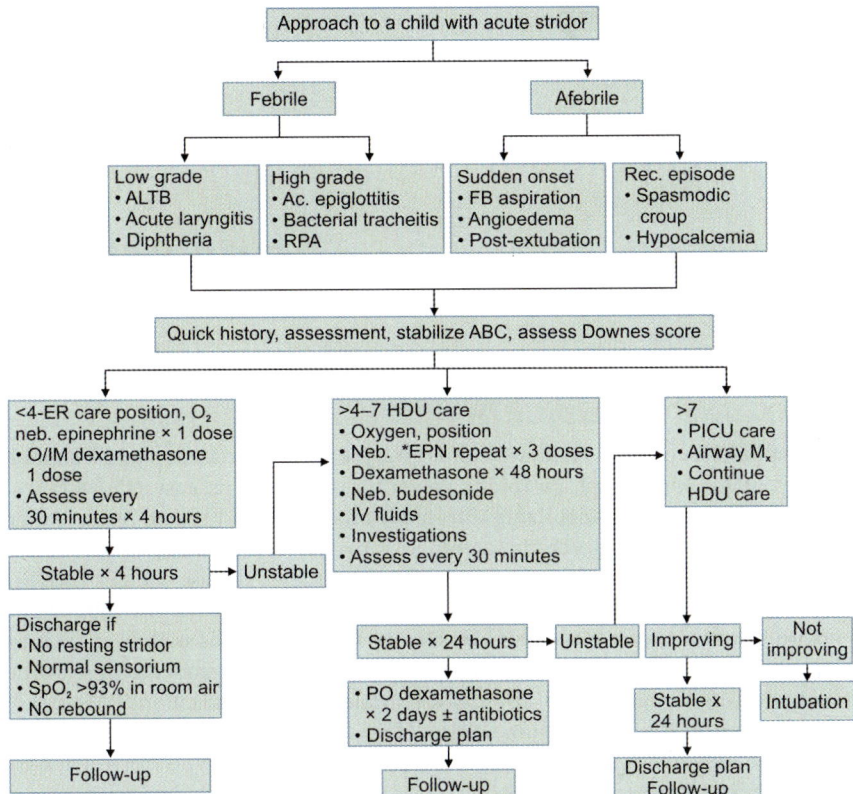

*Epinephrine
(ALTB, acute laryngotracheobronchitis; FB, foreign body; HDU, high dependency unit; PICU, pediatric intensive care unit; RPA, retropharyngeal abscess)

CONCLUSION

Acute stridor is a danger sign of differing etiology, should be perceived and severity assessment done at the earliest and treated with intensive supportive therapy and intubation if needed.

FURTHER READING

1. Downes JJ, Godinez RI. Acute upper airway obstruction in the child. In: American Society of Anesthesiologists Refresher Courses in Anesthesiology, Volume 8. Philadelphia: Lippincott; 1980.
2. Everard ML. Acute Bronchiolitis and Croup. Pediatric Clin N Am. 2000;56:119-33.

Chapter 19

Acute Asthma

Carol Sara Cherian, S Sushamabai

ABSTRACT

Acute asthma is a common pediatric emergency. Prompt recognition and treatment will save death and reduce morbidity. Severity assessment is easy clinically with pulmonary score (PS), categorizing into mild, moderate, and severe exacerbation. Red flag signs indicate acute life-threatening asthma (ALTA). Intensive bronchodilator therapy with short-acting beta-agonists (SABA) as metered dose inhaler (MDI) is recommended for mild exacerbation. In moderate exacerbation, SABA nebulization is advised intermittently but should be changed to continuous nebulization if the response is poor. Early steroid therapy is mandatory to hasten recovery. Other bronchodilators in the order of priority are ipratropium nebulization, IV SABA, IV aminophylline, and IV magnesium sulfate. Mechanical ventilation is the last choice and is to be judiciously applied. Supportive therapy with fluids and electrolytes and oxygen therapy carry equal significance. If treated appropriately, prognosis is very good. All children should be followed up for asthma education and preventive therapy.

DEFINITION

Acute asthma is exacerbation of respiratory distress due to progressive airway obstruction in an asthmatic child. A child with three or more episodes of cough, difficult breathing, and wheeze (triad of asthma) can be considered asthmatic with other causes of recurrent wheezing being excluded.

PATHOPHYSIOLOGY

Asthma is a chronic inflammatory disease of the airways due to hyper-responsiveness resulting in bronchospasm, mucosal edema, and mucous plugging. The blood gas changes in acute exacerbation are:
- Hypoxemia—because of airway obstruction and ventilation perfusion mismatch.
- Initial hypocarbia—due to reflex tachypnea secondary to hypoxemia; normal pCO_2 levels indicate significant airway obstruction.

- Hypercarbia is an ominous sign resulting from increased dead space because of alveolar hyperinflation and progressive muscle fatigue.

Goals of therapy are to:
- Correct hypoxemia
- Relieve bronchospasm and airway inflammation
- Detect and treat complications.

PATIENT APPROACH

Initial 5 minutes: Quick assessment to detect disease severity and for stabilization.
- Look for *red flag signs*: Altered sensorium, apnea, cyanosis, bradycardia, sweating, exhaustion, hypotension, silent chest, and blood oxygen saturation (SpO_2) less than 92%.
- Stabilize airway, breathing, circulation (ABC), mechanical ventilation if apneic.

Subsequent 5–15 minutes: Proceed to detailed history and clinical examination. Diagnosis of asthma is essentially clinical. Assess the disease severity by PS as in Table 19.1.

Decide treatment area and protocol

PS	Asthma exacerbation	Treatment area
0–3	Mild	Home/emergency room
4–6	Moderate	High-dependency unit
>6	Severe	Pediatric ICU

Pulmonary Score: 0–3 (Mild)
- Salbutamol MDI (100 µg/puff), 6 puffs (<6 years) or 12 puffs (>6 years) in 20 minutes; repeat three doses; reassess at 1 hour. Repeat MDI 1–4 hourly till PS is decreasing. If better, monitor for 6 hours. If stable in room air at 6 hours, advice home therapy with salbutamol MDI (6–12 puffs) every 6 hourly × 4 days.

Table 19.1: Pulmonary score.				
Score	Respiratory rate		Wheeze	Accessory muscle activity
	<6 yrs	>6 yrs		
0	<30	<20	Nil	Nil
1	30–45	20–35	End expiratory	Mild
2	>45–60	>35–50	Entire expiratory	Moderate
3	>60	>50	Inspiratory and expiratory/ silent chest	Severe

- Add oral corticosteroids (OCS)—prednisolone 1 mg/kg every 12 hours if past history of severe exacerbations or lack of improvement in 1 hour after salbutamol MDI. Continue at home for 4 days.
- Follow-up after 1 week for detailed evaluation, education and to consider the need for controller therapy.

Pulmonary Score: 4–6 (Moderate)

- Humidified O_2 to keep SpO_2 92–95%.
- Nebulized salbutamol 0.15 mg/kg (minimum dose 2.5 mg or 0.5 mL <1 year, 1 mL >1 year) with 3 mL normal saline and O_2 every 20 minutes for three doses. Continue with one dose every 1–4 hours as per response.
- Add ipratropium 0.5 mg to salbutamol nebulization, three doses every 20 minutes, followed by one dose 6 hourly.
- Prednisolone 1 mg/kg/dose q 12 hr (continue for 4–7 days).
- Intravenous fluids to correct dehydration; continue IV maintenance fluids till adequate oral intake.
- Observe for 12 hours; taper drugs as per response (assess by PS and SpO_2) 4–6 hourly.
- Discharge for home therapy with salbutamol as MDI + prednisolone as in mild episode if SpO_2 is stable in room air for 12 hours and tolerating adequate oral feeds.

Pulmonary Score>6 (Severe)

- Humidified oxygen to keep SpO_2 92–95%.
- Continuous salbutamol nebulization 5–15 mg in 6 mL saline in 1 hour; repeat till adequate response or untoward effects as tachycardia (exceeding 180/min).
- Nebulized ipratropium 0.5 mg in 3 mL saline 6 hourly.
- Intravenous methylprednisolone 1 mg/kg q 6 hr on day 1, q 12 hr on day 2, and then daily or IV hydrocortisone 5 mg/kg 6 hr; add proton pump inhibitors or ranitidine.
- Continue IV maintenance fluids with potassium 40 mEq/L; monitor serum potassium 12 hourly.
- Assess after 1 hour; if improvement, taper salbutamol nebulization 1 to 4 hourly and then 6 hourly; observe for 24 hours.
- If no improvement, administer IV salbutamol 15 µg/kg in 10 minutes followed by 1 µg/kg/min continuous infusion *or* IV terbutaline 2–10 µg/kg bolus followed by 0.1–0.4 µg/kg/min as continuous infusion; increase by 0.1–0.2 µg/kg/min every 30 minutes up to a maximum of 6 µg/kg/min depending on clinical response or untoward effects.

Note: Cardiac monitoring is mandatory in children on continuous SABA nebulization or infusion.

ACUTE LIFE-THREATENING ASTHMA (FLOWCHART 19.1)

- Deterioration or nonresponse after continuous SABA nebulisation with continuous intravenous infusion indicates acute life-threatening asthma (ALTA).
- Reassess the orders written and the medicines administered by the nurse.
- Consider chest skiagram to detect complications like collapse, pneumonia, air leak (pneumothorax, pneumomediastinum); treat the complications.
- Evaluate serum electrolytes (K, Na), blood sugar, and arterial blood gas; correct the electrolyte imbalances and hyperglycemia.
- Consider further intensive bronchodilator therapy or mechanical ventilation.

Intensive Bronchodilator Therapy

- Continue all medicines as in severe episode.
- Give adrenaline 0.01 mL/kg (1:1000) subcutaneous, intramuscular (IM) or intravenous (IV) followed by intravenous aminophylline 10 mg/kg loading dose followed by maintenance dose (1 mg/kg/hr <9 years, 0.7 mg/kg/hr >9 years); skip the bolus dose if already on theophylline; reduce terbutaline infusion to half the dose while aminophylline is added.
- If no improvement, add IV 50% magnesium sulfate (1 mL = 500 mg) 25–75 mg/kg up to a maximum dose of 2.5 g in 30 mL saline over 20 minutes followed by continuous infusion at the rate of 30 mg/kg/hr.
- Continuous cardiac and drug monitoring is mandatory; while on aminophylline and magnesium sulfate infusion, maintain serum magnesium levels to 1.5–2.5 mmol/L.
- Heliox, if available, can be administered.

Mechanical Ventilation

- Absolute indications—cardiac or respiratory arrest.
- Relative indications—rapid deterioration in mental status or severe exhaustion.
- Isolated abnormalities in blood gas analysis are not indications if clinically stable.
- Risks of mechanical ventilation in acute severe asthma are:
  - Aggravation of bronchospasm by endotracheal tube acting as a foreign body.
  - Barotrauma and hypotension due to positive pressure ventilation.
- Rapid sequence intubation and ketamine anesthesia are advised (Refer chapters 8, 9, 10, 16).
- As the child improves, start weaning and stopping drugs in the order last in, first out. Taper IV infusion of bronchodilators and continuous

Flowchart 19.1: Algorithm for acute asthma management.

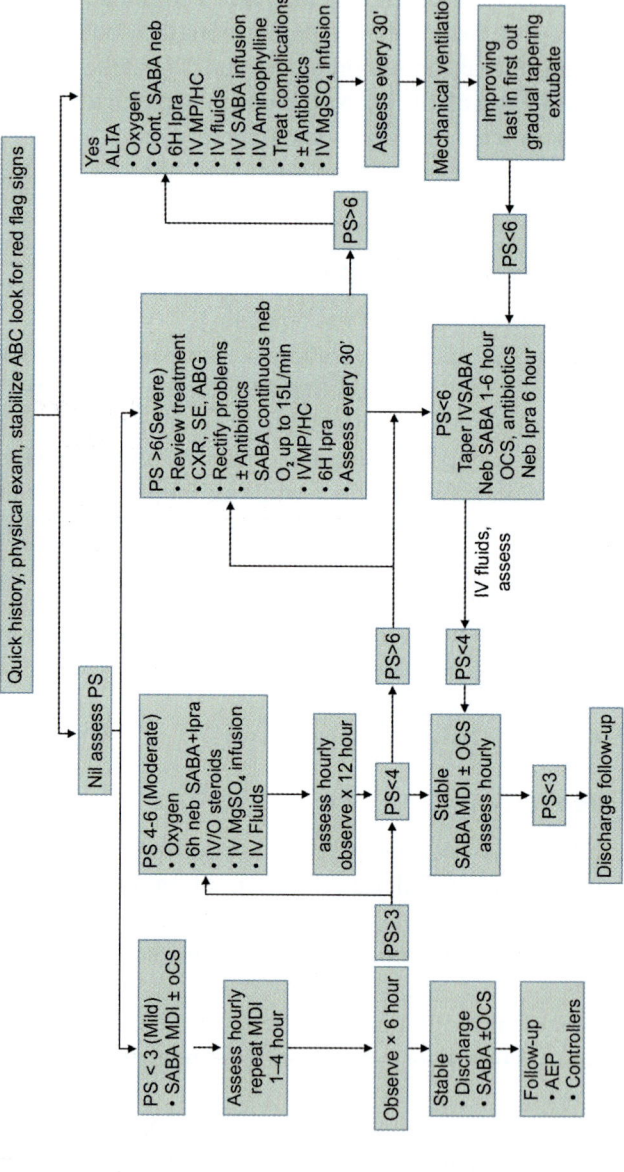

(AEP, asthma education program; HC, hydrocortisone; Ipra, Ipratropium; MDI, metered dose inhaler; MP, methylprednisolone; Neb, nebulization; OCS, oral corticosteroids ; SABA, short-acting beta agonists)

nebulization 1–6 hourly as per response; switch over to MDI and oral drugs; observe for 24 hours while on MDI + oral medicines.
- Discharge for home therapy and advise regular follow-up for asthma education.

Discharge Criteria
- Pulmonary score less than 3 in room air.
- Comfortable with SABA MDI.
- Tolerates oral feeds.

Prognosis

Good in pediatric intensive care units; death is unusual in hospital setting even with extreme measures of treatment.

CONCLUSION

Acute asthma should be promptly diagnosed and assessed for severity scoring with PS clinically and treated with intensive bronchodilator, steroid and supportive therapy to prevent death.

FURTHER READING

1. Robinson PD, Asperon PV. Asthma in childhood. Pediatr Clin N Am. 2009;56.

Chapter 20

Acute Bronchiolitis

S Sushamabai

ABSTRACT

Acute bronchiolitis is an inflammatory disease of the lower airways manifesting with features of cough, tachypnea, chest indrawing, and wheeze. The etiology is viral, joined infection with more than one virus produces severe episode. Severity rating can be done by ability to feed, respiratory rate, chest retraction, blood oxygen saturation (SpO_2), and chest skiagram. Chest X-ray (CXR) is mandatory to rule out differential diagnosis. Treatment is mainly supportive—propped up position, suction, O_2, fluid and electrolyte maintenance. Nebulization with salbutamol/adrenaline/3% saline and steroid therapy have not revealed any consistent benefit. Continuous positive airway pressure (CPAP) or intermittent positive pressure ventilation (IPPV) may be needed in resistant cases. Indications for antiviral agents and antibiotics are highlighted.

INTRODUCTION

Bronchiolitis is an acute inflammatory disease of the lower respiratory tract in infants (peak age 6 months) leading to obstruction of the small airways.

Pathogens: Respiratory syncytial virus (RSV), human metapneumovirus, influenza, parainfluenza, adenovirus, and *Mycoplasma pneumoniae*.

PATHOGENESIS

Edema and obstruction of the bronchioles causing hypoxia, hypercarbia, and respiratory failure.

CLINICAL PRESENTATION

- Preceding upper respiratory infection (URI), family history of contact with URI, and progressive cough.

Table 20.1: Grading of severity in bronchiolitis.

Parameter	Mild	Moderate	Severe
Ability to feed	Normal	Short of breath during feeds	Poor feeding (<50% of usual)
Respiratory effort	Little Rate <60/min	Moderate chest wall retractions; Rate >60–70/min	Marked chest retractions, grunting, apneic episodes; Rate >70/min
Oxygen saturation	>92% in room air	<92%, correctable with oxygen	<92%; may or may not be correctable with oxygen
Chest skiagram	(1) hyperinflation	(1) + (2) peribronchial thickening	(1) + (2) + (3) atelectasis, parenchymal infiltrates/collapse
Care area	Home	High dependency unit	Pediatric ICU *Stabilize the patient before investigations*

- Increasing respiratory distress manifesting as tachypnea, chest retractions, and hyperinflation.
- Extensive wheeze, crackles, and apparent hepatosplenomegaly.
- Cyanosis, apnea, absent wheeze, and drowsiness indicate severe illness.
- Severity is more with combined infection, overcrowding, and passive smoking.

PATIENT APPROACH

Assess the severity by history, physical examination, and relevant investigations *(Table 20.1)*.

DIFFERENTIAL DIAGNOSIS

- Foreign body aspiration
- Pertussis (may coexist causing severe respiratory distress)
- Myocarditis
- Vascular rings
- Congestive cardiac failure
- Tracheoesophageal fistula
- Gastroesophageal reflux
- Anaphylaxis
- Tuberculosis
- Immunodeficiency disorders
- Cystic fibrosis
- Asthma (in older children).

INVESTIGATIONS

- *Chest skiagram:* Anteroposterior and lateral views—features of bronchiolitis are hyperinflation, lung infiltrates, and atelectasis; cardiomegaly may indicate congenital heart disease, myocarditis or cardiomyopathy. Bedside USG chest is found to be superior to CXR in early detection of pathognomonic lung findings of bronchiolitis
- Complete blood count: Leukocytosis with lymphocytosis supports the diagnosis of pertussis.
- Arterial blood gas in respiratory failure to decide mechanical ventilation.
- Other investigations based on differential diagnosis.

INDICATIONS FOR HOSPITALIZATION

- Moderate and severe bronchiolitis
- Mild episode in high-risk babies (age <3 months, preterm birth, previous mechanical ventilation, underlying cardiovascular, and pulmonary or immune deficiency disorders).

TREATMENT—MAINLY SUPPORTIVE

1. *Those with proven efficacy:*
   i. 30° elevated position for head and chest.
   ii. Avoid agitation.
   iii. Saline nasal drops 4 hourly followed by, gentle nasal, and oral suction.
   iv. Humidified oxygen via nasal cannula/blow by to keep SpO_2 more than 92%; weaning when SpO_2 is constantly more than 94% in room air. Warm humidified O_2 through high flow nasal cannula (HFNC) at 10L/min can hasten recovery.
   v. Correction of dehydration followed by IV maintenance fluid therapy till stable (SpO_2 >94% in room air, sucking well). Early administration of ORS 10% excess for maintenance requirement (if needed through NG tube) can prevent dehydration and promote recovery faster.
2. *Those with inconsistent results:*
   i. 3% saline nebulization 4 mL q 4 hr
   ii. Adrenaline + dexamethasone nebulization 0.5 mL/kg with saline q 4 hr
   iii. Salbutamol (q 4 hr) + ipratropium nebulization (q 6 hr).

All the above in *group 2* produce short-term benefit by decreasing airway edema. Discontinue if untoward effects like tachycardia, tachypnea, and worsening of desaturation occur.

Oral or IV steroids may be tried in infants suspected to be asthmatic (family history of parents or siblings having asthma, patient revealing atopy <6 months age). Adding a single dose of dexamethasone orally (1 mg/kg) along with nebulized epinephrine and 3% saline during episodes of increased respiratory distress is found to reduce the duration of hospital stay and the need for ventilator therapy.

Specific Therapy

- *Respiratory syncytial virus infection:* Ribavirin small particle aerosol as intermittent therapy (2 gm in 2-3 hours 3 times daily) is beneficial for high risk patients with RSV infection. Is recommended in infants with acute bronchiolitis having underlying cardiac disease, chronic pulmonary, liver, renal, endocrine, and metabolic problems.
- Oseltamivir therapy therapy (dose:<15 kg = 30 mg BD; >15-23 kg= 45 mg BD; >23- 40 kg=60 mg BD; >40 kg= 75 mg BD; maximum dose 150 mg BD;. For infants<1yr:
- <3 m =12mg BD;>3 m- 5 m =20 mg BD; 6 m- 11m=25 mg BD); for all the duration of therapy is 5 days. in proved or suspected cases of severe influenza virus infection or having risk factors.
- Macrolides (azithromycin for 5 days) if chlamydia/mycoplasma/pertussis infection is suspected.
- Add broad-spectrum antibiotics if superadded bacterial pneumonia is suspected (high fever, toxic appearance, lung infiltrates, peripheral blood smear(PBS) revealing toxic granules or polymorphonuclear leukocytosis).

MONITORING

Severity scoring, cyanosis, pulse rate, SpO_2, and high fever.

COMPLICATIONS

Apnea, respiratory failure, air leak syndrome, and secondary bacterial infections.

INDICATIONS FOR CPAP OR MECHANICAL VENTILATION

- Apneic episodes
- Falling SpO_2
- Drowsiness
- Hypotonia
- Fatigue.

Continuous Positive Airway Pressure

Applied through nasal prongs or nasopharyngeal CPAP (endotracheal tube through nose up to tragus of the ear), levels of 5–8 cm water, FiO_2 titrated to maintain SpO_2 more than 92%.

Intermittent Positive Pressure Ventilation

Indicated if failure to improve on CPAP.

Discharge Criteria

Improvement in tachypnea and work of breathing, O_2 saturation stable in room air, feeding adequately, and no cyanosis.

CONCLUSION

Acute bronchiolitis is an inflammatory disease of viral etiology affecting the lower airways, affecting young infants; characterized by cough, tachypnea and wheeze; the main treatment being supportive therapy with suction, O_2 fluid and electrolyte therapy, occasionally requiring respiratory support.

FURTHER READING

1. Unaise VV, Cherian CS, S Sushamabai, et al. Clinical profile of acute severe bronchiolitis in children. Souveneir, State Pedicon, IAP, 2015 November 21, 22. p. 94.

Chapter 21

Pneumonia

Carol Sara Cherian, S Sushamabai

ABSTRACT

Pneumonia is the inflammation of lung parenchyma usually indicating bacterial infection. The chapter deals with the etiology, clinical classification, and management as per revised WHO criteria 2014. Children with fast breathing ± chest in drawing are categorized as pneumonia. Community-acquired pneumonia can be treated at home with oral amoxicillin 40 mg/kg q 12 hr (co-amoxiclav if drug resistance is suspected) for 3–5 days. Children having added danger signs require hospitalization, IV ampicillin + gentamicin/3rd generation cephalosporins and supportive measures. The duration of therapy is 7–10 days (IV + oral). For *Staphylococcus* pneumonia, inj. gentamicin (7 days) with cloxacillin/clindamycin/vancomycin (3–6 weeks) is advised. Treatment in infants less than 2 months and more than 5-year age groups, chlamydial and mycoplasmal infections and hospital-acquired pneumonias are specified. Investigations and supportive therapy are also included.

INTRODUCTION

Pneumonia is the inflammation of the lung parenchyma characterized by consolidation or lung infiltrate. It is the leading cause of death in children less than 5 years of age mainly due to underdiagnosis and undertreatment.

ETIOLOGY

- Infectious: Viruses, bacteria, and fungi
- Noninfectious: Aspiration of foreign body/gastric contents, eosinophilia, chemicals, drugs, and radiation exposure.

Age-wise distribution of microorganisms causing pneumonia throughout the world is shown in Table 21.1.

Table 21.1: Microorganisms causing pneumonia.

Age	Viruses	Bacteria
≤2 months	Human metapneumovirus (HMPV), respiratory syncytial virus (RSV)	Group B Streptococcus, Gram-negative bacteria, Staphylococcus aureus
3 months to 2 years	RSV, influenza, parainfluenza, HMPV, adenovirus	Haemophilus influenzae b, Streptococcus pneumoniae, S. aureus, Group A Streptococcus
3 years to 5 years	All viruses except RSV	Pneumococci, Mycoplasma, Chlamydia, Group A Streptococcus, S. aureus

Etiological agents (especially bacterial) are based on whether the pneumonia is:
- Community-acquired—typical or atypical
- Hospital-acquired (nosocomial)
- Opportunistic
- Aspiration-related

CLINICAL PRESENTATION

Pneumonia is essentially a clinical diagnosis.

Symptoms

- Fever, chills, cough, breathing difficulty, chest pain, and irritability (in young babies).
- Unusual presentations—acute abdomen, ileus, diarrhea, vomiting, and delirium.

Signs

Fast breathing, grunting, chest retractions, decreased chest movements, impaired percussion, poor air entry or bronchial breathing, and increased vocal resonance.

MANAGEMENT

Table 21.2 reveals the clinical classification and treatment of under-five children based on revised WHO classification for community-acquired pneumonias.

Table 21.2: Classification and treatment of childhood pneumonia more than 2 months to 5 years age.

Signs and symptoms	Classification	Route, dose, duration	Remarks
Cough and cold only	No pneumonia	Home remedies (ginger, honey, saline nasal drops)	Home therapy
Fast breathing* ± chest indrawing	Pneumonia	PO amoxicillin 40 mg/kg/dose q 12 hr × 5 days#	Home therapy
Pneumonia with any danger sign**	Severe pneumonia	IV/IM ampicillin 50 mg/kg/dose q 6 hr + gentamicin 7.5 mg/kg/day OD × 7 days or 3rd generation cephalosporins$	High-dependency unit care, O_2, IV fluids, monitoring. Inj. ampicillin can be changed to amoxicillin (O) when afebrile, stable.
	Staphylococcus pneumonia	Ceftriaxone (IV)$ till afebrile × 2 days, change to cefpodoxime 10 mg/kg/day (O) div q 12 hr + cloxacillin*** 25–50 mg/kg/dose q 6 hr/clindamycin 10 mg/kg q 6 hr/vancomycin 20 mg/kg/dose q 8 hr; change to oral cloxacillin/clindamycin/co-amoxiclav as the child improves	Pediatric intensive unit care, look for empyema or pus collection, treat accordingly
Persistent high fever, Hypoxia/shock	Pneumonia with septic shock/Postmeasles pneumonia not responding by 48 hrs, necrotizing pneumonia	Piperacillin–Tazobactam 90 mg/kg/dose q 6 hr+ vancomycin (IV) 30 mg loading dose foll by 20 mg/kg/dose q 8 hr/teicoplanin 12 mg/kg q 12 hr × 3 doses foll by 6 mg/kg OD/linezolid 10 mg/kg/dose q 8hr	PICU care, intensive organ supportive therapy

*≥60/min—<2 months age, ≥50/min—3 months to 1 yr age, ≥40/min—2 years to 5 years age. Severe infection; RR>70/min—newborn to 1 year, >50/min—1 year to less than 5 years.
**Cyanosis, drowsiness, poor feeding, convulsions, stridor, and grunting.
Duration 3 days in HIV low prevalent areas; consider co-amoxiclav if amoxicillin resistance is suspected.
$ Ceftriaxone 50 mg/kg/dose q 12 hr/cefotaxime 50 mg/kg q 6 hr
***Co-amoxiclav (IV foll by oral) is a good substitute to cloxacillin.
Note—all IV antibiotics should be followed by oral for a total period of 7–10 days. Staphylococcus pneumoniae total duration 3–6 weeks

Indications for Chest Skiagram (Posteroanterior and Lateral Views) (Fig. 21.1)

- Severe pneumonia with suspicion of empyema or pneumothorax
- Suspected staphylococcal pneumonia

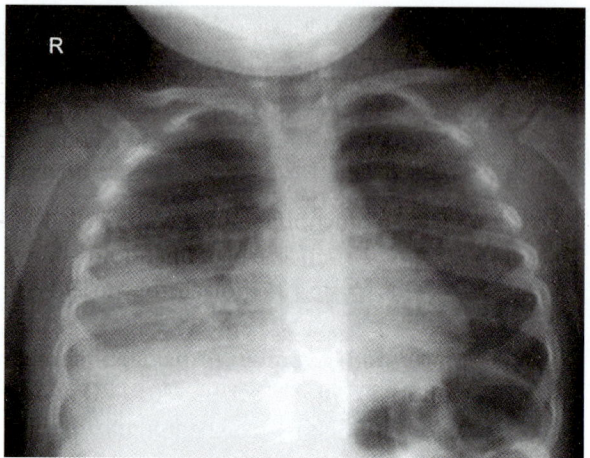

Fig. 21.1: Chest X-ray posteroanterior—pneumonia right lower zone: uniform opacity with no mediastinal shift.

- Poor response to antibiotics (within 48 hours)
- Persistent cough more than 30 days
- To assess the cardiac status.

Other Investigations

- Complete blood count—leukocytosis with neutrophilia, toxic granules in neutrophils, and elevated ESR are supportive.
- Blood/lung/tracheal aspirate culture—may be helpful but difficult to collect.
- Mantoux test and gastric aspirate for acid-fast bacilli to diagnose tuberculosis.
- Ultrasonography or CT chest to detect empyema.
- Sputum examination is possible in older children only.

Treatment in other Situations

- *Infants less than 2 months age:* IV 3rd-generation cephalosporins + gentamicin 5 mg/kg/dose q 24 hr × 7 days
- *Chlamydial or mycoplasmal infections at any age:* Add azithromycin (O) 10 mg/kg/day single dose daily × 5 days
- *Children more than 5 years:*
  - *first line*: IV Benzylpenicillin 50,000 u/kg/dose q 6 hr followed by procaine/oral penicillin 7–10 days *or* IV ampicillin 50 mg/kg/dose (max 2 g) q 6 hr followed by oral for total 7–10 days
  - *second line*: IV Ceftriaxone 50 mg/kg q 12 hr followed by oral for total 7–10 days.

- *Hospital-acquired pneumonias:*
  Piperacillin + tazobactam 300–400 mg/kg/day div q 6–8 hr
  or Cefoperazone + sulbactam 50 mg/kg/dose q 8 hr
  or Meropenem 60–120 mg/kg/day div q 8 hr (Max dose 6 gm/24 hr)
  or Cefepime 50 mg/kg/dose q 8 hr. Total duration of therapy (IV+Oral) should be 10-14 days.

ADJUNCTS

- Oxygen to keep SpO_2 92–95%
- Drainage of pus if empyema (Chapter 22)
- Fluid and electrolyte support
- Oral zinc (elemental) 10–20 mg/day × 2 weeks
- Treatment of malnutrition
- Preventive measures
- Proper immunization.

COMPLICATIONS OF PNEUMONIA

- Local—empyema, pericarditis, mediastinitis, and liver abscess
- Systemic—sepsis, meningitis, and shock
- Death due to overwhelming infection—usually late or inappropriate treatment.

CONCLUSION

Pneumonia is a serious bacterial infection of lungs, can be diagnosed by simple clinical parameters, and should be treated at the earliest as per updated national guidelines.

FURTHER READING

1. Kelly MS, Sandora TJ. Community-acquired pneumonia. In: Kleigman RM, Stanton BMD, St. Geme J, Schor NF (Eds). Nelson Textbook of Pediatrics, 20th edition. New Delhi: Elsevier India Pvt Ltd; 2016. pp. 2088-94.
2. Lassi ZS, Das JK, Haider SW, et al. Systematic review on antibiotic therapy for pneumonia in children between 2 and 59 months of age. Arch Dis Child. 2014;99:687-93.
3. Ministry of Health and Family Welfare, Government of India. (1994). Control of Acute Respiratory Infections. National Child Survival and Safe Motherhood Program. New Delhi. p 15-16.
4. World Health Organization. (2014). Revised WHO Classification and Treatment of Childhood Pneumonia at Health Facilities. Available from http://apps.who.int/iris/bitstream/handle/10665/137319/9789241507813:%20eng.pdf;jsessionid=A8C3A4D78D92EE2DA4114ED4DE4663F9?sequence=1 [Accessed September 2018].

Chapter 22

Empyema

S Sushamabai

ABSTRACT

Empyema is the accumulation of pus in the pleural cavity and is usually a complication of delayed or improper antibiotic therapy of bacterial pneumonia. Empyema is suspected in pneumonia if there is persistent high fever, recurrence of fever after apparent recovery, increasing chest pain, and respiratory distress or toxemia. Diagnosis can be confirmed by chest X-ray (CXR) and ultrasonography (USG) or CT of chest. The chapter reveals the etiology, clinical presentation, diagnostic approach, and investigations. Empirical antibiotic therapy with ceftriaxone, cloxacillin, and gentamicin or amikacin should be started at the earliest pending culture and sensitivity reports of pus or blood. If methicillin-resistant *Staphylococcus aureus* (MRSA) infection is suspected, linezolid should be replaced for cloxacillin. The minimum duration of antibiotic therapy is 3 weeks. The details of thoracocentesis, intercostal chest drainage (ICD), and intrapleural fibrinolytic therapy are also discussed.

INTRODUCTION

Empyema is the accumulation of pus in the pleural cavity, usually a complication following inadequate antibiotic therapy in pneumonia.

ETIOLOGY

- Common: Pneumonia
- Less common:
  - Trauma, crush injuries
  - Mediastinitis, liver abscess.

ORGANISMS

- Common: *Streptococcus pneumoniae, Staphylococcus aureus,* and *Haemophilus influenzae b*
- Rare: Gram-negative bacteria, *Group A Streptococcus*, fungi, tuberculosis, and anaerobes.

SYMPTOMS

- High fever, chest pain, abdominal pain, and breathing difficulty.
- Reappearance of high fever in a child getting treatment for pneumonia.

SIGNS

- Tachypnea, grunting, poor chest expansion, chest indrawing, and mediastinal shift to opposite side (no shift if pus is loculated).
- Dullness on percussion, reduced breath sounds (bronchial breathing in infants), and vocal resonance on the affected side.

INVESTIGATIONS

- *Chest skiagram:* Uniform opacity with mediastinal shift to the opposite side; pneumatoceles are characteristic of *Staphylococcus* pneumonia *(Figs. 22.1A to C)*; lateral decubitus film with the affected side as dependent reveals even small amount of pleural fluid.

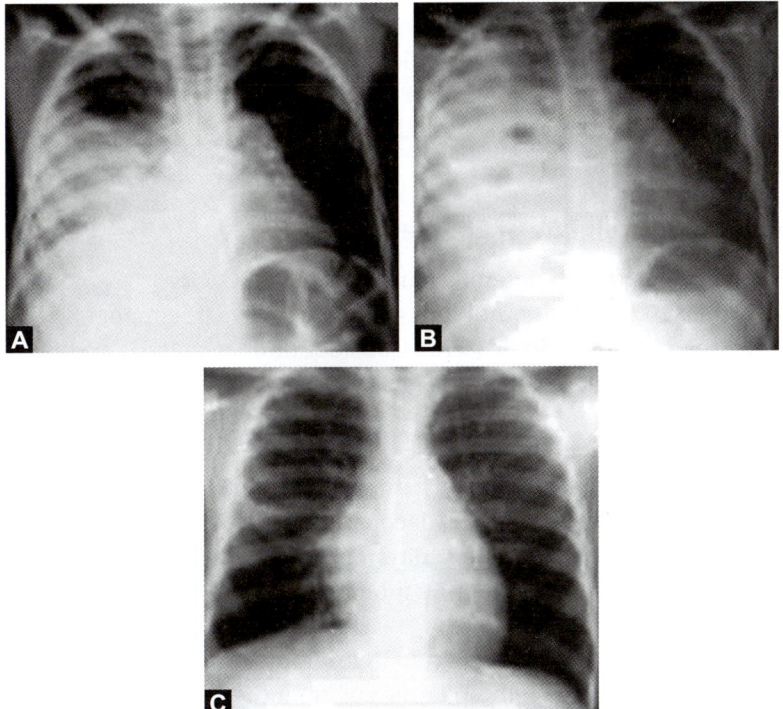

Figs. 22.1A to C: Chest X-ray in *Staphylococcus* pneumonia. (A) Empyema (R); (B) Pneumatoceles (R); (C) Complete resolution.

- *Ultrasonogram:* Quick and useful to detect the fluid quantity, confirm loculation, and guide aspiration of pus.
- *CT chest:* Better detection of loculation and quantity of pus.
- *Pleural fluid study:* Aspirate maximum amount; do microscopy after Gram staining—look for bacteria and neutrophils:
    - Neutrophils more than 100,000/mm^3, pH less than 7.20 (send in syringe with ice packs as for arterial blood gas), and lactate dehydrogenase more than 1,000 IU are diagnostic features of empyema and indicators for aspiration.
    - Biochemistry: Elevated proteins and reduced glucose.
    - Pleural fluid culture may reveal microorganisms.
    - Antigen detection for pneumococci and *H. influenzae* are available.
- *Blood culture:* Can isolate bacteria in 20% cases.
- *Complete blood count:* Leukocytosis more than 15,000/mm^3 suggests pneumococcal infection. Leukopenia heralds poor prognosis; and ESR will be high.

TREATMENT

Specific

Empirical antibiotic therapy: Ceftriaxone + Cloxacillin + Gentamicin/Amikacin—provides coverage for wide group of pathogenic bacteria. Change according to the culture reports or as per response. For staphylococcal infection, add clindamycin/cloxacillin/vancomycin. For MRSA, consider linezolid.

Aspiration or Drainage of Empyema

Quantity assessed by CXR lateral decubitus view/USG/CT.
- Less than 10 mm fluid: Antibiotics and supportive treatment
- More than 10 mm fluid, pH >7.2: Consider thoracocentesis additionally
- More than 10 mm fluid, pH <7.2, Gram stain positive: Antibiotics + tube thoracostomy
- Frank pus ± loculation: Antibiotics + tube thoracostomy
- Frank pus + multiple loculations: Intrapleural fibrinolytics/video-assisted thoracoscopic surgery (VATS)/decortications
- Duration of ICD: Maximum 7 days or earlier if no pus drainage for 48 hours; before removal, keep the tube blocked for 24 hours to assess pus collection.
- Daily monitoring of the ICD tube: Observe the air column movement inside the tube; assess the pleural pus quantity by chest radiograph or USG, CT chest may be needed in rare situations especially when diagnosis is dubious.

- Intrapleural fibrinolytic therapy:
    - Streptokinase 15,000 U/kg in 50 mL normal saline (NS) daily × 3–5 days
    - Urokinase 40,000 IU/kg in 40 mL NS 12 hourly × 6 doses
    - Alteplase (tissue plasminogen activator) is a newer drug advised.

Streptokinase can cause anaphylaxis but is cheaper; both streptokinase and urokinase are administered through the chest tube and clamped for 4 hours and then drained out, clearance is assessed by USG and skiagram; hemorrhage and lung gangrene are rare complications.

Supportive Therapy

- Oxygen if required
- Fluid and electrolyte maintenance
- Nutritious diet
- Analgesics and antipyretics
- Chest physiotherapy:
    - Blowing a balloon
    - Deep breathing
    - Incentive spirometry.

PROGNOSIS

Usually good; average recovery time is 2 weeks, and complete lung resolution takes years to establish.

CONCLUSION

Empyema is a serious complication of pneumonia and should be treated with appropriate antibiotics, thoracocentesis, and if required, with intrapleural fibrinolytic therapy.

Chapter 23

Pneumothorax and Pneumomediastinum

Carol Sara Cherian, S Sushamabai

ABSTRACT

Pneumothorax and pneumomediastinum are emergency situations due to the accumulation of air in the pleural cavity and mediastinum, respectively. The former causes respiratory compromise and subsequent cardiac compromise, whereas the latter primarily produces cardiac compromise. The chapter deals with the etiology, clinical features, and management of these emergencies. Needle aspiration, followed by tube thoracotomy, is the emergency procedure for relieving tension pneumothorax. Tracheotomy and mediastinal decompression are life-saving in pneumomediastinum.

PNEUMOTHORAX

Pneumothorax is the accumulation of air in the pleural space. Common causes are:
- *Primary spontaneous:* Rupture of subpleural blebs—more in thin-built young adult males.
- *Secondary spontaneous:*
    - Acute severe asthma
    - Staphylococcal pneumonia with pneumatoceles
    - Lung abscess
    - Foreign bodies in the lung
    - Cystic fibrosis
    - Malignancy
- *Chest trauma*
- *Iatrogenic*: Pleural tap, thoracotomy, and mechanical ventilation.

Pathogenesis

Positive intrapleural pressure created by air leads to underlying lung collapse and produces mediastinal shift to the opposite side thus compromising the normal lung function and cardiac output.

Clinical Presentation

- *Young infants:* Restlessness, increasing respiratory distress, cyanosis, sweating, and shock.
- *Older children:* Sudden severe chest pain, respiratory distress, sweating, and shock.

Physical Examination

- Tachypnea, tachycardia, and cyanosis
- On the affected side: Decreased chest movements and expansion, hyper resonance. on percussion, and decreased breath sounds
- Tracheal and mediastinal shift to the opposite side.

Investigations

- *Chest skiagram (Fig. 23.1):* Features are hyperlucent chest without bronchovascular markings and collapsed lung on the affected side; evidence of underlying lung disease will be obvious in most situations.
- *Ultrasonogram of the chest*
- *CT scan chest*
- *Arterial blood gas:* Reveals normal to severe hypoxemia, hypercarbia, and acidosis depending on the degree of pneumothorax and mediastinal shift leading to respiratory compromise.
- *Barium study:* Differentiates air-filled diaphragmatic hernia from pneumothorax.

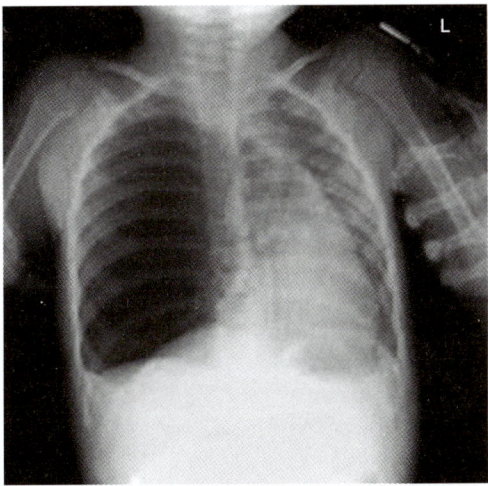

Fig. 23.1: Chest X-ray PA—Pneumothorax (R).

Treatment

Asymptomatic: Treat the cause; spontaneous resolution occurs within a week. Daily monitoring is needed by clinical assessment and chest skiagram.

Symptomatic: Provide initial stabilization:
- 100% oxygen, fluid and electrolyte balance.
- Needle aspiration with 23 G scalp vein set at 2nd intercostal space is immediately life-saving; should be followed by closed thoracotomy using intercostal drainage tube connected to underwater seal till air accumulation stops.
- Monitor for lung re-expansion daily: Clinically and by chest radiograph.
- Treat the precipitating cause.
- Administer analgesics for pain.
- Before removal of the thoracotomy tube, clamp the tube for 12 hours, assess reaccumulation of air by chest skiagram.
- Chemical pleurodesis in recurrent episodes may be considered.

PNEUMOMEDIASTINUM

Pneumomediastinum is the presence of air or gas in the mediastinum.

Common Causes

- Lower respiratory infections
- Acute severe asthma
- Acute respiratory distress syndrome
- Chest trauma
- Esophageal perforation
- Foreign body inhalation
- Other causes: Vomiting, adenotonsillectomy, dental extraction, high flow oxygen therapy, diabetic ketoacidosis, normal menses and delivery, and helium inhalation.

Pathogenesis

Intrapulmonary alveolar rupture causes escape of air through the perivascular sheaths which enters the mediastinum and produces compression of the mediastinal structures.

Clinical Features

- Dyspnea and cough
- Stabbing chest pain radiating to neck
- Abdominal pain and sore throat

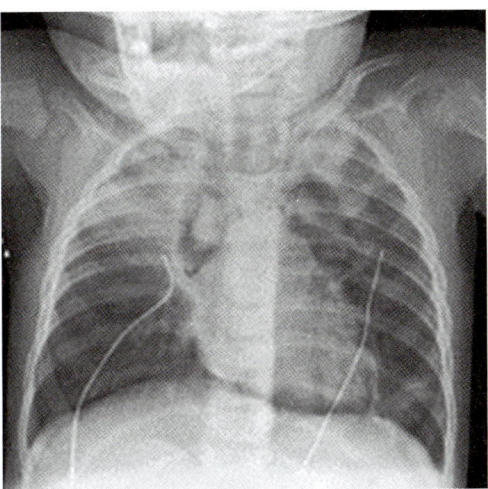

Fig. 23.2: Chest X-ray pneumomediastinum with pneumopericardium.

- Associated subcutaneous emphysema can be a clue to diagnosis.
- Hamman sign or mediastinal crunch (crunching sound heard over left sternal border during systole) is the clinical diagnostic sign but can be confused with pleural rub.
- Extreme accumulation of air can lead to cardiac compromise and shock in neonates.

Diagnosis

Chest skiagram posteroanterior/anteroposterior (PA/AP) reveals distinct cardiac borders (Fig. 23.2); in the lateral view retrosternal air and clearly defined posterior mediastinal structures will be seen.

Treatment

- Treat the primary cause
- Oxygen therapy
- Maintain fluid and electrolyte balance.
- Provide analgesics to relieve chest pain.
- Tracheotomy and mediastinal decompression if evidence of tracheal compression or cardiac compromise.

CONCLUSION

Pneumothorax and pneumomediastinum are life-threatening emergencies; the former requires tube thoracotomy and the latter tracheotomy and mediastinal decompression.

Chapter 24

Acute Respiratory Distress Syndrome

S Sushamabai

ABSTRACT

Acute respiratory distress syndrome (ARDS) is a potentially fatal lung inflammation with pulmonary edema encountered in a variety of pulmonary and extrapulmonary critical illnesses. The chapter deals with the etiology, clinical presentation, diagnostic approach, and management. Chest skiagram (the pathognomonic features are small volume lung with diffuse infiltrates, air bronchogram, and widespread atelectasis) and CT chest are diagnostic. Treatment should be for the underlying disease along with lung protective mechanical ventilation and multiorgan support.

INTRODUCTION

Acute respiratory distress syndrome is lung inflammation with alveolar epithelial and endothelial damage and protein-rich pulmonary edema; diagnostic criteria are:
- Acute lung disease which is persistent
- PaO_2/FiO_2 less than 200 ($PaO_2/FiO_2 <300$ is acute lung injury)
- Diffuse infiltrates in chest radiograph.

CAUSES

Can be pulmonary or extrapulmonary *(Table 24.1)*.

Table 24.1: Causes of acute respiratory distress syndrome.

Pulmonary (primary)	Extrapulmonary (secondary)
Pneumonia	Sepsis and shock
Aspiration	Poisoning
Drowning	Acute pancreatitis
Chemical inhalation	Burns
Embolism	Trauma
Contusion of chest	Surgery
Radiation injury	Transfusion related

PATHOPHYSIOLOGY

Diffuse alveolar damage, surfactant depletion, alveolar edema, small airways collapse and obstruction occur; posterior dependent parts of lungs are more affected, net result is overall hypoxia, hypercarbia, and acidosis.

CLINICAL STAGES

- Initial exudative phase (0–7 days)
- Subsequent fibroproliferative stage.

CLINICAL PRESENTATION

- Overlapping features of initial insult (primary or secondary) with those of ARDS will be seen.
- Severe respiratory distress, tachypnea, and chest indrawing.
- Decreased breath sounds, crackles, and wheezes.
- Cardiac compromise subsequent to lung injury.

INVESTIGATIONS

Chest Skiagram

- Small volume lungs with diffuse alveolar infiltrates *(Fig. 24.1)*
- Air bronchogram and widespread atelectasis.

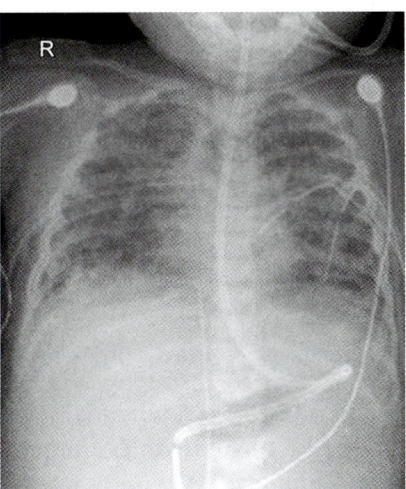

Fig. 24.1: Chest X-ray in acute respiratory distress syndrome—note the small volume lung with diffuse infiltrates.

CT Scan Chest

Increased densities in the dependent parts of the lungs.

Other Investigations

- Depending on suspected etiology, culture of body fluids.
- Complete blood count, arterial blood gas (ABG), serum electrolytes (SE), renal function test (RFT), liver function test, and coagulation profile—to assess the severity and plan the treatment protocol.

MANAGEMENT

- Treat the precipitating condition.
- No specific therapy for ARDS.
- Supportive management with mechanical ventilation utilizing lung protective strategies: tidal volume (V_T) 6 mL/kg, FiO_2 less than 0.6, SaO_2 86–90, optimal positive end-expiratory pressure (PEEP) (8–12 cm H_2O), peak inspiratory pressure less than 30 H_2O, and permissive hypercapnia of pCO_2 up to 80 mm Hg while pH is 7.15–7.2.
- Consider high frequency ventilation if PEEP needed is more than 12 cm H_2O.
- Continuous monitoring of vitals, SpO_2, and ventilator settings.
- Frequent monitoring of ABG, SE, RFT, and coagulation profile as needed.
- Fluid and electrolyte balance—treat shock and burns; after initial fluid bolus try maintenance therapy with negative balance using furosemide infusion 0.1–0.5 mg/kg/hour along with spironolactone.
- Proper sedation and analgesia.
- Early enteral nutrition.

Other Modalities of Treatment

- High frequency oscillatory ventilation
- Prone positioning (expert anesthesia team needed)
- Nitric oxide (NO) 10 ppm to produce pulmonary vasodilatation
- Surfactant therapy
- Extracorporeal membrane oxygenation.

CONCLUSION

Acute respiratory distress syndrome is a potentially fatal lung inflammation and should be aggressively treated with lung protective mechanical ventilation and multiorgan support.

C. Fluid refractory shock	Persistent shock after 60 mL/kg of isotonic saline infusion
D. Dopamine resistant shock	Persistent shock after fluid bolus and dopamine infusion.
E. Catecholamine resistant shock	Persistent shock after fluid bolus and direct acting catecholamine infusion (epinephrine, norepinephrine).
F. Refractory shock	Persistent shock after fluid bolus inotropes, vasopressors, vasodilators and correctable causes being rectified.

*Resting heart rate <1yr >180 min, ≥ 1 yr ≥160/min.
**Resting respiratory rate <2m ≥ 60/min, 3m-1yr≥ 50min, > 1yr to 5yr ≥ 40/min.

Hypotension—systolic blood pressure <5th percentile for age (in mm Hg)

<60 in term neonates (0–28 days)
<70 in infants (1 to 12 months)
≤70 + (2 × age in years) in children >1 year to 10 years
≤ 90 in children >10 years age

Pathophysiologic categorization	Clinical situations
A. Hypovolemic shock	Diarrhea, vomiting, blood loss, diuresis, (D. mellitus, D. insipidus), occult fluid loss (burns, nephrotic syndrome, dengue shock syndrome)
B. Distributive shock	Sepsis, anaphylaxis, neurogenic problems (head/spine injury) due to inadequate vasomotor tone
C. Cardiogenic shock	Congenital heart disease, myocarditis, cardiomyopathy, arrhythmias, and poisoning
D. Obstructive shock	Cardiac tamponade, tension pneumothorax, and duct-dependent lesions in early neonatal period

Chapter 25

Shock

S Sushamabai

ABSTRACT

Shock is an acute syndrome of circulatory dysfunction leading to defective oxygen and nutrient supply to the tissues. Hypovolemic shock is the most common type usually following diarrhea. The chapter deals with the clinical classification, systematic approach, fluid resuscitation (NS 20 mL/kg × 3 boluses followed by colloid—fresh frozen plasma (FFP) or dextran 40% 10-20 mL/kg), golden hour (1st hour) empirical antibiotic therapy in septic shock, investigations, and judicious administration of catecholamines and vasodilators. Roles of catecholamines, hydrocortisone, and vasodilators are detailed. In refractory shock, intensive monitoring, organ support, ventricular assist device (VAD) and extracorporeal membrane oxygenation (ECMO) may be needed.

INTRODUCTION

Shock is an acute syndrome of circulatory dysfunction characterized by defective supply of oxygen and nutrients to the body tissues to meet the metabolic demands. Remember that:
- Shock does not mean hypotension
- Shock becomes difficult to treat if BP falls
- Child in shock can have low, normal or high BP
- Untreated shock leads to irreversible tissue damage and death.

Clinical categorisation	Signs
A. Compensated shock	Tachycardia*,tachypnea**, Prolonged CRFT (>3 seconds), Weak peripheral pulses, Normal central pulses, Normal BP
B. Decompensated shock	All in (A) with hypotension# Absent peripheral pulses, Weak central pulses, oliguria

Section 5

CARDIOVASCULAR SYSTEM

- Septic shock, the most common type in pediatrics is a combination of hypovolemic, distributive, and cardiogenic shock.
- Warm shock (due to vasculoplegia) is characterized by warm flushed extremities, bounding pulses, and flash capillary refill time (CRFT) (<1sec).
- Cold shock characterized by cold extremities; weak or absent peripheral pulses and prolonged CRFT more than 3 seconds are due to hypovolemia and is the most common in children.

MANAGEMENT

Success in therapy of shock depends on early recognition and multipronged aggressive approach in the *first hour* of therapy (*Golden hour* therapy).

Golden Hour Therapy—observe six goals:
- Oxygenation
- Correction of fluid and electrolyte imbalance
- Improving cardiac output
- Control of infection
- Monitoring to rectify complications
- Prevention and management of multiple organ dysfunction syndrome (MODS).

PATIENT APPROACH

- Parallel history, quick assessment (color, alertness, vitals, and CRFT).
- Airway, breathing, circulation stabilization.
- Suspect shock in a sick looking child.
- Presence of fever with rash or evidence of infection—septic shock.
- Diarrhea/vomiting/blood loss—hypovolemic shock.
- Unexpected dehydration and shock can indicate:
    - Metabolic emergencies—diabetes
    - Congenital adrenal hyperplasia } Hypovolemic shock
    - Addison disease, Dengue shock.
- Acute urticaria, angioedema, injections, vaccination, exposure to allergens and ingestion of food items—distributive shock.
- History of heart disease, tachycardia, cyanosis, cardiomegaly, pulmonary crackles—cardiogenic shock.
- Poisoning and envenomation—cardiogenic shock.

THERAPY

- High flow oxygen by nasal cannula or mask; proceed to continuous positive airway pressure (CPAP) or mechanical ventilation if Glasgow coma scale is less than 8 or refractory shock.
- Get IV access (IO if >90 seconds delay); start normal saline (NS) 20 mL/kg in 1 hour (Ringer's lactate in diarrhea); push rapid in 5–10 minutes if in hypotension; restrict fluid to 10 mL/kg/hr in cardiogenic shock, increase to 30 mL/kg/hr in septic shock.
- Get the second IV access; send blood samples two—one for cultures, other for laboratory evaluation [complete blood count (CBC), C-reactive protein (CRP), packed cell volume (PCV), peripheral smear for malaria, platelet count, random blood sugar (RBS), lactate, serum electrolytes (SE), renal function test (RFT), liver function test (LFT), coagulation profile, and arterial blood gas (ABG)].
- Send samples for other cultures (cerebrospinal fluid, urine, pus).
- Consider CXR, ECG, USG, ECHO, CT, MRI and for toxicology screening as per situation.
- Urine collection device to assess the output.
- Start empirical antibiotics—1st dose administration in septic shock:
  - Neonate: Cefotaxime + ampicillin + gentamicin + acyclovir
  - Infants and children: Ceftriaxone + amikacin + (cloxacillin/vancomycin if serious pneumonia).
  - Any age: Intra-abdominal sepsis—III/IV generation cephalosporin + metronidazole/clindamycin/piperacillin–tazobactam.
  - Any age: nosocomial infection—III/IV generation cephalosporin/piperacillin–tazobactam + amikacin (+ vancomycin if indwelling device).
  - Any age: Immunocompromised—select any from the above as per situation + empirical antifungal drug.
- Continue NS bolus up to 200 mL/kg especially in septic shock till signs of shock disappear or evidence of over hydration like respiratory distress and/or hepatomegaly appear.

Note: After each bolus, in all category, monitor heart rate, respiratory rate, CRFT, mental status, extremity warmth, hepatomegaly, and lung crackles.

- More than three boluses of fluid should ideally be administered by central venous pressure (CVP) monitoring.

Further Management

- Continue maintenance fluid therapy with 5% DNS/$^1/_2$ DNS /NS for 24 hours, after golden hour therapy, if signs of recovery are revealed as shown in Box 25.1.

- Add replacement therapy for ongoing loss as ORS in diarrhea for each stool loss.
- Detect and treat metabolic derangements as perceived from laboratory reports.
- Consider shift to recovery ward provided the recovery signs are stable on maintenance fluid therapy for 24 hours without O_2 therapy.

Fluid Refractory Shock

- Continue O_2, IV NS 10–20 mL to 30 mL/kg/hr.
- Colloid administration 10 mL/kg in 2 hours after three boluses of NS (hexastarch, 40% dextran, albumin/FPP); packed RBC if Hb is less than 10 g or hematocrit is less than 30%.
- Administer dopamine (dobutamine in myocardial dysfunction); if no response change to epinephrine in cold shock or norepinephrine warm shock (Table 25.1).

Catecholamine-resistant Shock

- Monitor and maintain CVP at 10–12 cm H_2O, central venous oxygen saturation ($SvO_2 > 70\%$), mean arterial blood pressure (MAP = diastolic BP + 1/3 pulse pressure)—1 month–6 months: more than or equal to 40 mm Hg;

Box 25.1: Signs of recovery from shock.
- Improvement in sensorium
- Warm peripheries
- CRFT< 3 seconds
- Decreasing heart rate
- Normal systolic BP
- Urine output >1mL/kg/hr

Table 25.1: Dose and administration of catecholamines.

Drug	Dose	Dilution	Delivery rate	Effect
Dopamine	3–20 µg/kg/min	6 × wt (kg) = mg to be added to 100 mL	1 mL/hr yields 1 µg/kg/min	↑Cardiac contractility
Dobutamine	1–10 µg/kg/min	As above	As above	↑Cardiac contractility Peripheral vasodilatation
Epinephrine	0.05–0.3 µg/kg/min	0.6 × wt (kg) = mg to be added to 100 mL	1 mL/hr yields 0.1 µg/kg/min	Tachycardia, ↑cardiac contractility, increased vasoconstriction
Norepinephrine	0.1–0.2 µg/kg/min	As above	As above	Potent vasoconstriction

Table 25.2: Vasoactive drugs in shock.

Drug	Effects	Dose	Comments
Nitroprusside	Vasodilator (mainly arterial)	0.5–4 µg/kg/min	Rapid effect. Risk of cyanide toxicity (>96 hours use)
Nitroglycerine	Vasodilator (mainly venous)	1–20 µg/kg/min	Rapid effect. Risk of ↑ intracranial pressure
Prostaglandin E1	Vasodilator. Maintains ductus arteriosus open in newborns	0.01–0.2 µg/kg/min	Hypotension, risk of apnea
Milrinone	↑Cardiac contractility ↑Cardiac diastolic function, peripheral vasodilatation	Load 50 µg/kg in 15 minutes, then 0.5–1 µg/kg/min	Main use in myocardial disease; arrhythmogenic
Levosimendan	↑Cardiac contractility, Coronary and systemic vasodilator	Load 6–12 µg/kg in 10 minutes followed by 0.05 to 0.2 µg/kg/min	Use in myocardial disease, septic shock less arrhythmogenic

7 months to 5 years: more than or equal to 45 mm Hg; more than 5–12 years: more than or equal to 50 mm Hg; and more than 12 years: more than 60 mm Hg)
- Mean arterial pressure indicates better organ perfusion than systolic blood pressure.
- Consider intubation and mechanical ventilation.
- Continue O_2, IV NS 10–20 mL/kg/hr + others.
- IV hydrocortisone 2–50 mg/kg/day div q 6 hr.
- Correct metabolic derangements as revealed below:
  - Hyperglycemia: Insulin as infusion or subcutaneous 0.25 U/kg q 6 hr.
  - Hypocalcemia: 0.5 mL/kg of 10% calcium gluconate equally diluted in normal saline over 10 minutes.
  - Hypo-/hypernatremia (Chapter 53).
  - Hypo/hyper kalemia (Chapter 53).
  - Acidosis: Fluid resuscitation, IV sodium bicarbonate 1 mEq/kg in 1 hour if pH is less than 7.
  - Cold shock with normal BP: Fluids + epinephrine infusion, add vasodilator—nitroprusside or milrinone.
  - Cold shock with low BP: Fluids + epinephrine; add norepinephrine and dobutamine/milrinone/levosimendan.
  - Warm shock + low BP: Fluids + norepinephrine; consider vasopressin or terlipressin (Table 25.2; vasoactive drugs).
- Rule out by radiology—pericardial effusion, pneumothorax, empyema or raised intra-abdominal pressure more than 12 mm Hg.
- Continue all other modalities of treatment.

Refractory Shock

Consider ECMO and VAD.

Monitoring

Vitals, I/O charts, GCS, SvO_2/SpO_2, ABG/VBG, blood sugar, platelets, SE, RFT, Hb, Hct, and prothrombin time.

Additional Therapies

- Organ support—mechanical ventilation and renal replacement therapy.

Flowchart 25.1: Algorithm for hemodynamic management of shock.

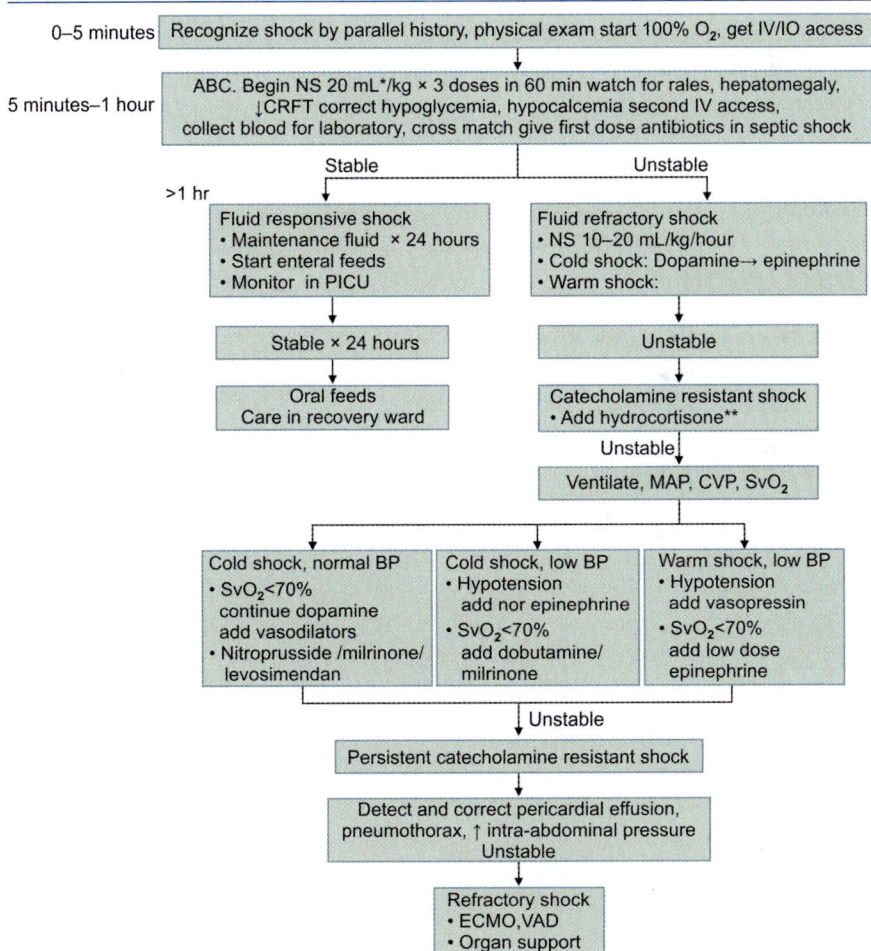

*10 mL/kg/hr in cardiogenic shock
**Adrenal insufficiency conditions
(ABC, airway, breathing, circulation; CRFT, capillary refill time; CVP, central venous pressure; ECMO, extracorporeal membrane oxygenation; IO, intraosseous; IV, intravenous; MAP, mean arterial pressure; NS, normal saline; PICU, pediatric intensive care unit; VAD, ventricular assist device)

- Blood components, vitamin K, H_2 receptor antagonists, and proton pump inhibitors.
- Early enteral feeds.
- Sepsis control—intravenous immunoglobulin and plasmapheresis.

PARAMETERS TO TAPER THERAPY

As revealed by signs of recovery.

POOR PROGNOSTIC FACTORS

- Low WBC count, low or falling platelet count
- Higher requirement for fluids
- Short history, less than 12 years age
- Rapid deterioration to multiorgan failure (ARDS, renal and or liver failure, coagulation abnormalities).

Flowchart 25.1 describes the algorithm for hemodynamic management of shock.

CONCLUSION

Shock is an acute syndrome of circulatory dysfunction which should be diagnosed at the early compensated stage and vigilantly treated with O_2, fluids, and vasopressors in the golden hour.

FURTHER READING

1. Kamnath SR, Jaykumar I, Matha S. Levosimendan. Indian Pediatr. 2009;46:593-6.

Chapter 26

Cardiac Arrhythmias

Carol Sara Cherian, S Sushamabai

ABSTRACT

Cardiac arrhythmias are diseases characterized by disturbances in heart rate or rhythm, mostly fatal if not treated in time. They can be primary (idiopathic) or secondary due to cardiac (congenital/acquired) or noncardiac (metabolic, drug-induced, endocrine, and hypo/hyperthermia) causes. The clinical presentation can be sudden death, shock, congestive cardiac failure (CCF) or seizure at any age. Should be suspected in fetal hydrops, in infants with sudden onset of restlessness and irritability, and in older children with palpitation and syncope. The broad groups are tachyarrhythmias, bradyarrhythmias, and extra systoles. The most common is supraventricular tachycardia, the features being heart rate 240–300/min, may present in cardiac failure, and ECG findings are diagnostic. The effective drugs are IV adenosine and IV amiodarone or procaine amide. If drugs fail, DC cardioversion or catheter ablation need be considered. Other conditions are also detailed.

INTRODUCTION

Arrhythmia indicates disturbances in heart rate or rhythm. Most of them are fatal diseases if not treated appropriately in time.

ETIOLOGY

- Primary idiopathic (50%)
- Secondary:
  - Metabolic (6 "H" and 4 "T"—Chapter 7)
  - Congenital heart disease
  - Acquired heart diseases, myocarditis, and cardiomyopathy
  - Drug-induced
  - Endocrine disorders
  - Maternal systemic lupus erythematosus (SLE)
  - Hyper-/hypothermia.

CLINICAL PRESENTATION

- At any age: Sudden death, shock, congestive heart failure, and seizures
- Fetus: Tachycardia and hydrops
- Infant: Abrupt episodes of restlessness and irritability
- Child: Palpitation and syncope.

Note: In children with syncope suspect the possibility of arrhythmias if family history of sudden death.

INVESTIGATIONS

- Complete blood count, random blood sugar, serum electrolytes, renal function test, and liver function test
- Chest X-ray
- ECG—14 leads with long lead II
- Echocardiography
- Others as per suspected etiology.

TYPES

- Tachyarrhythmias: Supraventricular tachycardia (SVT), ventricular tachycardia (VT), and atrial fibrillation (AF)
- Bradyarrhythmias: Complete heart block (CHB) and sinus node dysfunction (SND)
- Irregular heartbeats: Extrasystoles and premature ventricular contractions (PVC).

Tachyarrhythmias

Supraventricular Tachycardia (Flowchart 26.1)

- Episodic onset, more common in young infants, and heart rate 240–300/min.
- May present with features of cardiac failure.
- Differentiate from sinus tachycardia by 14-lead EEG with long leads.
- In SVT, P waves may be absent or have abnormal axis (negative in leads II, III, aVF) and narrow QRS (<0.08 seconds) (Fig. 26.1).

Treatment

- Assess whether hemodynamically unstable (hypotension, heart failure).
- *If stable:*
  - *Vagal maneuvers:*
    - Small children—place an ice bag over the face for 10–15 seconds.
    - Older children—Valsalva maneuver, straining or breath holding.

Flowchart 26.1: Algorithm for treatment of supraventricular tachycardia (SVT).

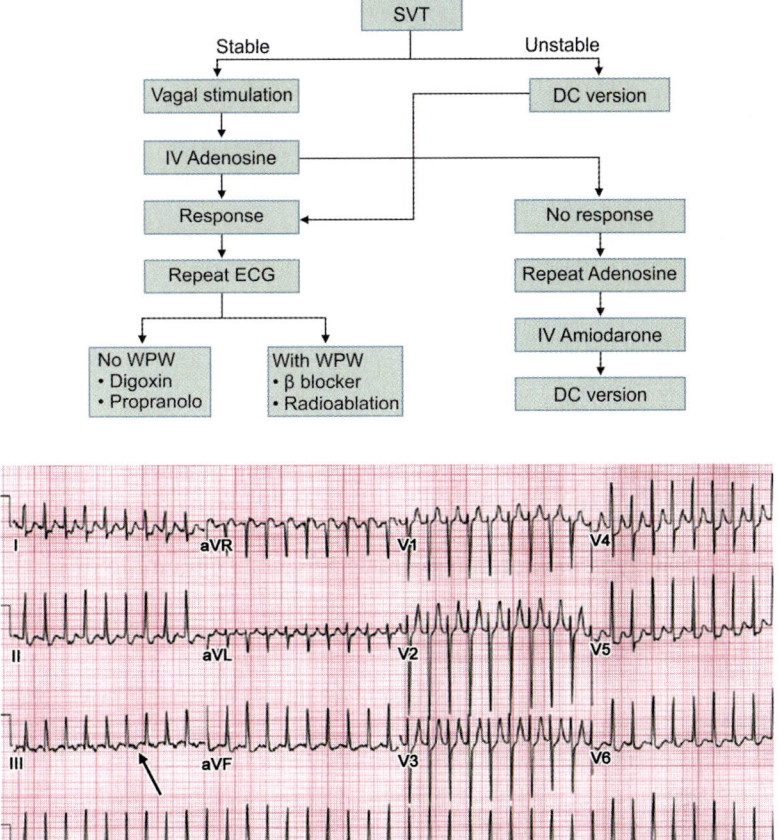

Fig. 26.1: ECG in supraventricular tachycardia showing abnormal P wave axis.

- *Pharmacological:*
    - IV adenosine 50 µg/kg rapid push followed by 50 µg/kg increments every 2 minutes flushed immediately with saline, maximum dose: 18 mg; bronchospasm and complete heart block may occur.
    - IV amiodarone 2.5–5 mg/kg in 30–60 minutes × 3 doses followed by 2–10 mg/kg/24 hr continuous infusion.
    - IV procainamide 10–15 mg/kg in 30–45 minutes followed by 20–80 µg/kg/min.
    - IV verapamil 0.1–0.2 mg/kg q 20 min × 2 doses (>1 year age only), maximum dose 5–10 mg.
- *If unstable or not controlled by pharmacological measures:*
    - IV adenosine as above; if no response
    - DC cardioversion (0.5–2 J/kg)
- *Catheter ablation* in refractory cases and in those requiring multiple agents

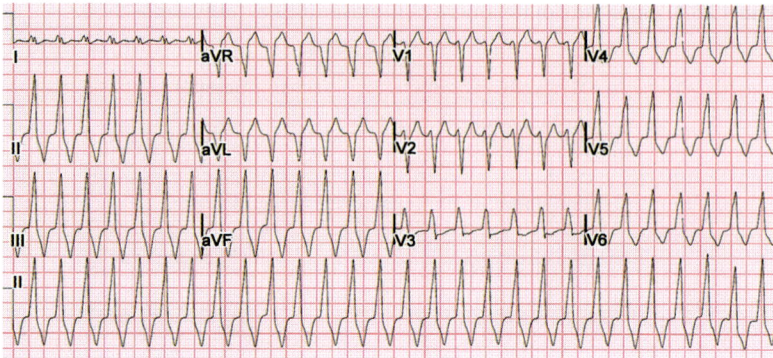

Fig. 26.2: Ventricular tachycardia.

Ventricular Tachycardia

It is defined as at least three PVCs, at more than 120 beats/min, and if not treated promptly, hypotension and ventricular fibrillation may occur.

Diagnosis: ECG revealing dissociated P waves, wide QRS more than 0.08 sec (>2 div) (Fig. 26.2).

Treatment

- *If stable:*
  - IV amiodarone, DC shock if no response.
- *If unstable:*
  - DC shock.

Catheter ablation or implantable cardioverter defibrillator (ICD) implantation after electrophysiologic study.

Ventricular Fibrillation or Pulseless VT (refer to Fig. 7. 4)

Immediate defibrillation with 2 J/kg to 4 J/kg along with anti-arrhythmia medication.

Long QT Syndrome

Heart rate corrected interval more than 0.44 seconds with symptoms (Fig. 26.3).

Treatment

- Beta-blockers, pacemaker, and ICD.

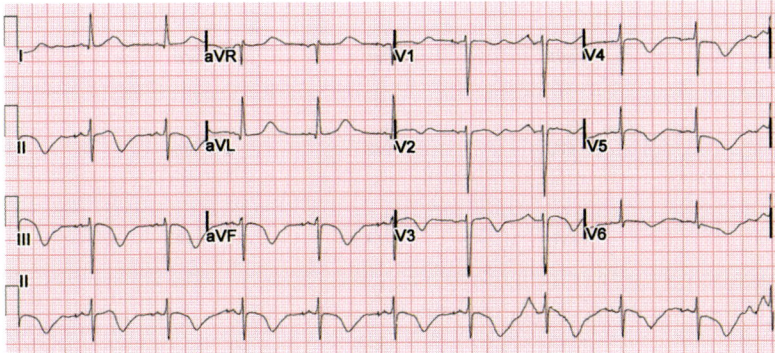

Fig. 26.3: Long QT syndrome.

Treatment of atrial flutter and atrial fibrillation: It is synchronized by DC cardioversion and followed by digoxin/beta-blockers/calcium channel blockers.

- *Continuation therapy—up to 1 year from last episode:*
  – No WPW:
    - Propranolol: 1–4 mg/kg/day div q 6 hr
    - Digoxin: 10 µg/kg/day div q 12 hr
    - Atenolol: 0.5–1 mg/kg/day once daily
    - Verapamil: 2–7 mg/kg/day div q 8 hr.
  – With WPW:
    - Avoid digoxin
    - Use propranolol or atenolol.

Bradyarrhythmias

Complete Heart Block

- Decreased heart rate (<60/min)
- High systolic BP
- Irregular large jugular venous pulsations
- Variable heart sounds, systolic and diastolic flow murmurs—may be revealed clinically
- ECG features are inconstant relationship between P waves and QRS complexes (Fig. 26.4).

Treatment

- *Medical*: IV atropine (0.01–0.03 mg/kg, maximum 0.5 mg)/isoproterenol/epinephrine if symptomatic.
- *Permanent pacemaker*: For those with heart rate less than 50 minutes or features of heart failure.

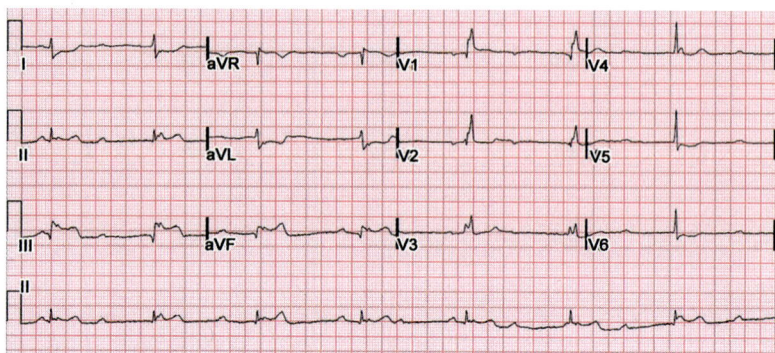

Fig. 26.4: Complete heart block.

CONCLUSION

Cardiac arrhythmias are disturbances in heart rate or rhythm; should be suspected in sudden death, shock, seizure, hydrops fetalis, palpitation restlessness, and syncope, but most of them can be diagnosed and treated.

Chapter **27**

Congestive Heart Failure

S Sushamabai

ABSTRACT

Congestive heart failure (CHF) is inadequate cardiac output to meet he metabolic demands of the body. The diagnosis is mainly clinical. All patients should have chest X-ray, complete blood count; electrocardiography (ECG), echocardiography (ECHO), serum electrolytes, and arterial blood gas (ABG). Treatment includes O_2, diuretics, digoxin, inotropes, angiotensin-converting enzyme (ACE) inhibitors, beta-blockers, isoprenaline and milrinone depending on the etiology and the nature of CHF. In resistant cases, ventricular assist devices (VAD) and heart transplantation should be considered.

INTRODUCTION

Congestive heart failure denotes inadequate cardiac output to meet the metabolic needs of the body. Infants are affected in 80% of the situations.

ETIOLOGY

Cardiac

- Acyanotic congenital heart diseases L→R shunt (ACHD): ventricular septal defect (VSD) and patent ductus arteriosus (PDA)
- Cyanotic congenital heart diseases high flow (CCHD): Transposition of the great arteries (TGA) and tricuspid atresia (TA)
- Obstructive lesions: Coarctation of aorta (COA)
- Cardiomyopathies
- Rheumatic heart disease
- Metabolic disorders.

Noncardiac

- Severe anemia
- Generalized edema as in acute nephritis, renal or hepatic failure, and iatrogenic fluid overload
- Severe respiratory disease.

Diagnosis of CHF is mainly clinical.

Symptoms—can be acute or insidious:
- Infants: Irritability, feeding difficulty, cough, dyspnea, excessive scalp sweating, and poor weight gain
- Children: Exercise intolerance, dyspnea of varying grades, recurrent cough, poor growth, and edema over face/legs/presacral region.

Signs

Resting tachypnea and tachycardia, edema, facial puffiness, raised jugular venous pressure, hypotension, cardiomegaly, S_3 gallop, murmurs of underlying disease, bilateral crackles, tender hepatomegaly, and growth failure.

DIFFERENTIAL DIAGNOSIS

Acute bronchiolitis, bronchopneumonia, episodic viral wheeze, foreign body obstruction of the airway, upper GI anomalies, renal failure, hepatic failure, and edematous malnutrition.

INVESTIGATIONS

- Hb, total count, differential leukocyte count, hematocrit—helpful to detect anemia and infection.
- Chest radiograph anteroposterior or posteroanterior—features are cardiomegaly; may reveal increased pulmonary vascularity.
- Echocardiography to assess the cardiac function and underlying defect.
- ECG 14 leads with long lead II.
- Renal function test, serum electrolytes, and ABG.

TREATMENT

- Admit in PICU; stabilize airway, breathing, circulation; and plan the investigations as per etiology.
- *Supportive therapy—to reduce the workload of heart:*
  - Rest till respiratory distress is controlled; sedation with triclofos/morphine may be required especially in young babies.
  - Propped up position 30 degree.
  - Oxygen 2–5 L/min by facemask or hood.
  - Reduce physical activity; gradual ambulation after controlling dyspnea.

- Salt (<6 g/day) and fluid (1/2 to 2/3 of maintenance) restriction.
- Correction of anemia—packed RBCs 10 mL/kg in 2 hours with IV furosemide 1 mg/kg if Hb is less than 7 g/dL or hematocrit is less than 30% followed by oral iron therapy to bring up Hb to 12 g.
- Nutritional support—add 10% extra calories to the normal requirement. If associated protein-energy malnutrition increase to 150 cal/kg/day. Consider NG tube feeds if sick and unable to feed.
- Reduce the preload by diuretics—IV furosemide 1–2 mg/kg along with oral potassium chloride 1 mEq/kg/day.
- Control of fever with paracetamol.
- Antibiotics for associated infections.
- *Specific drug therapy for CHF*
    - *IV inotropes:*
        - Dopamine (CHF + hypotension) for 48 hours; taper in 24 hours.
        - Dobutamine (CHF + normotension) for 48 hours; taper in 24 hours.
        - Combination: dopamine +dobutamine—start with dopamine (hypotension/poor renal perfusion); add dobutamine when BP normalizes; continue combined infusion (5–7.5 µg/kg/min of each drug) till improvement.
        - Milrinone in resistant cases as an adjunct to dopamine/dobutamine as IV infusion 0.25–1 µg/kg/min. Can cause hypotension.
    - *Digoxin:*
        - Rapid digitalization IV or oral (Table 27.1)
        - Slow digitalization by oral maintenance dose (one-fourth of total digitalizing dose div q 12 hr) depending on the clinical situation.
        - *ACE inhibitors (ACEI)*
        - Enalapril 0.08–0.5 mg/kg/day div q 12 hr PO.
    - *Beta-blockers:*
        - Carvedilol 0.1 mg/kg/day div q 12 hr increase in 2 weeks interval up to 0.5–1 mg/kg/day PO; may cause hypotension, oliguria, and wheeze. Refer Tables 27.2 and 27.3 for drug therapy in CHF.
- *Treatment of underlying disease:*

Table 27.1: Digoxin for rapid digitalization.

Age group	Oral digitalizing dose—total	Frequency (all age groups)	Remarks
Newborn	30 µg/kg	Half the dose immediately, half dose q 8 hr for 2 doses	Reduce to 75% for IV digitalization (div q 12 hr × 2 doses)
Infants and children	40 µg/kg	as above	in rheumatic carditis, myocarditis. ECG monitoring before 2nd and 3rd doses

Table 27.2: Disease-specific drug therapy in congestive heart failure.

Disease	IV inotrope	Digoxin	ACEI	Beta-blocker	Others
ACHD L→R shunt	+	+	++	+	–
CCHD ↑ pulmonary flow	+	++	+	–	–
Coarctation of aorta	+	++	+	–	–
Dilated cardiomyopathy	+	++	++	++	–
Myocarditis	++	+	++	+	IVIG
PPHN	++	+	–	–	Isoprenaline, Milrinone
Rheumatic carditis	+	+	++	–	–
Open heart surgery	+	+	+	–	

(ACHD, acyanotic congenital heart diseases; ACEI, angiotensin-converting enzyme inhibitor; CCHD, cyanotic congenital heart diseases; IVIG, intravenous immunoglobulin; PPHN, persistent pulmonary hypertension of the newborn)

Table 27.3: Therapy in congestive heart failure (CHF) according to the severity.

Critically ill CHF	Recovering CHF/chronic CHF
• Stabilize airway, breathing, circulation • Supportive therapy • IV Inotrope × 48 hours • Oral slow digitalization • Angiotensin-converting enzyme inhibitor (ACEI) or beta-blockers • Others	• Digitalization(IV/oral), rapid or slow • Maintenance dose digoxin • Diuretics • ACEI, beta blockers • IV inotrope intermittently • others

- Specific therapy to the underlying heart disease—congenital or acquired.
- Intravenous immunoglobulin or steroid therapy in myocarditis; myocardial biopsy and treatment accordingly.

• *Ventricular assist devices and heart transplantation.*

CONCLUSION

Congestive heart failure is serious dysfunction of the heart which can be diagnosed clinically, confirmed by investigations, and treated with drugs or in resistant cases, VAD or heart transplantation.

Chapter 28

Hypercyanotic Attacks (Tet Spells)

S Sushamabai

ABSTRACT

Hypercyanotic attacks or "Tet spells" are life-threatening aggravation of cyanosis leading to hypoxia in children with cyanotic congenital heart disease of reduced pulmonary flow. They can mimic seizures, aspiration of feeds or breath-holding spells. Child needs urgent stabilization and pediatric intensive care unit (PICU) treatment with O_2, morphine, volume expansion (NS/RL), maintenance fluids, sodium bicarbonate for acidosis, propranolol, correction of hypoglycemia, and packed cell transfusion for anemia in repeated spells. In resistant cases, intubation and sedation are needed. Surgical correction to improve the pulmonary flow is advised if spells exceed 30 minutes.

INTRODUCTION

"Tet" spells are abrupt episodes of irritability with crying, hyperpnea, deepening cyanosis, limpness, and gasping respirations terminating in loss of consciousness; seen in infants below 2 years of age with cyanotic congenital heart disease of reduced pulmonary flow.

ETIOPATHOGENESIS

Aggravation of already compromised pulmonary blood flow and hypoxia in cyanotic congenital heart diseases with low pulmonary blood flow (tetralogy of Fallot and pulmonary atresia).

DIFFERENTIAL DIAGNOSIS

- Seizures
- Aspiration of feeds
- Breath holding spells

Diagnosis is mainly clinical; have a high index of suspicion to diagnose Tet spells in babies less than 6 months age.

INVESTIGATIONS

These should be carried out after stabilization.
- Complete blood count, serum electrolytes, renal function test, liver function test, and arterial blood gas—to detect anemia, dyselectrolytemia, organ failure, and acidosis.
- Chest X-ray, ECG, and echocardiography—to confirm the cardiac problem.
- Others as per differential diagnosis.

TREATMENT (FLOWCHART 28.1)

- Place the child in knee chest position; this provides increase in systemic vascular resistance so that the pulmonary blood flow increases.
- Give 100% oxygen by head box or nasal prongs.
- Subcutaneous morphine 0.2 mg/kg to relieve pain.
- Start IV fluids—Normal saline or Ringer's lactate 20 mL/kg in 1 hour followed by maintenance fluid therapy to correct hypovolemia so as to increase the pulmonary blood flow.

Flowchart 28.1: Algorithm for management of hypercyanotic spells.

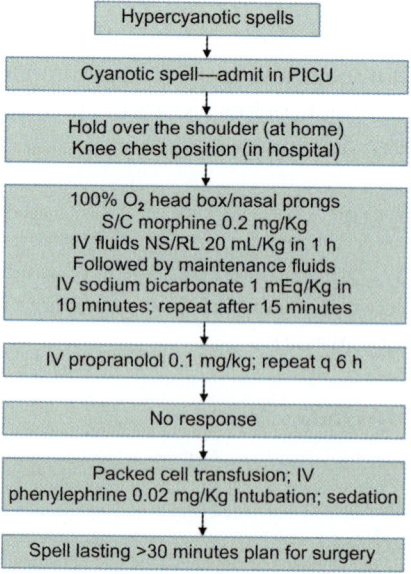

(NS, normal saline; PICU, pediatric intensive care unit; RL, Ringer's lactate; S/C, subcutaneous)

- IV sodium bicarbonate 1 mEq/kg equally diluted in distilled water in 10 minutes to correct the metabolic acidosis.
- Detect and correct hypoglycemia.
- Consider packed cell transfusion to maintain packed cell volume more than 45% in anemic babies with repeated spell episodes.
- IV propranolol 0.1 mg/kg diluted 4 times, each one-fourth volume in 5 minutes; repeat q 6 hr; continue with oral propranolol 1 mg/kg q 6 hr.
- Alternatively IV esmolol can be given.
- IV phenylephrine or norepinephrine infusion may be tried.
- Resistant spells may respond to intubation and sedation.
- Plan for surgical correction.
- Oral iron therapy to prevent anemia will reduce the frequency and intensity of hyper cyanotic spells.

CONCLUSION

Life-threatening hypercyanotic spells in children with cyanotic congenital heart disease should be promptly detected and treated with drugs and in resistant cases surgically.

Chapter 29

Viral Myocarditis

S Sushamabai

ABSTRACT

Myocarditis is a serious manifestation of certain viral infections and may end in rapid progression to death in infants to chronic cardiomyopathy in older children. Clinical presentation can be sudden death, shock, cardiac arrhythmias or congestive heart failure (CHF). Critically ill children should be cared in pediatric intensive care unit (PICU) with airway, breathing, circulation (ABC) stabilization, O_2, maintenance fluids, and dopamine infusion. Intravenous immunoglobulin and pulse dose methylprednisolone followed by gradual tapering are beneficial in sick babies. In refractory cases, extracorporeal membrane oxygenation (ECMO), ventilator support, and heart transplantations are required. In patients presenting with CHF, dobutamine, angiotensin-converting enzyme (ACE) inhibitors, and reduced maintenance dose of digoxin and diuretics are advised. Amiodarone (arrhythmias), isoprenaline infusion (heart block), milrinone infusion (shock), cardiac pacing, and beta-blockers are further treatment modalities advised.

INTRODUCTION

Viral myocarditis is inflammation of the myocardium due to viral infections and mostly affects infants.

COMMON ORGANISMS

Coxsackie B, enteroviruses, adenovirus, influenza, Epstein–Barr, and cytomegaloviruses.

CLINICAL PRESENTATION

It can be of varying severity.
- Cardiogenic shock (fulminant myocarditis)—mostly in newborns
- Congestive cardiac failure and cardiac arrhythmias—in infants
- Unexplained respiratory distress, chest pain, and exertional dyspnea ± cardiomegaly—in older age group children.
- Inappropriate or unexplainable tachycardia.
- Sudden cardiac death—at any age.

DIFFERENTIAL DIAGNOSIS

- Other causes of myocarditis (sepsis, rheumatological disorders)
- Acute bronchiolitis
- Congenital heart diseases [Anomalous left coronary artery arising from the pulmonary artery (ALCAPA) and coarctation of the Aorta (CoA)] and endomyocardial fibroelastosis
- Metabolic—carnitine deficiency, mitochondrial disorders, and glycogen storage disease
- Diabetes mellitus

Clues for the diagnosis of viral myocarditis:
Onset with flu-like illness, respiratory distress, associated tachycardia, tachypnea, hypotension, cardiomegaly, S_3 gallop, and cardiac murmurs indicate viral myocarditis.

INVESTIGATIONS

- Complete blood count, C-reactive protein, and arterial blood gas
- Enzymes elevated—serum glutamic-oxaloacetic transaminase, lactate dehydrogenase, creatine phosphokinase muscle/brain, and cardiac troponin 1
- Chest X-ray: Cardiomegaly and features of pulmonary venous congestion.
- 14-lead ECG with rhythm strip—sinus tachycardia, arrhythmias, low voltage complexes, ST elevation, T inversion, and various types of heart block.
- Echocardiography—left atrial and left ventricular enlargement and impaired ejection fraction less than 60%.
- Others—viral serology and myocardial biopsy.
- MRI—*gold standard*: Reveals the earliest abnormalities in myocarditis.

PATIENT APPROACH (REFER CHAPTERS 25 TO 27)

Assess and categorize (A—shock, B—heart failure/others)

A—Shock (fulminant form):
- Admit in PICU
- ABC stabilization:
  - 100% O_2, IV access (2 lines), and Ringer's lactate 10 mL/kg in 1 hour.
  - Dopamine infusion, dobutamine when the BP is stable.
  - Continue maintenance fluids.
  - Digoxin, ACE inhibitors, diuretics, as recovery starts.
  - Investigations as per differential diagnosis.
  - Intravenous immunoglobulin (2 g/kg in 2 days)/corticosteroids (prednisolone/methylprednisolone 1–2 mg/kg/day).
  - Taper biweekly; low maintenance dose 3–6 months.

- Refractory cases—ventilator support, ECMO, and heart transplantation as per availability.

B: Heart failure/other problems—most common presentation:
- Admit in PICU
- Oxygen, IV access, and parallel investigations.
- Dobutamine—5 µg/kg/min increase up to 12 µg/kg/min for 48 hours.
- Angiotensin-converting enzyme inhibitor—captopril 0.5 mg/kg (1st dose), increase up to 3–4 mg/kg/day in three divided doses (over 3 days).
- Digoxin in reduced maintenance dose (RMD 7.5 µg/kg/day).
- Diuretics—IV furosemide 3 mg/kg/day in three divided doses, change to oral as recovery is revealed.
- Anticoagulants—warfarin for intracardiac clots or embolism.
- Amiodarone—for arrhythmias.
- Isoprenaline infusion in heart block.
- Milrinone infusion for shock.
- Cardiac pacing.
- Beta-blockers (carvedilol) 0.1–0.4 mg/kg/day in 2 div. doses.

Management of viral myocarditis is shown in Flowchart 29.1.

Flowchart 29.1: Management of viral myocarditis.

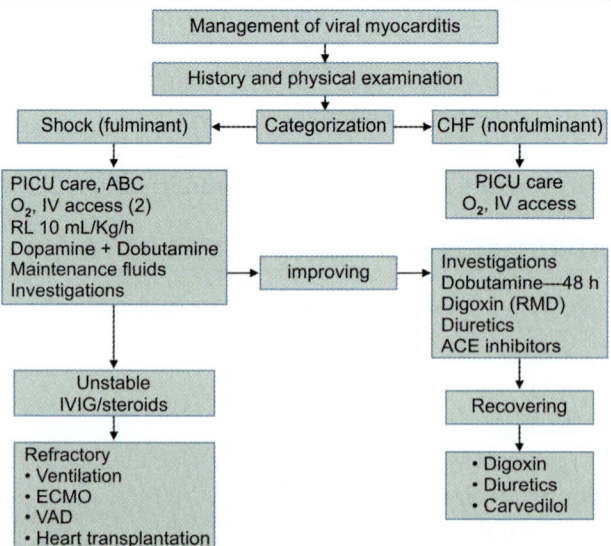

(ABC, airway, breathing, circulation; ACE, angiotensin-converting enzyme; ECMO, extracorporeal membrane oxygenation; IVIG, intravenous immunoglobulin; RL, Ringer's lactate; VAD, ventricular assist devices)

CONCLUSION

Viral myocarditis is an occasional serious illness which should be anticipated in any viral infection since drug therapy and cardiac pacing are effective.

FURTHER READING

1. Ahmed MZ. Viral Myocarditis: diagnosis and treatment. Souvenir, Summer Pedicon 2012. IAP Kerala sessional conference.

Chapter 30

Rheumatic Carditis

S Sushamabai

ABSTRACT

Rheumatic carditis is a serious complication of group A beta-hemolytic streptococcal infection resulting in death or chronic valvular heart disease. The clinical presentation can be classical or subclinical (rarely). Patients with carditis require pediatric intensive care unit (PICU) care with O_2, 45° propped up position, diuretics, paracetamol for pain and fever, and urgent echocardiography study for the diagnosis of carditis and its severity. The ideal drug for rheumatic fever prophylaxis is IM benzathine penicillin G; PO penicillin V/amoxicillin/azithromycin/cephalexin/erythromycin are the other options. All children with previous episode of rheumatic fever should have secondary prophylaxis with any one of these drugs; the duration depends on the severity of carditis. The additional drugs are aspirin for arthritis, prednisone for carditis and diuretics, digoxin and angiotensin-converting enzyme (ACE) inhibitors for heart failure. The duration for rest depends on the severity of carditis and cardiac failure.

INTRODUCTION

Rheumatic carditis is a nonsuppurative sequelae of group A streptococcal infection (GAS). If not treated in time, rapid progression to cardiac decompensation and death or chronic valvular heart disease and severe disability can occur in later years.

CLINICAL PRESENTATION

Classical onset is seen in majority, features being:
- Chest pain, effort intolerance, and breathlessness in the school going age group.
- Past history of recurrent sore throat and migratory polyarthritis of large joints.
- Tachy or bradycardia, cardiomegaly, muffling of first heart sound, and cardiac murmurs of mitral and/or aortic regurgitation.

- Pericardial rub, hepatomegaly, and peripheral and pulmonary edema in severe carditis.

Subclinical onset:
- Fever ± migrating polyarthritis without cardiac symptoms or signs.
- Cardiac involvement is detected only by echocardiography.
- Severe persistent arthritis and monoarthritis are rare manifestations; hence in such doubtful cases echocardiography is mandatory.
- Arthritis of spine, hips, shoulders, and small joints of hands are not features of rheumatic fever.

PATIENT APPROACH

- Admit in PICU if features of classical carditis are present. Keep in 45° propped up position if evidence of cardiac failure.
- Administer oxygen.
- IV furosemide 1 mg/kg/dose q 12 hr.
- Paracetamol for joint or chest pain.
- Proceed for urgent echocardiography: Experienced cardiologist can detect rheumatic carditis and the severity.
- Other investigations suggested and the supportive values are:
  - Complete blood count—leukocytosis with neutrophilia, ESR more than 30 mm/hr.
  - C-reactive protein—more than 8 mg/dL.
- Essential criteria for evidence of streptococcal infection are (any one):
  - Throat swab culture positivity.
  - Antistreptolysin O titer more than or equal to 4-fold rise in titer.
  - Rapid antigen and streptozyme tests positivity.
- Others:
  - Chest X-ray to detect cardiomegaly and pulmonary edema.
  - ECG 14 leads + rhythm strip—look for I and II degree atrioventricular block, junctional rhythm, and bradycardia.

DIFFERENTIAL DIAGNOSIS

- Viral myocarditis
- Viral pericarditis
- Infective endocarditis
- Mitral valve prolapse
- Kawasaki disease
- Juvenile idiopathic arthritis
- Innocent cardiac murmurs.

SUBSEQUENT MANAGEMENT

Antibiotic Therapy

To eradicate GAS infection from upper respiratory tract—primary prophylaxis:
- Penicillin V (Oral): 20–50 mg/kg/day div q 6 hr ×10 days *or*
- Benzathine penicillin G single IM (6L IU <27 kg, 12 L IU ≥27 kg) *or*
- Amoxicillin PO 25–50 mg/kg/day div q 8 hr × 10 days *or*
- Erythromycin PO 40 mg/kg/day div q 6 hr × 10 days *or*
- Azithromycin PO 12.5 mg/kg/day OD × 5 days *or*
- Cephalexin PO 15–20 mg/kg/dose q 12 hr × 10 days.

Anti-inflammatory Therapy

- Should be started after confirmation of diagnosis as:
    - Patients with carditis but no cardiomegaly or CCF—aspirin 50–70 mg/kg/day in 4 div doses for 3–5 days, followed by 50 mg/kg/day in 4 div doses for 3 weeks, and then 25 mg/kg/day for 2–4 weeks.
    - Patients with carditis + cardiomegaly ± CCF—prednisone 2 mg/kg/day div q 6 hr for 2–3 weeks followed by 1 mg/kg/day for 2–3 weeks and then tapering by 5 mg/day every 2–3 day; add aspirin 50 mg/kg/day div q 6 hr for 6 weeks when prednisone is being tapered.
    - If reappearance of inflammatory features on termination of therapy—increase aspirin or steroids till the clinical features disappear and till the ESR/CRP become normal; taper and stop after that.

Supportive Therapy

- Rest—refer Table 30.1
- Fluid and salt restriction
- Oxygen for respiratory distress
- Diuretics—furosemide 1 mg/kg IV OD or BD or 2–3 mg/kg/day orally daily.
- Digoxin—slow digitalization with 0.075 mg/kg/day.
- Angiotensin-converting enzyme inhibitors—captopril 1–4 mg/kg/day div q 6 hr.

Table 30.1: Guidelines for rest in rheumatic carditis.

Severity of carditis	Rest at home (weeks)	Restricted activity (weeks)	Schooling (weeks)
Nil	2	4	6
Mild	2	6	8
Severe	4	8	12
Severe + CCF	Till CCF is controlled	8	12

Table 30.2: Chemoprophylaxis for recurrence of rheumatic fever.

Drug, route and dose (choose any one as per situation and patient compliance)		Disease category	Duration
Benzathine penicillin IM	0.6 million U <27 kg 1.2 million U ≥ 27 kg every 3–4 week	Rheumatic fever without carditis	5 years or until 18 years of age whichever is longer
or Penicillin V PO	250 mg BD	Rheumatic fever with carditis but without residual heart disease, no valvular disease	10 years or until 25 years age whichever is longer
or Sulfadiazine PO	0.5 g OD <27 kg 1 g OD ≥27 kg		
For patients allergic to penicillin/sulfa: Erythromycin PO	250 mg BD	Rheumatic fever with carditis/ persistent valvular disease/ following valve surgery/balloon mitral valvotomy	Lifelong prophylaxis; get expert consultation to discontinue after 40 years of age

Prevention of recurrence—secondary prophylaxis:
Continuous chemoprophylaxis to all children diagnosed as rheumatic fever with or without carditis to prevent recurrence as in Table 30.2.

CONCLUSION

Rheumatic carditis is still prevalent, can have subclinical presentation, drug therapy for carditis and streptococcal eradication and prevention of infection should be carried out.

FURTHER READING

1. National Centre for Disease Control, Directorate of General Health Services, Ministry of Health & Family Welfare, Government of India. (2016). National Treatment Guidelines for antimicrobial use in infectious diseases. Version 1.0 (2016). Available from http://pbhealth.gov.in/AMR_guideline7001495889.pdf [Accessed on September 2018].

Chapter 31

Pericardial Effusion

S Sushamabai

ABSTRACT

Pericardial effusion is the accumulation of fluid in the pericardial space leading to cardiac tamponade and death. The common causes are viral (Echo, Coxsackie) and bacterial (*Haemophilus influenzae B*, pneumococcal, and *Mycobacterium tuberculosis*) infections and rheumatologic disorders. The child may present in shock or with stabbing chest pain, cough and respiratory distress, distended jugular veins, muffled heart sounds, and pericardial rub. The gold standard for diagnosis is echocardiography. Chest X-ray (CXR), electrocardiography (ECG), and pericardial fluid study are supportive. The patient should be stabilized; broad-spectrum antibiotics for bacterial infection, nonsteroidal anti-inflammatory drugs (NSAIDs) ± steroids for viral and rheumatic etiology, anti TB + steroids for TB, and anakinra for idiopathic recurrent pericarditis are recommended. Surgical intervention may be needed occasionally.

INTRODUCTION

Pericardial effusion is the accumulation of fluid inside the pericardial space which is nondistensible. The fluid can be serous, purulent or hemorrhagic depending on the etiology.

COMMON CAUSES

- Infections:
  - Viral: Coxsackie, Epstein–Barr
  - Bacterial (pyogenic—*H. influenzae B*, pneumococci, *Mycobacterium TB*)
  - Fungal
  - Parasitic
- Rheumatic pancarditis
- Collagen diseases
- Malignancy (leukemia, lymphoma)

- Uremia
- Postoperative
- Trauma.

PATHOPHYSIOLOGY

Fluid inside the pericardial space results in cardiac tamponade (abrupt impairment of function of cardiac chambers due to the fluid pressure) and shock.

CLINICAL PRESENTATION

- Depends on the etiology.
- Can present as cardiogenic shock when fluid accumulation is rapid.
- Chest pain of stabbing nature (manifested in young infants as irritability and crying), dyspnea, cough, abdominal pain, vomiting, tachycardia, narrow pulse pressure, jugular venous distension, muffled or distant heart sounds, and pericardial friction sound in the early stage. Pulsus paradoxus (>10 mm Hg fall of systolic BP during inspiration—assessed by auscultatory BP determination).

DIFFERENTIAL DIAGNOSIS

- Pleurodynia
- Cardiomyopathy
- Mediastinal tumors
- Pericardial cyst
- Gastroesophageal reflux.

PATIENT APPROACH

- *History and physical examination:*
  - Assess the severity: shock and cardiac tamponade reveals severe form.
  - Find out the possible etiology.
- *Investigations:*
  - Chest X-ray (Fig. 31.1): Reveals cardiomegaly of "Erlenmeyer flask" shape
  - Electrocardiography: Low voltage, ST and T changes.
  - Echocardiogram: *Gold standard*—features are echo-free space behind the posterior left ventricular wall, compression, and collapse of the right atrium and/or ventricle.
  - Others to detect the etiology: Complete blood count, cultures, Mantoux test, antistreptolysin O titer, and pericardial fluid study (Chapter 121).

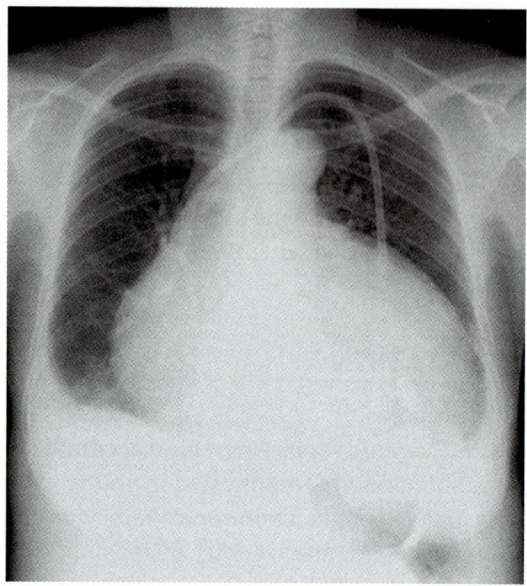

Fig. 31.1: Pericardial effusion.

- *Treatment:*
    - Admit in PICU, stabilize ABC.
    - Treatment of specific etiology:
        - Antibiotics in purulent pericarditis (IV ceftriaxone+ cloxacillin or vancomycin as empirical, change as per culture and sensitivity report)
        - NSAIDs ± steroids in viral and rheumatic diseases
        - Anti-TB (as per RNTCP) + steroids in TB effusion
        - Anakinra in idiopathic recurrent pericarditis
        - Surgical intervention.

CONCLUSION

Pericardial effusion is a serious disease leading to cardiac tamponade and death, can be diagnosed by echocardiography and treated with steroids and drugs for the underlying disease.

Chapter 32

Hypertensive Crisis

S Sushamabai

ABSTRACT

Hypertensive crisis or emergency is the situation characterized by end organ damage (eyes, brain, heart, and kidneys) secondary to BP (systolic and/or diastolic) above 95th percentile. In hypertensive urgency, there is no end organ damage with high BP. Most cases in children are secondary to renal diseases. Pharmacologic therapy should be IV drugs—labetalol, nicardipine, esmolol, sodium nitroprusside, hydralazine, and fenoldopam to reduce the BP 30% in first 12 hours, 30% in next 12 hours, and rest in 24 hours, below 90th percentile, and thereafter continuing with oral preparation. Underlying cause should be treated always.

INTRODUCTION

Hypertensive crisis or emergency is the dangerous situation due to systemic hypertension leading to end organ damage manifested as any of the following:
- Blurring of vision, papilledema (retinopathy)
- Headache, dizziness, convulsions, and paralysis (encephalopathy)
- Neck stiffness and coma [intracranial hemorrhage (ICH)]
- Cough, dyspnea, edema, and hepatomegaly (cardiac failure)
- Edema, oliguria, and hematuria (renal failure).

Hypertension (HT) is defined as mean systolic and/or diastolic BP more than or equal to 95th percentile for age, sex, and height percentiles.

SEVERITY CLASSIFICATION

- *Stage I:* BP between 95th and 99th percentile plus 5 mm Hg.
- *State II:* BP more than 99th percentile plus 5 mm Hg.

CLASSIFICATION ACCORDING TO DURATION

- *Acute:* Less than 6 months duration
- *Chronic:* More than 6 months duration.

Age-wise approximate values for hypertension (in mm of Hg):
- Birth: 90/60
- 1 week to 1 month: 105/70
- More than 1 month: 100 + (age in year × 3)/70 + (age in year × 1.5)

Consider hypertensive crisis in all children with stage II hypertension and with stage 1 hypertension having symptoms or end organ damage.

ETIOLOGY

Primary (Essential)

No detectable cause clinically or after investigations to explain the high BP.

Secondary

- *Renal:* Congenital/acquired
- *Vascular:* Coarctation of aorta (COA) and vasculitis
- *Endocrine:* Cushing syndrome, hyperthyroidism, congenital adrenal hyperplasia (CAH)
- *Drugs/toxin:* Topical/inhaled/oral medicines, appetizers, excess vitamin D intake, and alternate system medicines
- Porphyria
- *Neurological:* Guillain–Barré syndrome, intracranial space-occupying lesions (ICSOL), ICH, and head injury.

DIAGNOSIS

- Often detected by routine vital assessment.
- By evaluation of specific symptoms.

PATIENT APPROACH

- Admit in pediatric intensive care unit. Stabilize airway, breathing, circulation.
- History and physical examination to assess HT as:
    - Primary (essential)
    - Secondary (symptomatic)
    - Hypertensive crisis
    - Hypertensive urgency (BP >95th percentile, asymptomatic)
    - Acute or chronic.

Note: BP has to be assessed on all 4 limbs manually; hypertension in upper limbs only indicates COA.

- Proceed for parallel investigations:
  - *First line:*
    - Complete blood count, platelet count, renal function test, and serum electrolytes.
    - Urinalysis and culture
    - Fasting lipid profile and fasting blood sugar to detect comorbid conditions
    - Chest X-ray, electrocardiography, and echocardiography to assess the cardiac status and anomaly
    - Fundus evaluation for hypertensive changes
    - Ultrasonography abdomen to assess renal and other problems
    - CT/MRI of brain to detect end organ damage
    - Hormone assay: Thyroid-stimulating hormone (TSH), free T_4, and plasma cortisol
    - Metabolic screening if inborn errors of metabolism are suspected.
  - *Second line:* Includes selected investigations which are:
    - Plasma renin
    - Plasma and urine catecholamines
    - Renovascular imaging.
- Treatment:
  - Pharmacologic therapy to reduce BP
  - Treatment of underlying disease.

Note: Nonpharmacologic therapy of life style modification is a must in essential hypertension.

Pharmacologic therapy: Should be controlled BP reduction as:
- 30% in first 12 hours
- 30% in next 12 hours
- Rest in next 24 hours (to reduce the BP below 90th percentile)
- Rapid reduction in 60 minutes is advised in dissection of aorta
- Start with IV infusion; continue orally as per etiology (Tables 32.1 and 32.2)
- Consider diuretics as per situation
- Oral drugs are to be started as continuation therapy 6 hours after IV dose
- In hypertensive urgency, administer oral drugs to reduce the BP to 90th percentile within 2–3 days.

Detect and treat the underlying cause for hypertension.

Table 32.1: Drug therapy in hypertensive crisis.

Drug	Specific indication, mode of action	Dosage, administration (IV)	Remarks, relative contraindications
Labetalol	Hypertension encephalopathy Intracranial bleeding Pheochromocytoma	0.2 to 1 mg/kg bolus up to 40 mg/dose. Infusion 0.25 to 3 mg/kg/hr	Asthma, overt heart failure
Nicardipine	Acute renal failure (Newer parenteral vasodilator)	Bolus 30 µg/kg up to 2 mg/dose; infusion 0.5–4 µg/kg/min	Can cause reflex tachycardia
Esmolol	Post coarctation repair	100–500 µg/kg/min	Profound bradycardia
Hydralazine	Direct vasodilator	0.25 mg/kg/dose, max 25 mg/dose; IV, IM Repeat q 4 hr	Contraindicated in subarachnoid hemorrhage
Sodium nitroprusside	Direct vasodilator	0.5–10 µg/kg/min	Cyanide toxicity >72 hours use, especially in renal failure
Fenoldopam	Selective dopamine agonist	0.2–0.8 µg/kg/min	Selectively increases renal blood flow

Table 32.2: Drugs for hypertensive urgency.

Drug	Specific indication, mode of action	Dosage, administration	Remarks, relative contraindications
Enalapril (O) Enalaprilat (IV)	Diabetes, congestive heart failure, dyslipidemia	Oral 0.1–0.6 mg/kg/day Divided q12 hr; IV 5–10 µg/kg/dose up to 1.25 mg/dose as bolus	Can be used in unilateral renal artery stenosis
Nifedipine (O)	Acute nephritis, nephrotic syndrome, asthma	0.5–3 mg/kg/day Div q 6 hr	
Amlodipine (O)	As for nifedipine	0.06–0.3 mg/kg/day q d.	Long half-life
Hydralazine (O)	Direct vasodilator	0.25 mg/kg/dose Up to 7.5 mg/kg/day div q 6 hr	Suspension unstable

CONCLUSION

Hypertensive crisis is not uncommon in children, is usually secondary and IV drugs should be used for immediate control followed by oral drugs till the underlying disease process is controlled.

Section 6

NERVOUS SYSTEM

Chapter **33**

Raised Intracranial Pressure

Manju George Elenjickal, S Sushamabai

ABSTRACT

Raised intracranial pressure (ICP) is rarely perceived in time in children because of the subtle clinical presentations in the early stage. The chapter deals with the definition, etiology, clinical features, and stepwise management. Child should be cared in pediatric intensive care unit (PICU), requires immediate stabilization, sedation, temperature control, euglycemia, fluid and electrolyte management, osmotherapy with mannitol + furosemide/3% saline and dexamethasone in selected situations. The etiology should be treated without delay. In refractory raised ICP, hyperventilation and decompressive craniectomy are advised.

INTRODUCTION

Raised intracranial pressure is the pathological state of rise in intracranial pressure above 20 mm Hg due to the addition of blood/CSF/brain tissue to the intracranial vault. The normal ICP is 6–8 mm Hg. The situation, though not uncommon in children, is rarely perceived in time because of the vague clinical manifestations and late diagnosis. Timely treatment is crucial in saving life as well as reducing the morbidity.

PATHOPHYSIOLOGY

- Brain blood supply depends upon mean arterial pressure (MAP) and ICP, the difference between the two being cerebral perfusion pressure (CPP).
- Fall in CPP results in cerebral ischemia.
- Rise in ICP causes brain herniation leading to death or significant morbidity.

ETIOLOGY

- *Neurological:* Head injury, meningitis, encephalitis, intracranial hemorrhage, brain abscess, brain tumors, dural sinus thrombosis, and pseudotumor cerebri.
- *Systemic:* Hypo/hypernatremia, diabetic ketoacidosis, hepatic/renal failure, metabolic encephalopathy, and systemic hypertension.

SYMPTOMS

- Headache and projectile vomiting more in the morning (due to the prolonged supine posture).
- In infants, seizures, irritability, bulging fontanel, and increasing head size are the features and the diagnosis may be delayed.
- Varying grades of altered sensorium.
- Features of brain herniation as:
  - Diplopia, defective vision, and squint (because of 3rd and 6th cranial nerve palsy) in central brain herniation.
  - Paralysis of varying degrees; hemiplegia occurs in uncal herniation.
  - Stiffness of neck—characteristic of cerebellar tonsillar herniation.

SIGNS

- Irritability, decreasing levels of consciousness (Chapter 34 Comatose child), squint (6th/3rd cranial nerve palsy), unequal pupils, and Cushing's triad (hypertension, bradycardia, irregular/chaotic breathing).
- In chronic cases, varying degrees of paralysis.
- Papilledema is a late sign in children.
- Symptoms and signs of underlying disease.

PATIENT APPROACH

- History and rapid clinical examination—to assess the severity and etiology of raised ICP, which will be disclosed in most patients.
- Admit in PICU; stabilize ABC.
- Rapid sequence intubation (RSI) if Glasgow Coma Scale (GCS) is less than or equal to 8 or rapid fall in GCS more than 3 points or evidence of brain herniation or Cushing's triad.
- Evaluate ICP and CPP if facilities are available; the normal CPP is between 40 mm Hg and 60 mm Hg in infants and children, respectively, and more than 60 mm Hg in adolescents.
- Parallel investigations to detect the etiology:
  - Complete blood count, renal function test (RFT), liver function test, serum electrolytes, random blood sugar, venous blood gas/arterial blood gas (VBG/ABG) and urinalysis.
  - CT/MRI brain, lumbar puncture (LP) after stabilization.
  - Others as per suspected etiology.
  - Fundus evaluation by the ophthalmologist.

SUBSEQUENT MANAGEMENT

General

- Head end elevation to 30° in neutral position; avoid if hypertension.

- Sedation by morphine 2–4 mg every 2–4 hourly/IV midazolam 0.1 mg/kg/dose q 8 hr since pain, discomfort, cough, and agitation can increase ICP further.
- Minimal handling.
- Monitor core temperature—control fever by paracetamol.
- Ensure normovolemia—two-thirds maintenance requirement with normal saline; avoid hypotonic solutions.
- Treat shock aggressively as per guidelines (Chapter 25); early administration of low-dose dopamine (10 µg/kg/min) with normal saline improves CPP.
- Treat hypo/hyperglycemia.
- Maintain serum Na between 145 mEq/L and 160 mEq/L; for patients with hyponatremia, 3% saline 5 mL/kg over 10 minutes followed by continuous infusion at 0.1–1 mL/kg/hr is advisable if hemodynamically unstable.
- In children with associated hypotension normal saline infusion with early administration of dopamine is advised.

Osmotherapy

- Intravenous mannitol 0.5–1 g/kg (2.5 mL–5 mL/kg of 20% solution) in 30 minutes followed by 0.25 g/kg/dose q 6 hr for 48 hours; maintain serum osmolality less than 320 mOsm/L to prevent renal toxicity; mannitol should be avoided in hypotension.
- Intravenous furosemide 1–2 mg/kg/dose q 6 hr, taper slowly as per recovery.
- Intravenous dexamethasone 1 mg/kg/dose loading dose followed by 1 mg/kg/day divided q 6 hr in intracranial tumor, brain abscess, and infections to reduce perilesional and vasogenic edema.

Specific Therapy

Should be started as early as possible for the underlying etiology—antibiotics in meningitis, resection of brain tumors, aspiration of abscess, etc.

Refractory raised ICP—to be considered when the above measures fail; treatment modalities being:
- Hyperventilation to bring down PCO_2 to 25 mm Hg for a brief period during which time further measures are undertaken.
- Pentobarbital infusion—loading dose 5–10 mg/kg in 30 minutes followed by 5 mg/kg every 30 min × 3 doses; then maintenance with 1 mg/kg/hr.
- Decompressive craniectomy by the end of 48 hours if medical therapy fails.
- Mild hypothermia 32–34°C for 24 hours.
- Treatment for nonconvulsive seizures ideally with bedside EEG evaluation. If facilities are not available, empirical anticonvulsant therapy with phenytoin has to be considered.

Flowchart 33.1: Algorithm for management of raised intracranial pressure.

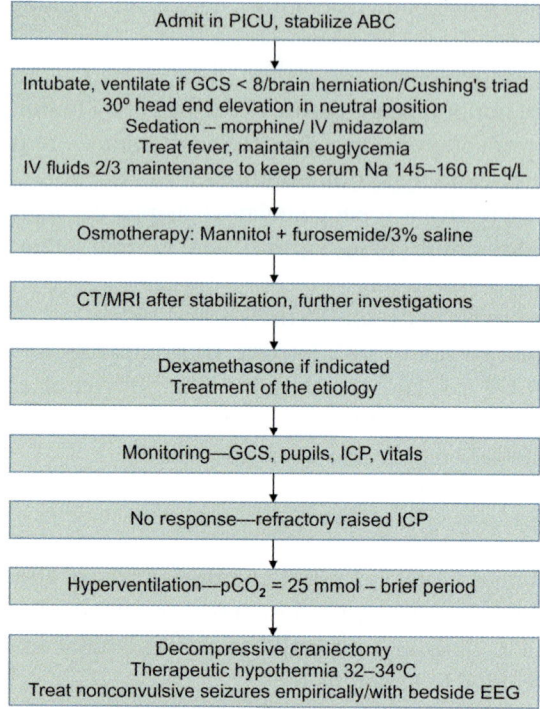

(ABC, airway, breathing, circulation; EEG, electroencephalography; GCS, Glasgow Coma Scale; ICP, intracranial pressure; PICU, pediatric intensive care unit)

MONITORING

- Vitals, GCS, pupils, I/O chart, and SpO_2 hourly.
- Continuous monitoring—CVP, ICP, and invasive arterial BP if conditions are feasible.
- Arterial blood gas 4–12 hourly, continuous capnography.
- Random blood sugar and serum Na 6 hourly.
- Daily RFT.
- Repeated cranial imaging as per the underlying condition.

The algorithm for management of raised intracranial pressure is described in Flowchart 33.1.

CONCLUSION

Raised ICP should be detected early in children from the subtle signs and treatment implemented so as to save the life.

Chapter 34

Comatose Child

S Sushamabai

ABSTRACT

Coma is a state of decreased consciousness from which the patient cannot be aroused by ordinary verbal, physical or sensory stimuli. The severity of coma can be graded by AVPU/GCS/FOUR Score assessment. The leading medical causes are sepsis, metabolic derangement, status epilepticus, poisoning, acute encephalitic syndrome, and cerebral malaria. Patient approach is initial rapid assessment for severity staging and probable cause of coma and immediate stabilization. Systematic patient approach and investigations should follow. Neuroimaging should be done once the child is stable. Supportive and specific therapy and monitoring are detailed.

INTRODUCTION

Coma is the state of decreased consciousness from which the patient cannot be aroused by ordinary verbal, physical or sensory stimuli.

GRADING OF COMA

AVPU score: This is one second assessment of sensorium (**A**—awake, **V**—verbal command response, **P**—response to pain, **U**—unresponsive)—stages **P** and **U** carry bad prognosis.

Glasgow Coma Scale (Box 34.1): Total score is 15. Interpret as shown below:

Score	Impairment
≤8	Severe
9–12	Moderate
13–14	Mild

Fall of 3 scores from the previous value also indicates bad prognosis; hence periodic evaluation is needed.

> **Box 34.1:** Glasgow coma scale.
>
> **Eye Opening**
>   1= does not open eyes
>   2= opens eyes in response to noxious stimuli
>   3= opens eyes in response to voice
>   4= opens eyes spontaneously
> **Verbal Output**
>   1= makes no sounds
>   2= makes incomprehensible sounds
>   3= utters inappropriate words
>   4= confused and disoriented
>   5= speaks normally and oriented
> **Motor Response (Rest)**
>   1= makes no movements
>   2= extension to painful stimuli
>   3= abnormal flexion to painful stimuli
>   4= flexion/withdrawal to painful stimuli
>   5= localized to painful stimuli
>   6= obeys commands

> **Box 34.2:** FOUR score: Full Outline of UnResponsiveness score.
>
> **Eye Response**
>   4= eyelids open or opened, tracking, or blinking to command
>   3= eyelids open but not tracking
>   2= eyelids closed but open loud voice
>   1= eyelids closed but open to pain
>   0= eyelids remain closed with pain
> **Motor Response**
>   4= thumbs-up, fist or peace sign
>   3= localizing to pain
>   2= flexion response to pain
>   1= extension response to pain
>   0= no response to pain or generalized myoclonus status
> **Brainstem Reflexes**
>   4= pupil and corneal reflexes present
>   3= one pupil wide and fixed
>   2= pupil or corneal reflexes absent
>   1= absent pupil, corneal, and cough reflex
> **Respiration**
>   4= not intubated regular breathing pattern
>   3= not intubated, Cheyne-Stokes breathing pattern
>   2= not intubated, irregular breathing
>   1= breathes at ventilator rate
>   0= breathes at ventilator rate or apnea

FOUR Score (Full Outline of UnResponsiveness): This scale is more objective to assess brainstem involvement than the other two (Box 34.2).

COMMON CAUSES OF COMA

- Infections—sepsis, meningitis, encephalitis, cerebral malaria, brain abscess, and cortical thrombophlebitis.
- Status epilepticus.
- Head trauma—accidental and battered child.
- Poisons and toxins—accidental ingestion and snake envenomation.
- Metabolic—hyper/hypoglycemia, hyponatremia, acidosis, renal or hepatic failure, hyperammonemia.
- Drug overdose.
- Hypo/hypertension.
- Raised intracranial pressure (ICP).

PATIENT APPROACH

(Refer Chapter 33, Raised ICP)

Initial Approach

- Admit in pediatric intensive care unit.
- Parallel history, assess vitals and sensorium, and stabilize airway, breathing, circulation:
  - Administer 100% O_2
  - Correction of shock—IV normal saline (NS) 20 mL/kg in 20-60 minutes (Chapter 25)
  - Intubate if GCS less than or equal to 8, SpO_2 less than 92% in 100% O_2, abnormal respiratory pattern, and signs of raised ICP or features of brain herniation as shown in Box 34.3.
- Assess capillary blood glucose; give dextrose if the value is less than 50 mg/dL.
- Send blood for complete blood count, random blood sugar, serum electrolytes, renal function test, liver function test, arterial blood gas, lactate, plasma ammonia, malarial parasite (RDT, smear), cultures, viral studies, toxicology screening, and urine for sugar and ketones (as per indications).

Box 34.3: Signs of raised intracranial pressure and brain herniation.

- Glasgow Coma Scale ≤8
- Abnormal pupillary size and/or reaction (uni/bilateral)
- Absent dolls eye movements
- Abnormal tone (hyper/hypo)
- Abnormal posturing—decorticate, decerebrate
- Hypertension, bradycardia, apnea (Cushing's triad)
- Abnormal respiration (hyperventilation, Cheyne–Stokes breathing, irregular breathing, and respiratory arrest)
- Papilledema (in older children)

- Administer 20% mannitol 5 mL/kg in 10–15 minutes. Alternately 3% saline is preferred for patients in shock.
- Consider short-term hyperventilation (to attain pCO_2 30–35 mm Hg) to bring down raised ICP rapidly.

Subsequent Approach

Detailed History

- Fever, headache, rashes, vomiting, irritability—indicate acute infection of brain or sepsis.
- Trauma, drug/toxin exposure, dog bite, and malaria endemic region or travel.
- Past medical and family history regarding seizures, drug intake or omission of drugs.

Clues in General Physical Examination

Look for	If present, think of
Pallor	Cerebral malaria, intracranial bleed, hemolytic uremic syndrome
Icterus	Hepatic encephalopathy, leptospirosis, malaria
Head and scalp hematoma	Traumatic/non-accidental injury
Dysmorphism, neurocutaneous markers	Seizures
Abnormal odor of exhaled breath	Diabetic ketoacidosis, hepatic coma, alcohol intoxication
Bradycardia, hypertension, apnea	Raised intracranial pressure leading to Cushing's triad
High BP	Hypertensive encephalopathy

- *Nervous system examination:* Should be in detail; quick assessment initially for:
    - Signs of brain herniation
    - Focal neurological deficit—proceed to corrective measures.
- *Examination of other systems*—to detect the etiology.

FURTHER INVESTIGATIONS

- CT/MRI brain, after stabilization
- Other imaging studies as indicated
- Cerebrospinal fluid studies (deferred till stable)
- Others (toxicology screening, coagulation profile).

Flowchart 34.1: Algorithm for management of comatose child.

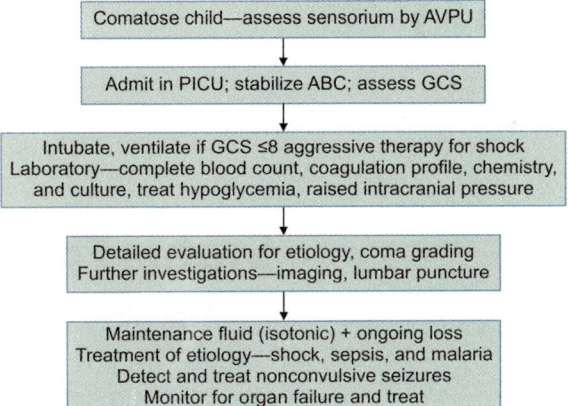

CONTINUING TREATMENT

- Maintenance fluids—2/3 isotonic (NS) + ongoing loss
- Empirical antibiotics for infection (ceftriaxone ± vancomycin)
- Acyclovir if suspected herpes encephalitis (CT, EEG, hemorrhagic CSF)
- Coma care—eyes, back, lungs, bladder, and bowel
- H_2 receptor antagonists to prevent stress ulcers
- Steroids—in meningococcemia with shock, acute disseminated encephalomyelitis, and enteric fever with encephalopathy
- Shock as per guidelines (Chapter 25)
- Seizures—lorazepam 0.1 mg/kg (IV), then fosphenytoin/others
- Raised ICP—Refer Chapter 33
- Dyselectrolytemia and acidosis (Chapter 53)
- Hepatic encephalopathy (Chapter 63)
- Renal failure (Chapter 59)
- Hyperammonemia (Chapter 54)
- Start early enteral feeds.

MONITORING (FLOWCHART 34.1)

- Glasgow Coma Scale, I/O chart, vitals, pupils, and blood glucose 6 hourly.
- Renal function tests daily.
- Others as indicated.

CONCLUSION

Coma in children should be assessed for severity staging and etiology and treated as an emergency.

Chapter 35

Status Epilepticus

Manju George Elenjickal, S Sushamabai

ABSTRACT

Status epilepticus (SE) is a pediatric emergency which may end up in death or neurological deficit. Prompt recognition and systematic management are effective in preventing the adverse outcome. The definition of SE is continuous seizure or recurrent seizure activity without regaining consciousness lasting more than 5 minutes. Etiology, prognostic factors, and stepwise management are discussed here. The first-line drugs for seizure control are IV lorazepam or midazolam; and, the second-line drugs can be IV fosphenytoin followed by IV phenobarbitone or IV sodium valproate or levetiracetam. In refractory status epilepticus aggressive treatment with third-line drugs—midazolam or propofol or thiopental as infusion should be tried under strict monitoring along with mechanical ventilation. Inhalation anesthesia should be tried as the last modality. Supportive management for hypoxia, hypoglycemia, temperature regulation, and fluid and electrolyte management to prevent organ damage with vigilant monitoring are detailed.

INTRODUCTION

Status epilepticus is a common pediatric emergency, which if not treated promptly, may result in death or permanent neuronal damage.

Definition: Continuous seizure activity or recurrent seizure activity without regaining consciousness, lasting more than 5 minutes; a child brought with seizure to hospital also is considered as SE.

COMMON CAUSES (BEYOND NEONATAL PERIOD)

- Febrile status epilepticus
- Metabolic problems—hypoglycemia, hypocalcemia, hypo/hypernatremia, and inborn errors of metabolism
- Intracranial infections—meningitis, encephalitis, and brain abscess
- Drugs (intoxication/missed dose) and poisons
- Intracranial bleeding

- Hypoxic episodes—submersion, anesthesia, and severe respiratory illness
- Head trauma—accidental/battered baby
- Space-occupying lesions—tuberculoma, brain tumors, and neurocysticercosis
- Hypertensive/hepatic/renal encephalopathy
- Deficiency diseases—folinic acid and pyridoxine.

MECHANISM OF STATUS EPILEPTICUS

- Imbalance between excitatory and inhibitory neuronal activity causes seizures.
- Subsequent increased cellular metabolism and reduced cerebral oxygen supply leads to widespread neuronal injury which may end up in death or disability.

CLINICAL PRESENTATION

- Common presentation is convulsive SE presenting as generalized tonic, tonic–clonic or clonic movements, and altered sensorium.
- Nonconvulsive SE has to be suspected in confusional state, behavioral problems, fluctuating impairment of consciousness, hallucinations, and psychotic symptoms; EEG is helpful for diagnosis.

PATIENT APPROACH

- Quick history and clinical examination to establish the diagnosis and assess the severity; the prognostic factors in SE are mentioned in Table 35.1.

Table 35.1: Prognostic factors in status epilepticus (SE).

I. Clinical	Initial compensated SE; convulsions <30 minutes	Late decompensated SE; convulsions >60 minutes
Pulse	Bounding, rapid	Weak, rapid/slow
BP	↑	N/↓
Temp	↑	↓
ICP	↑	↑↑
II. Biochemical		
PaO_2	↓	↓↓
$PaCO_2$	↑	>50 mm Hg
HCO_3	↓	↓↓
Blood glucose	N/↑	↓↓
Serum sodium	N	↓
Serum potassium	N	↑
Blood lactic acid	↑	↑↑

- Admit in PICU. Goals of therapy are—(1) stabilization, (2) seizure control, (3) treatment and prevention of complications, and (4) treatment of etiology.

Stabilization—ABCD (0–10 minutes)
- **A**irway: Keep the patient in midline/left lateral position, oral suction, and airway placement.
- **B**reathing: Provide 100% O_2, intubate and ventilate if needed.
- **C**irculation: Secure two IV/IO access; send blood for complete blood count, sugar, liver function tests, renal function test, serum electrolytes (Na, K, Ca, Mg), and arterial blood gas; save 50 mL of serum and urine samples for future analysis including toxicology; start IV bolus normal saline 20 mL/kg in 1 hour.
- **D**extrose: Assess capillary blood sugar; administer 10% dextrose 2 mL/kg if hypoglycemic (blood glucose <50 mg/dL).

Seizure Control (10–30 minutes)
Under strict monitoring:
- *Early status—First-line drugs: Benzodiazepines (caution—respiratory depression)*
    - IV lorazepam 0.1 mg/kg (maximum 4 mg); may be repeated after 5–10 minutes *or*
    - IV midazolam 0.2 mg/kg (maximum 10 mg); may repeat after 5–10 min; if no IV access—IM, intranasal or buccal midazolam can be given (0.2–0.5 mg/kg) *or*
    - IV diazepam 0.15 mg/kg (maximum 10 mg); may repeat after 5–10 min *or* rectal diazepam 0.2–0.5 mg/kg/dose.

    Add pyridoxine 50 mg IM in infants.
- *Established status—Second-line drugs:*
    - IV fosphenytoin 30 mg/kg in 30 minutes at the rate of 3 mg/kg/min; therapeutic concentration is achieved by 2 hours; maintenance dose 6 mg/kg/day div q 12 hr.
    - If no response, start IV phenobarbital 10 mg/kg at the rate of 10 mg/kg/min (caution—respiratory depression, hypotension especially after benzodiazepines).
    - Other *Second-line drugs* are IV sodium valproate (25 mg/kg in 30 minutes followed by 30–60 mg/kg/24 hr), IV levetiracetam (20–60 mg/kg load followed by 10 mg/kg/dose q 6 hr, maximum dose 80 mg/kg/day, not exceeding 3 g/day) depending on the situation.

Caution: Sodium valproate can cause liver dysfunction, pancreatitis, and bleeding; Levetiracetam side effects are—neuropsychiatric symptoms, albuminuria, and leukopenia.
- *Refractory status epilepticus (RSE)* is considered if seizures persist after the third drug—*Start Third-line drugs*. Monitoring includes EEG at least twice daily at this stage; drugs can be:
  - IV midazolam infusion (0.1 to 0.2 mg/kg bolus followed by 0.05–0.5 mg/kg/hr titrated to effect, increase infusion rate by 2 µg/kg/min to a maximum of 20 mg/hr)
  - IV propofol (1 mg/kg bolus, then 1–15 mg/kg/hr infusion)
  - IV thiopental (5 mg/kg 1st hour, then 1–2 mg/kg/hr).

Caution: Intubation, ventilation, pressor support, and strict monitoring to safeguard against multiorgan dysfunction are needed for the above drugs.

Drug tapering: Patient is seizure-free, burst suppression is observed in EEG for 24 hours.
- Weaning of drugs should be reduced two hourly while on IV infusion.

Other drugs in RSE:
- IV lignocaine—2 mg/kg followed by 2–4 mg/kg/hr
- PO topiramate—5–10 mg/kg loading dose, then same or lower dose div q 12 hr in focal SE (Table 35.2).

Continuing seizures: Inhalation anesthesia—isoflurane is preferable; halothane can increase intracranial pressure (ICP).

Treatment and Prevention of Complications

- Identify and treat medical complications, e.g. antibiotics for infections, mannitol for raised ICP, fluid and electrolyte therapy.
- Intracranial pressure monitoring if possible.
- CT/MRI and cerebrospinal fluid studies once the child becomes stable.
- Plan long-term management.

Treatment of Etiology

In most situations, etiology will be made out by clinical assessment and investigations; treat the cause.

Table 35.2: Algorithm for management of status epilepticus (SE).

Time/Stage	Actions	Outcome
0–10 min Early status	Confirm seizure; stabilize ABC, position, airway, suction, oxygen; RSI, ventilate, IV/IO access, blood samples, IV fluid - NS ± glucose. ↓ **Seizures +** ↓	→ **No seizures** ↓ Send investigations Treat etiology Plan long-term management (Mx)
10–30 min Early SE Start first-line drugs	ICU admission, monitoring, IV lorazepam/IV midazolam + Inj. pyridoxine + supportive measures ↓	→ **No seizures** ↓ Further Mx as above.
30–60 min Established SE Start second-line drugs	**Seizures +** ↓ IV Fosphen **Seizures+** ↓ Add pheno *or* IV valproate *or* IV levetiracetam ↓	→ **No seizures** ↓ Fosphen maintenance dose, investigate, treat as per etiology. ↓ → **No seizures** ↓ Maintenance drugs, investigate, treat as per etiology
Beyond 60 min Failure of second-line drugs—**RSE** Start third-line drugs	**Seizures +** ↓ IV midazolam infusion *or* IV propofol infusion *or* IV thiopentone infusion Intubate, ventilate Supportive measures, monitoring, EEG ↓	→ **No seizures** ↓ Taper drugs 2 hourly once there is burst suppression for 24 hours, investigate, treat as per etiology
	Seizures + ↓ Other drugs – IV lignocaine - Oral topiramate Monitoring ↓ **Seizures +** Inhalation anesthesia	→ **No seizures** ↓ Taper drugs, investigate, treat as per etiology

(ABC, airway, breathing, circulation; NS, normal saline; RSI, rapid sequence intubation; RSE, refractory status epilepticus)

CONCLUSION

Status epilepticus is continuous seizure or recurrent seizure activity lasting for more than 5 minutes, needs early prognostication and stepwise aggressive management with IV anticonvulsants or inhalation anesthesia along with vigilant supportive therapy.

FURTHER READING

1. Abend NS, Huh JW, Helfaer MA, et al. Anticonvulsant medications in the pediatric emergency room and intensive care unit. Pediatr Emerg Care. 2008;24(10):7005-718.
2. Kirmani BF, Crisp ED, Kayani S, et al. Role of intravenous levetiracetam in acute seizure management of children. Pediatr Neurol. 2009;41(1):37-9.

Chapter 36

Encephalitis

Manju George Elenjickal, S Sushamabai

ABSTRACT

Encephalitis is inflammation of the brain parenchyma usually due to viral infections, the most common being herpes simplex, Japanese B, enteroviruses, varicella-zoster and mumps. Usual clinical presentations include fever, headache, altered sensorium, and seizures. Signs of meningeal irritation, focal neurologic deficits, and clinical features of underlying illness will be coexisting. The chapter elaborates the pathogens, clinical presentation, patient approach, differential diagnosis, investigations, and management. Details of supportive therapy and antiviral drug administration are also included.

INTRODUCTION

Encephalitis is the inflammation of the brain parenchyma usually due to infections. Common pathogens are:
- Viral: Herpes simplex virus (HSV), Japanese B (JE), Varicella-zoster virus (VZV), Epstein–Barr virus (EBV), influenza, mumps, enteroviruses, and rabies
- Bacterial: As part of pyogenic or TB meningitis
- Protozoal: Malaria.

CLINICAL PRESENTATION

- Fever (varying grades), headache, altered sensorium (drowsiness, irritability, coma), behavioral changes, and seizures.
- Signs of meningeal irritation, focal neurologic deficits + features of underlying infection (rashes in measles and EBV; parotid swelling in mumps; vesicles in VZV and hand-foot-mouth disease; diarrhea in enterovirus infections; myalgia in influenza) may be present.
- Early grand mal seizures, psychotic episodes, tremors, rigidity, hypo- and hyperreflexia are features of JE.
- Less than 10% do present with serious illness.

PATHOPHYSIOLOGY

- Specific neuronal damage due to direct viral invasion or post-infectious immunological reaction.
- Inflammatory cell infiltration and edema of the brain and subsequent defective neurotransmission.

DIFFERENTIAL DIAGNOSIS

Meningitis (pyogenic, tuberculous meningitis), acute disseminated encephalomyelitis (ADEM), brain abscess, stroke, and intracranial space-occupying lesions (ICSOL).

PATIENT APPROACH

- Suspect encephalitis in a patient with altered sensorium, seizures, and behavioral changes preceded by fever.
- Admit in PICU, stabilize ABC; proceed to intubation and mechanical ventilation if Glasgow Coma Scale less than or equal to 8, getting continuous seizures or having cardiorespiratory compromise; supportive therapy is the main treatment.
- Send blood for complete blood count, smear for malarial parasite (MP), culture, paired serum (on D1 and D14) for viral antibody studies; keep in refrigerator at 4°C and send the serum samples and cerebrospinal fluid (CSF) with appropriate clinical details to the nearest recognized laboratory as notified by the health authorities.
- Cerebrospinal fluid study at the earliest if no contraindication for lumbar puncture; supportive findings for diagnosing encephalitis are—CSF with raised pressure, clear with predominantly mononuclear leukocytosis, elevated proteins and normal sugar; presence of RBCs is supportive of HSV encephalitis.
- Send samples for viral PCR (HSV) or antibody titer as per facility available.
- Electroencephalogram study at the earliest; CT/MRI brain (contrast enhanced) as soon as the child is stable; repeat if needed.
- Other investigations—chest skiagram, tuberculin test, and cultures based on the suspected diagnosis.
- Fluid and electrolyte therapy—correction of dehydration, maintenance fluid two-thirds of daily requirement, ideal fluid being NS with added potassium; assess blood sugar, prevent or treat hypo/hyperglycemia and hyponatremia
- Treatment of brain edema, seizures (Chapters 33 and 35)
- Monitoring, vasopressor therapy if needed
- Adequate nutrition—enteral nutrition should be started as early as possible to prevent stress ulcers and to promote fast recovery.

SPECIFIC THERAPY

- HSV encephalitis—acyclovir 10 mg/kg/dose as infusion 8 hourly for 14 days (21 days in newborns); suspect HSV infection when focal seizures, focal neurologic deficits, behavioral changes, EEG revealing periodic lateralized epileptiform discharges (PLEDs) and CT revealing hypodensity in frontotemporal regions and hyperintensity in mesial temporal lobe in T2 weighted images in MRI.
- Acyclovir is also indicated in VZV encephalitis
- Oseltamivir is advised in influenza virus encephalitis.

CONCLUSION

Encephalitis is inflammation of brain parenchyma due to protean causes; the main line of management is vigilant supportive therapy and antiviral therapy if suspected.

Chapter 37

Acute Bacterial Meningitis

S Sushamabai

ABSTRACT

Bacterial meningitis is a serious infection involving meninges along with brain parenchyma. Death and disability can be prevented by timely diagnosis and updated management. The common bacterial pathogens are *Haemophilus influenzae b, Streptococcus pneumoniae,* and meningococci. Usual type of clinical presentation is the insidious onset with classical symptoms and signs but rarely can present as rapidly progressive form with shock and disseminated intravascular coagulation (DIC). Empirical antibiotics are IV ceftriaxone ± vancomycin ± ampicillin or chloromycetin for 7–21 days. IV dexamethasone for 2 days, first dose 20 minutes prior to antibiotics in children more than 2 months age is recommended to prevent deafness. Details of supportive therapy are also discussed.

INTRODUCTION

Bacterial meningitis is the primary infection of meninges, a serious illness of all age groups, often associated with brain parenchymal involvement. Common bacterial pathogens from 1 month to 12 years age group are:
- *H. influenzae b*, *S. pneumoniae,* and *Neisseria meningitides.*
- *Pseudomonas aeruginosa, Staphylococcus aureus,* coagulase-negative Staphylococci, *Salmonella,* and *Listeria monocytogenes* in immunocompromised persons.

PATHOPHYSIOLOGY

- Bacterial infection produces vascular inflammation and occlusion resulting in cerebral infarction, brain edema and raised intracranial pressure (ICP).

CLINICAL PRESENTATION

Usual—Insidious Onset

- Fever of varying durations with nonspecific symptoms like irritability, lethargy, poor feeding, vomiting, and body ache.
- Photophobia, altered sensorium of varying degrees, seizures, and paralysis are more specific symptoms of brain affection.
- Neck stiffness and Kernig's and Brudzinski's signs are the specific signs of meningeal irritation but may not be elicitable in infants less than 1 year age and in those with severe malnutrition.
- Bulging fontanel (<1 yr age), 3rd and 6th nerve palsy (revealed by anisocoria, ptosis, medial squint), facial palsy, and focal motor deficits (hemiplegia, monoplegia) of varying extents are usual.
- Signs of raised ICP (Chapter 33) and brain herniation should be looked for in all patients for immediate life-saving intervention.
- Papilledema is a late sign in older children, often indicates complications like brain abscess; it is not seen in young infants with open fontanel.
- Respiratory and gastrointestinal symptoms unrelated to the nervous system complaints often coexist.

Rare Presentation

Sudden rapidly progressive form with shock and DIC.

DIFFERENTIAL DIAGNOSIS

Viral encephalitis, TB meningitis, cerebral malaria, leptospirosis, subarachnoid hemorrhage, rickettsial disease, Kawasaki disease, juvenile idiopathic arthritis, enteric fever, malignancies of the brain, and dural sinus thrombosis.

APPROACH

- Suspect bacterial meningitis in any child having fever without focus and in all critically ill children.
- Admit in pediatric intensive care unit, stabilize Airway, Breathing, Circulation, Dextrose (ABCD).
- Send blood for complete blood count, peripheral smear for malaria and card test, culture, serum electrolytes, renal function test, liver function test, and blood lactate.
- Lumbar puncture and cerebrospinal fluid studies after stabilization (Chapter 116).
- Cerebrospinal fluid findings in bacterial meningitis are high pressure, turbid appearance, polymorphonuclear leukocytosis, raised protein, low sugar (<50% of the blood sugar collected simultaneously), and presence of bacteria in Gram stain.

- Isolation of bacteria in culture may be negative in those with prior antibiotic therapy.
- In partially treated bacterial meningitis, CSF may reveal mononuclear leukocytosis and normal glucose level.
- Investigations to rule out the differential diagnosis, coexisting infections, and complications are CXR, urine and blood culture, tuberculin test, MRI brain, and others as per clinical situation.
- *Start empirical antibiotic therapy*—after sending specimens for culture:
    - IV ceftriaxone 100 mg/kg/24 hr as single dose or as div q 12 hr *or*
    - IV cefotaxime 300 mg/kg/24 hr div q 6 hr ±
    - IV vancomycin 15 mg/kg/dose q 6 hr if 3rd-generation cephalosporin resistance is suspected.
    - Add IV ampicillin 200 mg/kg/day div q 6 hr if *Listeria monocytogenes* infection is suspected.
    - In patients allergic to cephalosporins, option is IV chloromycetin 100 mg/kg/day div q 6 hr.
    - Change the antibiotics as per culture reports and clinical response.
- *Supportive therapy:*
    - Fluid and electrolyte balance: Correction of dehydration/shock as per guidelines; isotonic maintenance fluid (NS) is advised at least for 24 hours after the child becomes hemodynamically stable.
    - Anticerebral edema measures (Chapter 33)—mannitol ± furosemide for 2 days if evidence of raised ICP; intubation and ventilation, if needed.
    - Seizure control (Chapter 35); ideal drug is fosphenytoin.
- *Steroid therapy:*
    - IV dexamethasone 0.15 mg/kg/dose × q 6 hr × 2 days in children more than 1 month age to prevent deafness; give first dose 20 minutes prior to the first dose of antibiotics (caution—dexamethasone may decrease the CSF penetration of vancomycin; addition of rifampicin to ceftriaxone + vancomycin is advised recently).

Duration of Antibiotic Therapy

- Meningococci—5–7 days; *H. influenzae b*—7–10 days; Pneumococci—10–14 days; Gram-negative bacterial infections or in complicated cases 21 days.
- Provide chemoprophylaxis for close contacts and vaccination for the patient after recovery.
- Follow-up is advised to detect sequelae including hearing defect.

CONCLUSION

Bacterial meningitis is serious infection of the brain parenchyma and meninges and requiring intensive antibacterial and supportive therapy along with short-term dexamethasone.

Chapter 38

Tuberculous Meningitis

S Sushamabai

ABSTRACT

Tuberculous meningitis (TBM) is an invariably fatal disease; death can be prevented by timely and proper treatment. Clinical presentation can be stage I (nonspecific symptoms and signs), stage II (stage of meningeal irritation), and stage III (stage of focal neurologic signs). The gold standard for diagnosis is cerebrospinal fluid (CSF) studies to demonstrate acid-fast bacilli (AFB) and culture retrieval of the organism. The specific therapy [as per Revised National Tuberculosis Control Program (RNTCP)] is streptomycin (2 months), isoniazid (9 months), rifampicin (9 months), and pyrazinamide (2 months) along with corticosteroid for the initial 2 months. Supportive measures for fluid and electrolyte maintenance, seizures, brain edema, raised intracranial pressure (ICP), and early rehabilitation are the other modalities of treatment.

INTRODUCTION

Tuberculous meningitis is the most dreaded form of tuberculosis disease, invariably ending in death unless early and proper treatment is provided. Since the illness is an important differential diagnosis of bacterial meningitis, clinical manifestations, differential diagnosis, investigations, and patient approach are similar.

CLINICAL STAGING

Stage I: Stage of nonspecific symptoms and signs—fever, headache, vomiting, general weakness, and cough. History of TB contact, recurrent or chronic cough, wheeze, presence of lymphadenopathy, hepatosplenomegaly, and pneumonia, etc. are supportive evidences for TB. High index of suspicion is needed for meningitis detection at this stage. Complete recovery is possible if treatment is given in stage I.

Stage II: Stage of meningeal irritation—typical clinical signs are present. Consider TBM as a differential diagnosis in all children with features of meningitis or encephalitis. Treatment at this stage though reduces mortality, morbidity is usual.

Stage III: Stage of focal neurologic deficits—features are varying degrees of coma, paralysis (multiple cranial nerve palsies of 2, 6, 7, early papilledema, monoplegia, and hemiplegia), decerebrate posturing, and early hydrocephalus. High mortality is usual; recovery will be associated with paralysis, deafness, blindness, seizures, and hydrocephalus.

Unusual presentations: Can be fever without focus, encephalopathy, radiculopathy, spinal paraplegia, and movement disorders.

Note: Patient approach is as in bacterial meningitis as initial stabilization, detailed history, physical examination, investigations.

CSF FINDINGS IN TB MENINGITIS

- Cerebrospinal fluid pressure is raised, fluid reveals ground glass appearance; cobweb formation may be observed if the CSF is kept undisturbed for 30 minutes.
- Total cell count ranges from 10/cmm to 500/cmm, with lymphocytic predominance.
- Protein content is high (400–5,000 mg/dL) with reduced glucose less than 40 mg/dL but never less than 20 mg/dL. CSF findings may be difficult to differentiate from viral meningitis and partially treated bacterial meningitis.
- TB polymerase chain reaction and AFB staining for bacilli, if positive, are helpful for confirmation of diagnosis.

Note: CSF obtained from ventricular tap may be normal.

RADIOLOGY

- Chest skiagram in 50% of patients with TBM may be normal.
- CT/MRI brain—can be normal in early stages; late stage findings are brain edema, early hydrocephalus, basilar enhancement, and focal ischemia.

Others

- Tuberculin skin test—found to be negative in 50% cases.
- Biopsy study of enlarged lymph nodes or granulomas helpful for diagnosis.
- Gene Xpert study from gastric lavage or induced sputum is fruitful only in those having intrathoracic TB.

SPECIFIC TREATMENT

As per revised national tuberculosis control program (RNTCP)- 2 SHREZ* +7 HRE

*IM streptomycin 20 mg/kg/day (superior to ethambutol 20 mg/kg/day) × 2 months
*Isoniazid 10 mg/kg/day OD × 9–12 months PO
*Rifampicin 15 mg/kg/day OD × 9–12 months PO
*Pyrazinamide 25 mg/kg/day OD × 2 months PO

Note: In HIV-infected children, therapy should be continued for the maximum period. If drug resistance is suspected, the best possible drug combination should be selected.

Corticosteroids

Prednisolone 1–2 mg/kg/day (equivalent dose of inj. dexamethasone preferred in very sick children) for 4–6 weeks followed by tapering in 4–6 weeks is effective in reducing inflammation and sequelae.

Other Supportive Measures

- Treatment of cerebral edema—IV mannitol and oral glycerin (Chapter 33)
- Seizure control (Chapter 35)
- Fever control
- Fluid and electrolyte balance
- Nutrition—early enteral feeding
- Physiotherapy
- Shunt surgery for hydrocephalus.

CONCLUSION

Tuberculous meningitis is a fatal disease and should be diagnosed at the early stage and specific treatment based on RNTCP should be implemented.

Chapter **39**

Guillain–Barré Syndrome

Manju George Elenjickal, S Sushamabai

ABSTRACT

Guillain–Barré syndrome *(GBS)* is the condition of acute flaccid paralysis (AFP) due to demyelinating neuropathy. The illness follows certain viral infections and vaccinations. The main clinical feature is rapidly progressing ascending paralysis (hypotonia and areflexia), the legs being more affected. Lower cranial nerve involvement in the form of bulbar palsy and facial weakness can occur and herald diaphragm paralysis and the need for mechanical ventilation. Sensory and autonomic manifestations are common. The most important differential diagnosis is paralytic poliomyelitis and hence AFP reporting is needed. The diagnosis is confirmed by cerebrospinal fluid (CSF) studies revealing albuminocytological dissociation, decreased nerve conduction velocity and magnetic resonance imaging (MRI) with gadolinium enhancement. Specific therapies are intravenous immunoglobulin (IVIG), intravenous (IV) methyl prednisolone or plasmapheresis in resistant cases. Mechanical ventilation is to be considered in respiratory paralysis. Good nutrition and early physiotherapy will speed up the recovery.

INTRODUCTION

Guillain–Barré syndrome (GBS) is the condition of acute flaccid paralysis *(AFP)* due to postinfectious polyneuropathy of autoimmune nature.

CLINICAL FEATURES

- Progressive symmetrical flaccid weakness of limbs, evolving over hours to days, legs being more affected.
- Lower cranial nerves are often affected; facial or bulbar palsy in the first week of illness herald the need for mechanical ventilation.
- Hypo- or areflexia.
- Mild sensory symptoms—tingling of limbs, pain in the neck, shoulder, back and spine are common.
- Autonomic involvement include: BP fluctuation, postural hypotension, cardiac dysrhythmias and pain of affected limbs.
- Transient bladder dysfunction may occur.

- Paralysis can be rarely of descending type "Miller–Fisher syndrome" presenting as acute external ophthalmoplegia, ataxia and areflexia.
- High fever, severe bladder involvement and altered sensorium are clinical features indicating search for other causes of flaccid paralysis.

PATHOGENESIS

- Demyelinating neuropathy of autoimmune nature.
- Follows certain viral and bacterial infections (*Campylobacter*, *Helicobacter* more common).
- Can be postvaccination.

DIFFERENTIAL DIAGNOSIS

Other Causes of Acute Flaccid Paralysis

- Postdiphtheritic paralysis
- Hypokalemia, hypophosphatemia
- Organophosphate poisoning
- Myasthenia gravis
- Traumatic acute cord compression
- Paralytic poliomyelitis
- Acute transverse myelitis
- Epidural abscess
- Drug induced—vincristine
- Dermatomyositis

Acute flaccid paralysis is sudden onset of weakness or flaccid paralysis anywhere in the body within the past 6 months in a child less than 15 years of age or a person of any age in whom polio is suspected.

PATIENT APPROACH

Suspect Guillain–Barré syndrome in any child with:
- Limping, sudden onset of inability to walk or sit up.
- Increasing general weakness following diarrhea or fever or acute respiratory infection when recovery is expected.
- Admit in pediatric intensive care unit (PICU).
- Quick assessment of vitals, sensorium, respiratory status for shallow breathing, cranial nerve paralysis as squint, pupillary abnormalities, pooling of secretions, facial palsy, deltoid weakness or diaphragm paralysis (detected by paradoxical respiratory movements and feeble voice). Assess vitals for brady- or tachycardia hypo- or hypertension.
- Stabilize airway, breathing and circulation (ABC), arrange for intubation and mechanical ventilation if the patient has facial palsy, feeble voice,

pooling of secretions, poor respiratory effort or evidence of diaphragm paralysis.

INVESTIGATIONS

- Cerebrospinal fluid studies—to detect albuminocytological dissociation characterized by:
  - Cerebrospinal fluid proteins more than twice the upper limit of normal with CSF cell count less than 10 WBC/mm^3.
- Magnetic resonance imaging of spinal cord—thickening of the cauda equina and intrathecal nerve roots with gadolinium enhancement.
- Nerve conduction studies—reveal low velocity.
- Electromyography study—evidence of muscle denervation.
- Antiganglioside antibodies—ganglioside-monosialic acid (GM1), ganglioside-disialic acid (GD1) will be elevated.
- Creatine phosphokinase (CPK)—normal or mild elevation.
- Serologic tests for Campylobacter jejuni and Helicobacter pylori though reveal the etiology, will not alter the treatment.

All children with suspected GBS should be reported to the AFP surveillance program. Two stool samples (24 hours apart) should be sent for viral studies so as to exclude the possibility of paralytic poliomyelitis.

TREATMENT

Specific

- Intravenous immunoglobulin 400 mg/kg/day × 5 days—in rapidly progressing type; should be started at the earliest to have best effect.
- Intravenous methylprednisolone 30 mg/kg/day × 3–5 days; taper with oral steroids in 2 weeks; effective in mild types only.
- Plasmapheresis in resistant cases.

Supportive

- Ventilatory support
- Fluid and electrolyte therapy in the acute stage
- Early enteral nutrition
- Physiotherapy.

CONCLUSION

Guillain–Barré syndrome is acute flaccid paralysis due to demyelinating neuropathy; simulates paralytic poliomyelitis; and can be diagnosed by CSF studies and treated with drugs or plasmapheresis.

Chapter 40

Acute Disseminated Encephalomyelitis

S Sushamabai

ABSTRACT

Acute disseminated encephalomyelitis *(ADEM)* is the condition of multifocal neurological deficits with encephalopathy. The etiopathogenesis is postinfectious (viral mainly) demyelination. Clinical presentation can be abrupt with rapid progression or slow insidious with seizures, paralysis, multiple cranial nerve palsy and cerebellitis. The gold standard for diagnosis is MRI scan. The specific drugs are methyl prednisolone and intravenous immunoglobulin (IVIG) and plasmapheresis in resistant cases. Supportive therapy is equally important. Empirical antibiotic and antiviral therapy should be continued till the diagnosis is confirmed and the possibility of bacterial and viral infections are excluded.

INTRODUCTION

Acute disseminated (demyelinating) encephalomyelitis *(ADEM)* is an initial inflammatory demyelinating event with multifocal neurologic deficits always accompanied by encephalopathy.

ETIOPATHOGENESIS

- Infection or vaccination triggers CNS autoantigen production due to molecular mimicry resulting in demyelination throughout the brain and spinal cord.
- Common preceding infections are mainly viral—herpes simplex, varicella, influenza, Epstein-Barr, enteroviruses, measles, mumps and rubella and also *Mycoplasma pneumoniae*.
- All vaccines—including oral polio can cause demyelination.

CLINICAL PRESENTATION

- *It can be of two types:*
  - *Abrupt onset* and rapid progression.
  - *Slow onset* with slow or rapid progression.

- Fever, headache, vomiting and altered sensorium of varying grades, behavioral problems, seizures including status epilepticus, meningeal signs.
- Encephalopathy is the hallmark of the illness ranging from confusion to deep coma and seizures.
- Focal neurological deficits—visual loss, multiple cranial nerve palsies, ataxia, varying grades of motor deficits.
- Sensory deficits, bowel and bladder dysfunction.

DIFFERENTIAL DIAGNOSIS

Brainstem or cerebellar tumors, acute cerebellar ataxia, drug overdose or poisoning, multiple sclerosis, autoimmune encephalitis, vasculitis, rheumatological disorders, tuberculous (TB) meningitis.

PATIENT APPROACH

- Admit in pediatric intensive care unit (PICU), stabilize airway, breathing and circulation (ABC).
- Control of seizures (Chapter 35).
- Treatment of coma (Chapter 34) if present.
- Simultaneous investigations—complete blood count (CBC), peripheral smear for malarial parasite (MP), serum electrolytes, renal function test (RFT), liver function test (LFT), coagulation profile.
- Cerebrospinal fluid studies to rule out CNS infections—findings suggestive of ADEM are—clear appearance, pleocytosis with lymphocytic or mononuclear predominance, moderate increase in proteins and normal sugar; additionally CSF studies for viral agents, TB, and anti-N-methyl D-aspartate receptors (NMDAR) antibodies should be considered in all such children.
- In the severe form of acute hemorrhagic leukoencephalopathy (Hurst disease) CSF will reveal polymorphonuclear leukocytosis.
- Electroencephalography (EEG) may reveal generalized or focal slowing or epileptiform discharges.
- Magnetic resonance imaging (MRI) brain is the gold standard for diagnosis—features are multifocal large lesions with variable enhancement in T2-weighted images involving white and gray matters throughout brain and spinal cord; in severe forms edema and mass effect will be observed.
- Anti-NMD antibodies may be present in a minority.

SPECIFIC TREATMENT

- Intravenous methylprednisolone 30 mg/kg/day for 3–5 days followed by oral prednisolone for 1 month in tapering dose.
- Intravenous immunoglobulin 2 g/kg administered in 2–5 days if no response to steroids.
- Plasmapheresis (5–7 exchanges on alternate days) in resistant cases.
- In severe disease rituximab or cyclophosphamide are advised.
- Empirical antibiotic and antiviral therapy should be given till the possibility of bacterial or viral meningoencephalitis is excluded by specific lab studies.

SUPPORTIVE MEASURES

- Fluid and electrolyte balance if comatose or critically ill.
- Early enteral feeds.
- Physiotherapy.

FOLLOW-UP

- Majority reveal complete recovery.
- Recurrent episodes can occur in a minority—such episodes may herald multiple sclerosis.
- Recurrences are treated similarly as the first episode.

CONCLUSION

Acute disseminated encephalomyelitis is post-infectious neuropathy with multifocal deficits, diagnostic confirmation is by MRI and the treatment options are methylprednisolone, IVIG, and plasmapheresis.

Chapter 41

Myasthenic Paralysis

Manju George Elenjickal, S Sushamabai

ABSTRACT

Myasthenic paralysis is progressive flaccid weakness of cranial nerve muscles. The pathogenesis is reduced number of acetylcholine receptors and can manifest as neonatal and juvenile forms. Organophosphorus poisoning, snake envenomation, tick paralysis, and botulism are important differential diagnosis. Neostigmine and edrophonium tests are confirmatory. Drug therapy includes neostigmine and pyridostigmine mainly. Myasthenic crisis is also described.

INTRODUCTION

Myasthenic paralysis is characterized by progressive fatigability of striated muscle mainly extraocular and palpebral muscles and those of swallowing striated muscles.

PATHOGENESIS

There is decreased number of acetylcholine (ACh) receptors due to:
- Congenital or familial defect.
- Circulating ACh receptor binding antibodies:
    - The result is neuromuscular blockade at the myoneural junction.

CLINICAL PRESENTATION

- Neonatal:
    - Congenital (usually familial).
    - Transient (transplacental passage of maternal antibodies).
    - The clinical presentation in the neonate can be hypotonia, apnea, dysphagia (manifested as sucking and swallowing difficulty), hyporeflexia and stridor.
- Juvenile:
    - Autoimmune (more common).

- Familial (due to deficiency of ACh receptors).
- Features are progressive ptosis, diplopia, dysphagia, facial weakness, rapid and easy fatigue as the day progresses; the weakness involves muscles innervated by multiple cranial nerves of the brainstem. Progressive weakness involving the limb girdle and distal muscles can occur.

DIFFERENTIAL DIAGNOSIS

- Organophosphate poisoning (Chapter 93-A), excluded by acute onset of symptoms and history of poison ingestion.
- Botulism—especially from honey ingestion, characterized by acute onset of diarrhea, vomiting, cranial nerve palsy and progressive symmetric flaccid paralysis.
- Snake envenomation—mainly krait bite. History of (h/o) snakebite or presence of bite marks is the clue (Chapter 94-A).
- Tick paralysis—acute paralysis of cranial nerves with Guillain–Barré syndrome (GBS) like weakness and respiratory paralysis. Diagnosis is by identifying the tick (usually over the scalp). Treatment is removal of the entire tick and supportive measures.

Note: In all these conditions, paralysis is of acute onset in an otherwise healthy child.

INVESTIGATIONS

- Electromyography (EMG) is diagnostic, but difficult to record in young children. The diagnostic findings are progressively decreasing muscle potentials on repetitive nerve stimulation. The affected muscle should be selected for the test.
- Motor nerve conduction (MNC) studies—reveal normal recording.
- Acetylcholine receptor (AChR) antibodies—can be retrieved in autoimmune disorder but will be negative in familial forms of reduced synthesis of acetylcholine or receptor deficiency.
- Antibodies against muscle-specific tyrosine kinase (MuSK) receptor in children negative for AChR antibodies should be assessed.
- Other tests—antinuclear antibody (ANA), thyroid function studies, creatine-kinase, electrocardiography (ECG), chest skiagram or computed tomography (CT), choline esterase inhibitor diagnostic tests. These investigations are important to exclude associated diseases.
- Muscle biopsy is having a limited role in diagnosing myasthenic disease.

CONFIRMATORY TESTS

Neostigmine test: For children less than 2 years age, should be done in pediatric intensive care unit (PICU) setting as detailed below:
- Start intravenous (IV) infusion for rapid administration of medicines if any adverse event following neostigmine occurs.
- Electrocardiogram monitoring is a must during the test to detect cardiac arrhythmias.
- Atropine sulfate 0.01 mg/kg for IV immediate administration should be kept ready to block the muscarinic effects.
- Administer neostigmine as IM 0.04 mg/kg; improvement in strength of fatigued muscles is observed within 20–40 minutes. If the result is negative or equivocal, one more dose can be repeated 4 hours after the first dose.

Edrophonium test for children more than 2 years age:
- Prerequisites are as for neostigmine test (PICU, IV infusion, ECG monitoring, IV atropine).
- Intravenous edrophonium chloride (Tensilon)—test dose of 0.01 mg/kg is given first to assess the drug tolerability. If well tolerated diagnostic dose of 0.01 mg–0.02 mg/kg is given IV every 30–45 seconds to the maximum tolerated dose of 0.1 mg/kg for children less than 30 kg to 0.2 mg/kg for those more than 30 kg. Improvement in ptosis (measured as distance between the upper and lower eyelids before and after administration of the drug), disappearance of diplopia and ability to swallow are observed from 10 seconds to 120 seconds after drug administration.
- Drug side effects are nausea, vomiting, light headedness and bradycardia.

TREATMENT

- Mild myasthenia—no treatment is needed.
- Severe forms—neostigmine methylsulfate IM (0.04 mg/kg/dose) q 4–6 hour till improvement followed by oral neostigmine bromide 0.4 mg/kg/dose q 4–6 hourly or pyridostigmine 1.6 mg/kg/dose q 6 hour.

Other Therapies

- Long-term steroids
- Thymectomy
- Intravenous immunoglobulin
- Plasmapheresis
- Rituximab (in refractory cases).

Prevention of acute paralysis is to be considered in a patient already on treatment by avoiding neurotoxic drugs like succinylcholine, pancuronium and aminoglycosides.

Myasthenic crisis is an acute or subacute severe increase in weakness in patients with myasthenia gravis, usually precipitated by infection, surgery or stress. Treatment should be intensive with IV choline esterase inhibitors, IVIG, plasma exchange, gavage feeding and occasionally mechanical ventilation. It has to be differentiated from *cholinergic crisis* due to overdose of anticholinesterase medications. The differentiating features in cholinergic crisis are the presence of muscarinic effects like abdominal cramps, diarrhea, salivation, sweating and bradycardia along with increased weakness and miosis. Treatment is temporary stopping of drugs and supportive care till recovery.

CONCLUSION

Myasthenic paralysis is progressive flaccid paralysis occasionally encountered in children with appropriate investigations and definite therapy.

Chapter 42

Subdural Empyema

S Sushamabai

ABSTRACT

Subdural empyema is a complication of pyogenic meningitis in infants, can follow sinusitis in adolescents. This complication should be suspected in babies on treatment for meningitis with persistent fever with or without vomiting and seizures. The signs are increasing head circumference, bulging fontanel, sutural separation and focal neurologic deficits. The diagnostic confirmation is by magnetic resonance imaging (MRI) brain with gadolinium. Subdural tap and the fluid study are detailed. Treatment is combination antibiotic therapy for 3 weeks and removal of subdural pus.

INTRODUCTION

Subdural empyema *(SDE)* is the collection of pus in the subdural space over the cranium. It is a complication of pyogenic meningitis in infants usually following *Haemophilus influenzae* type b infection.

CLINICAL FEATURES

- Suspect SDE if the patient has persistent fever ± vomiting or seizures in spite of adequate antibiotic therapy for pyogenic meningitis.
- The signs are increasing head circumference, bulging fontanels and sutural separation.
- Increased transillumination of the cranium is a diagnostic sign.

DIAGNOSTIC INVESTIGATIONS

- Cerebrospinal fluid (CSF) studies to diagnose clearance or persistence of meningitis in infants (should be avoided in older children—can cause brain herniation).
- Magnetic resonance imaging (MRI) head with gadolinium administration is confirmative to detect pus in the subdural space.

DIFFERENTIAL DIAGNOSIS

- Brain abscess
- Subdural hematoma
- Superior sagittal sinus thrombosis.

TREATMENT

- Antibiotic therapy for meningitis, empirical as combination of ceftriaxone + vancomycin + metronidazole or as per culture report × 3 weeks.
- Aspiration of subdural fluid (SD tap).

Subdural Fluid Tap

Indications—in an infant while on treatment for meningitis:
- Features of raised intracranial pressure (ICP)
- Impaired sensorium
- Persistent fever or seizures
- Focal neurologic deficit
- To differentiate between effusion and hematoma.

PROCEDURE

- Obtain informed consent.
- Preparation—shave the head, clean the area [anterior fontanel (AF) and scalp around].
- Keep the baby in supine position; bring the head near the table edge and keep it slightly extended; site for tap is 2.5 cm lateral to the midpoint of AF.
- An assistant should restrain the baby firmly.
- Clean and drape the skin over the site, administer local anesthetic.
- Insert a 20/21-gauge (G) lumbar puncture (LP) needle 90° to the skin and slowly advance the needle with a "Z"-like movement up to 1–1.5 cm deep till a sudden popping sensation is obtained while the dura is pierced.
- Tapping should be bilateral.
- Remove the stylet and collect 15–20 mL subdural fluid from both sides.
- Send for analysis (cell count, culture, biochemistry) immediately.
- Seal the punctured area, apply gentle firm pressure over the puncture site for 5 minutes, keep the child head elevated with a pillow or in sitting position for 1 hour.

- Diagnostic features of subdural empyema are—elevated pressure, proteins and cell count [polymorphonuclear cell (PMN) predominance] and presence of bacteria on Gram staining; culture may be positive.

CONCLUSION

Subdural empyema is an occasional complication of pyogenic meningitis in infants and can be confirmed by MRI scan and should be treated with aspiration and antibiotics.

Chapter **43**

Acute Stroke in Children

Manju George Elenjickal, S Sushamabai

ABSTRACT

Acute stroke is sudden unexpected impairment of blood supply to the brain leading to derangement of brain function. Clinical manifestations of acute stroke are often subtle in children leading to late diagnosis and improper treatment culminating in more adverse outcome as compared to adults. Since the pediatrician is the first to be consulted in this situation, a basic knowledge regarding the diagnosis and management of stroke in children is mandatory. The chapter deals with the classification, clinical presentation, predisposing factors, differential diagnosis, investigations and management. Medical management is early neuroprotective therapy and treatment of predisposing factors and underlying etiology followed by rehabilitation.

INTRODUCTION

Stroke is sudden unexpected episode of disordered blood supply to the brain resulting in brain dysfunction. It is a neurologic emergency and is an important cause of acquired brain injury in newborns and children. Pediatric stroke differs from adults because of the:
- Subtle and vague clinical presentation causing delay in diagnosis.
- Diverse etiology requiring extensive investigations.
- Subsequent worsened outcome.

Early diagnosis and specific treatment can reduce the adverse neurologic outcome.

CLASSIFICATION

- Arterial ischemic stroke (AIS)
- Cerebral sinovenous thrombosis (CSVT)
- Hemorrhagic stroke (HS).

CLINICAL PRESENTATION

It can be from *subtle* features to *apoplectiform* onset:
- *Subtle* is the usual mode of presentation in CSVT and AIS, features being:
  - Altered sensorium, seizures and focal neurologic deficits as hemiplegia, cranial nerve palsy and diplopia—isolated or in combination.
  - Diffuse neurologic signs like headache and papilledema.
- *Apoplectiform* onset is characteristic of HS—presents as instantaneous or *thunderclap* headache, loss of consciousness and nuchal rigidity along with the other features observed in subtle form.

PREDISPOSING FACTORS

- Hypoxic-ischemic encephalopathy—mainly in newborns.
- Infections of the brain—bacterial, viral.
- Dehydration—diarrhea, sepsis, diabetic ketoacidosis (DKA).
- Head trauma
- Cardiac—cyanotic and acyanotic congenital heart defect (CHD), arrhythmias, postintervention phase problem.
- Vasculitis syndromes
- Nephrotic syndrome
- Coagulopathies (congenital and acquired)
- Dyslipidemias
- Hematologic—sickle cell anemia, thrombotic disorders (inherited, drug induced), hematological malignancies (leukemia or lymphoma).
- Arterial and venous malformations of the brain.

DIFFERENTIAL DIAGNOSIS

- Migraine
- Seizures
- Brain tumors
- Hypertension
- Infections—meningitis, encephalitis
- Acute demyelination
- Hyperglycemia
- Bleeding disorders
- Inborn errors of metabolism.

PATIENT APPROACH

Detailed History and Physical Examination

- Have an index of suspicion of stroke in any child brought with altered sensorium, seizures and focal neurologic deficits, headache, speech and vision problems.
- Admit in pediatric intensive care unit (PICU); airway, breathing and circulation (ABC) stabilization as per situation, rapid sequence intubation (RSI) and ventilation if cardiorespiratory compromise or refractory shock.
- Investigations after stabilization:
  - Computed tomography or diffusion weighted magnetic resonance imaging (MRI), magnetic resonance (MR) angiography as per clinical diagnosis.
  - Computed tomography may be initially negative in 50% of cases; repeat evaluation may be needed if stroke is strongly suspected; CT venography or MR venography is needed to diagnose CSVT; in neonatal stroke, cranial USG is ideal; CSF studies to rule out subarachnoid hemorrhage or meningitis.
- Hematological studies—complete blood count (CBC), peripheral smear, coagulation profile, serum electrolytes (SE), renal function test (RFT), liver function test (LFT), lipid profile and special investigations.
- Electrocardiogram and echocardiogram for all children suspected of AIS.
- Emergency neurosurgical intervention.

Neuroprotective Therapy

- *It should be implemented while waiting for the neurosurgical intervention:*
  - Aggressive therapy of infection (sepsis, meningitis, mastoiditis).
  - Correction of dehydration; for maintenance fluid therapy, use isotonic fluid ideally normal saline (NS) to maintain serum sodium (S. Na) 145–150 mEq/L.
  - Control of blood glucose.
  - Control of seizures—early administration of fosphenytoin (Chapter 35).
  - Control of fever
  - Maintenance of normal BP
  - Regular fundus examination to assess optic neuropathy
  - Treatment of raised intracranial pressure (ICP) (Chapter 33).
- Treatment of predisposing factors or etiology:
  - Antibiotics for infection.
  - Corticosteroids or immunosuppressive therapy in vasculitis.
  - Anticoagulation with heparin in cardiogenic causes.

- Antiplatelet therapy in vasculitis (Chapter 87).
    - Blood transfusion for sickle cell anemia.
- Follow-up and rehabilitation therapy.

CONCLUSION

Acute stroke is not uncommon in children, but diagnosis is often delayed and early neuroprotective therapy provides better outcome.

Chapter 44

Intracranial Hemorrhage

S Sushamabai

ABSTRACT

Intracranial hemorrhage (ICH) is the collection of blood inside the cranial cavity. Though a neurosurgical emergency, patients initially report to the general pediatrician so that initial stabilization, diagnostic work up and timely neurosurgical reference are the duty of the attending pediatrician. Initial quick assessment, ABC stabilization including mechanical ventilation and intravenous (IV) access, computed tomography (CT) brain after stabilization are the priorities. ICH can be traumatic or nontraumatic. The bleeding can be intracerebral or extracerebral, accidental or nonaccidental. Immediate treatment for traumatic brain injury is neuroprotective medical therapy till surgical intervention is highlighted. Management of nontraumatic ICH includes therapy for the precipitating cause additionally.

INTRODUCTION

Intracranial hemorrhage indicates bleeding inside the cranial cavity which may be traumatic or nontraumatic.

CLASSIFICATION

Within the Brain

- Intraparenchymal
- Intraventricular.

Outside the Brain

- Epidural (Fig. 44.1)
- Subdural (Fig. 44.2)
- Subarachnoid.

Note: Epidural and subdural hemorrhages are usually post-traumatic.

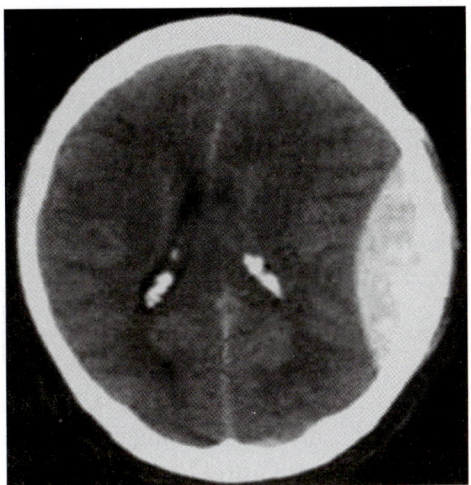

Fig. 44.1: Epidural hemorrhage.

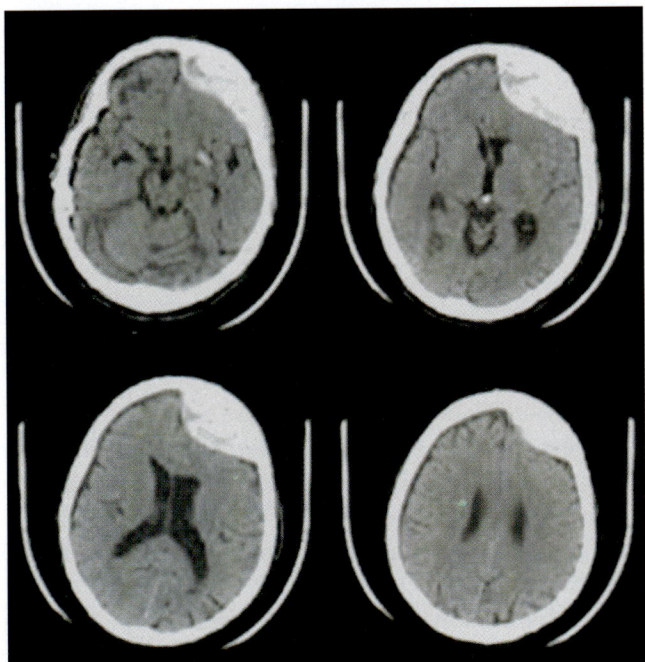

Fig. 44.2: Subdural hemorrhage.

PATHOPHYSIOLOGY

- Cranial vault is a rigid structure. Intracranial blood collection of any type and quantity will be at the expense of compression of brain.
- The problems encountered in ICH are raised intracranial pressure (ICP), those subsequent to the quantity and rapidity of bleeding and the basic cause of ICH.
- The clinical presentation will depend on all these factors.

ETIOLOGY

- Spontaneous:
  - Vessel wall defects [arteriovenous (AV) malformations are the most common followed by aneurysms, angiomas, vasculitis, neoplastic lesions with unstable vasculature].
  - Hemorrhagic disorders [hemophilia, immune thrombocytopenic purpura (ITP), leukemia, hemolytic uremic syndrome (HUS), infections, hepatic or renal failure, vitamin K deficiency, disseminated intravascular coagulation (DIC), drug-induced].
  - Systemic hypertension.
- Traumatic brain injury (TBI):
  - Accidental—traffic, blasts, falls, drowning, hit.
  - Nonaccidental—assaults, child abuse, battered child.

CLINICAL PRESENTATION

- Irritability (infants), headache, vomiting, altered sensorium of varying grades.
- Seizures.
- Focal neurologic deficits—hemiplegia, monoplegia, cranial nerve palsy.
- Features of the inciting event.
- The symptoms and signs will be immediate mostly.
- Initial alertness followed by gradual deterioration can occur in epidural hematoma and diffuse brain swelling. Hence lack of symptoms does not exclude ICH.
- Coma can be severe [Glasgow Coma Scale (GCS 3-8), moderate (GCS 9-12) and mild (GCS 13-14).
- Signs of brain herniation and raised ICP—anisocoria, Cushing triad, 6th nerve palsy, down and out position of the eye globe, ptosis, papilledema, if present, prognosis is grave.

PATIENT APPROACH

- Quick history, assessment, intensive care unit (ICU) admission, ABC stabilization.

- History may not be fruitful; may be misleading in child abuse.
- While being stabilized proceed for investigations:
  - Complete blood count, peripheral smear, coagulation profile, renal function test (RFT), liver function test (LFT), serum electrolytes (SE), blood glucose (BG), blood gas, others in relation to the history and etiology.
- Cranial CT after stabilization—indications are:
  - All children with severe and moderate coma.
  - Mild coma (GCS 13–14) in children less than 2 years age.
  - Loss of consciousness more than 5 min, focal neurologic deficit, seizures, depressed skull fracture, basilar skull fracture, fall from height more than 3 meters, suspected child abuse, traffic accidents even if the GCS is full.

Note: Computed tomography brain is sensitive to pick up recent intracranial (IC) bleeds, quick and easy; MRI brain reveals old and recent bleeds but is technically more difficult.

- Arrange for neurosurgical procedures to evacuate epidural and subdural hematoma.
- Start neuroprotective therapy for minimizing the adverse effects:
  - Head elevation 30° and neutral positioning.
  - Therapy for the underlying cause, e.g. factor therapy for hemophilia, vitamin K ± FFP (fresh frozen plasma) for reversal of anticoagulation, platelet transfusion in thrombocytopenia.
  - Fluid and electrolyte balance using isotonic fluid—normal saline (NS) to maintain serum sodium (S. Na) more than 145 mEq/L.
  - Treatment of raised ICP (Chapter 33).
  - Maintain normal body temperature with paracetamol if there is fever.
  - Treat seizures; detect nonconvulsive seizures by 12 hourly electroencephalogram (EEG) and treat.
  - Maintain normal BP; if hypertensive the ideal drug is nicardipine.
  - Intracranial pressure (ICP) monitoring if facilities are available; maintains ICP below less than 20 mmHg.
- Follow up MRI or MR angiography to detect the extent of clearance of hemorrhage and to diagnose the vascular abnormality.
- Specific therapy for the underlying neurosurgical problem.
- Follow-up and rehabilitation therapy.

CONCLUSION

Intracranial hemorrhage, though a neurosurgical emergency, the initial management may have to be done by a pediatrician very often.

Chapter 45

Head Injury

S Sushamabai

ABSTRACT

Children are more vulnerable for traumatic brain injury (TBI) which includes primary and secondary damage to the brain. The causes of TBI can be accidental or nonaccidental; types of head injury are external, internal or combined. Primary internal injuries manifest within seconds, can be concussion, contusion and hemorrhage. Secondary injuries evolve within hours to days. Patient approach is by quick parallel assessment and stabilization. Clinical grading of TBI is by Glasgow Coma Scale (GCS) as mild, moderate and severe. All children with head injury should be monitored for 24 hours. Investigations, stabilization, neuroprotective medical therapy for rapid recovery and prevention of secondary brain insults are discussed. Neurosurgical intervention should be carried out at the earliest.

INTRODUCTION

Head Injury includes a wide spectrum of traumatic damage to the various structures of the head. In practice, the term indicates *traumatic brain injury (TBI)*. Children sustain greater brain damage after TBI because of:
- Relatively large head.
- Incomplete myelination.
- Immaturity of the brain.

Causes of traumatic brain injury:
- Accidental:
  - Traffic injuries
  - Falls and hits
  - Submersion injuries
  - Sports
  - Disasters.
- Nonaccidental:
  - Assaults
  - Battered child
  - Child abuse.

TYPES OF HEAD INJURY

- External:
  - Open wounds
  - Contusion
  - Hematoma
  - Fractures (depressed fracture skull, basal fracture).
- Internal:
  - Primary (Within seconds)—concussion, contusion, hemorrhage.
  - Secondary (Within hours to days)—endogenous evolution of brain damage, raised intracranial pressure (ICP) subsequent to extracerebral insults (shock, hypoxia, hypercarbia).

GOALS OF THERAPY

- Rapid detection and correction of primary brain insults.
- Detection and correction of other organ injuries.
- Prevention and modification of secondary brain insults.

PATIENT APPROACH

Quick history along with assessment and stabilization.

All children with TBI should be observed in an ICU (pediatric or neurosurgery or pediatric surgery) for at least 24 hours.

History

- May not be clear or available in a child found lone unconscious or an accident victim.
- Often misleading in child abuse, sexual abuse or battered baby.
- Usual symptoms are fall or hit followed by repeated vomiting, rapid loss of consciousness and seizures.
- Consider the possibility of late onset coma several hours after head injury in epidural hemorrhage.
- Neurological deficits as cranial nerve or limb paralysis may be present or appear later.

Assessment and Parallel Stabilization

- *Grade the severity of TBI:*
  - Look for respiratory compromise—revealed by irregular or shallow breathing, apnea. Proceed to rapid sequence intubation (RSI) (protecting cervical spine) and mechanical ventilation.
  - Assess the cardiovascular status—pallor, external bleeding, tachycardia, feeble pulse, hypotension, prolonged CRFT. Secure two

intravenous (IV) access, push normal saline (NS) bolus, vasopressor support if persistent shock after 3 boluses of NS.
- Assess the sensorium by GCS—value 3–8 severe, 9–12 moderate and 13–14 indicate mild coma respectively.
- After stabilization evaluate for other injuries—cervical spine, bone fractures and rupture viscera.
- Seek neurosurgery, critical care medicine, orthopedic and pediatric surgery consultations.

Investigations while Stabilization

- Complete blood count (CBC), peripheral smear, coagulation profile, serum electrolytes (SE), renal function test (RFT), liver function test (LFT), blood sugar, arterial blood gas (ABG), blood grouping, typing, others as per situation.
- Cranial computed tomography (CT) and other imaging studies as soon as the child is stabilized.
- Repeat CT or magnetic resonance imaging (MRI) may be needed to assess the prognosis.

Subsequent Treatment

- Continue airway, breathing and circulation (ABC) stabilization.
- Neuroprotective therapy for prevention of secondary brain insults:
  - Neutral head position, 30° head elevation, O_2 administration.
  - Fluid therapy—correction of dehydration and shock by NS bolus, maintenance fluid therapy with NS to keep S. Na 145–160 mEq/L.
  - Vasopressor therapy (dopamine is ideal) if fluid refractory shock after 3 boluses of NS.
  - Prevent early post-traumatic seizures in severe TBI by fosphenytoin administration.
- Maintain normothermia (paracetamol for fever).
- Avoid agitation, sedation with benzodiazepines or narcotics if needed (Chapter 46).
- Maintain normal BP—best antihypertensive is IV nicardipine.
- Intracranial pressure monitoring, maintain ICP less than or equal to 20 mm Hg.
- Maintain $PaCO_2$ around 35 mm Hg—mild hyperventilation ($PaCO_2$ = 25–30 mm Hg) is beneficial in decreasing ICP.
- Treatment of raised ICP—20% mannitol 0.25–1 g/kg in 20 minutes q 4–6 hourly or 3% saline 5–10 mL/kg IV. Hypertonic saline is ideal if the child is in shock. To be given as continuous infusion at 0.1–1 mL/kg/hr.
- Maintain euglycemia—both hypo- and hyperglycemia should be corrected.

- For refractory raised ICP consider pentobarbital infusion, decompressive craniotomy, hypothermia, hyperventilation, lumbar cerebrospinal fluid (CSF) drainage, etc. in consultation with the neurosurgeon.
- Neurosurgical procedures for increasing size of hematoma.

Monitoring

Vitals, intake and output (I/O) chart, GCS, pupils, paralysis of eye and limb muscles, electroencephalography (EEG), serum sodium (S. Na), RFT, blood sugar.

Follow-up Care

- Children with TBI can have postconcussive symptoms of headache, dizziness, memory loss, cognitive problems, sleep problems, and personality changes for variable period (up to 2 years).
- Rest, proper sedation, reduced academic work and television watching and individualized support for learning activities should be provided.

CONCLUSION

Traumatic brain injuries are more common and serious in children; they should be evaluated and observed at least for 24 hours even if apparently normal.

Chapter 46

Pain Management and Sedation

Manju George Elenjickal, S Sushamabai

ABSTRACT

Pain in children is under-recognized and undertreated. Proper pain management results in better quality of life and nullifies catecholamine-induced adverse problems. Diagnosis of pain in young children is usually made by parents that may not be correct. Wong–Baker FACES Pain Rating Scale is a good objective method to assess pain severity in developmentally normal children. Pain causes tachycardia, tachypnea, hypertension, ventilator dyssynchrony and hypoxemia. Pain management is needed in various systemic diseases, procedures and topical application of painful lesions. The pharmacologic modality for pain as per the World Health Organization (WHO) guidelines is a stepwise increase in opioid and nonopioid drugs as a combination therapy. For topical analgesia of skin or mucosa, 5% lidocaine cream or 0.5% lidocaine infiltration are advised. For CT/MRI, chloral hydrate or a combination of IV ketamine and IV midazolam are effective.

INTRODUCTION

Pain is a sensation of discomfort due to the stimulation of specialized nerve endings. Pediatric pain is under-recognized and under-reported both by children and parents and undertreated by doctors and parents. Apart from humane considerations, pathological problems are aggravated or created if pain and anxiety are not properly controlled. This is due to the release of endogenous catecholamines producing:
- Hypertension
- Tachycardia
- Tachypnea
- Ventilator dyssynchrony
- Hypoxemia.

In chronic diseases, amelioration of pain improves the quality of life.

DIAGNOSIS

- Parental reporting irrespective of age and cognitive or expressive ability.
- Older children (> 8 years of age)—direct verbalization is possible.
- Infants and young children—features are irritability, incessant or inconsolable crying, facial expression, fisting, poor feeding and sleep, paucity of limb movements.
- Physiologic indicators: Tachycardia, changes in respiratory rate, falls in blood oxygen saturation level (SpO_2) and rise in BP.
- Pain rating scales—the face, legs, activity, cry, consolability *(FLACC)* scoring system is one widely accepted. Face's scale based solely on facial expression is very simple to use (Fig. 46.1).
- The child is asked to point the cartoon face to rate the degree of pain.
- Difficult to assess in cognitively impaired children as in Down syndrome, autism, etc.

Note: Do not underdiagnose pain in a calm-appearing child.

Table 46.1 shows the drugs used for pain management, dose, frequency, route of administration and adverse effects.

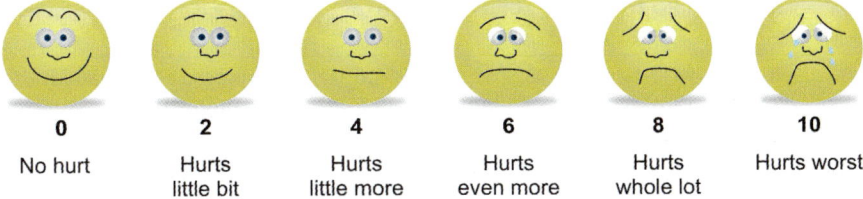

0	2	4	6	8	10
No hurt	Hurts little bit	Hurts little more	Hurts even more	Hurts whole lot	Hurts worst

Fig. 46.1: Wong-Baker Faces Pain Rating Scale.
Note: Older children and adolescents will be able to rate the pain.

Table 46.1: Drug therapy for pain management.[1-3]

Drug	Dosage	Comments
Acetaminophen	PO 10–15 mg/kg q 4 hr[1] IV 10–15 mg/kg q 4–6 hr[1] PR 20–30 mg/kg/ q 4 hr or 40 mg/kg q 6–8 hr[1] Maximum daily dosing: 90 mg/kg/24 hr (children) 60 mg/kg/24 hr (< 2 years) 30–45 mg/kg/24 hr (neonates)	Fulminant hepatic failure can occur if ceiling dose is exceeded[1]
Aspirin	PO 10–15 mg/kg q 4 hr. Maximum daily dosing: 120 mg/kg/24 hr (children)	Prone for Reye syndrome; prolonged antiplatelet activity can cause bleeding[1]

Contd...

Contd...

Drug	Dosage	Comments
Ibuprofen	PO 8–10 mg/kg/dose PO q 6 hr[2]	Anti-inflammatory activity with very good safety profile in children[2]
Naproxen	PO 5–7 mg/kg/dose q 8–12 hr[2]	Good anti-inflammatory agent, longer duration analgesia than ibuprofen[2]
Ketorolac	IV loading dose 0.5 mg/kg (max 30 mg), then 0.25–0.3 mg/kg/dose (max 15 mg) q 6 hr, maximum 5 days	Anti-inflammatory, advised for short-term analgesia in which oral dosing is not feasible[2]
Celecoxib	PO 3–6 mg/kg /dose q 12–24 hr[2]	Anti-inflammatory; can reveal cross-reactivity with sulfa allergies[2]
Choline magnesium salicylate	PO 10–20 mg/kg/dose q 8–12 hr[2]	Less bleeding and gastritis when compared with other NSAIDs[2]
Nortriptyline, amitriptyline, desipramine	PO 0.1–0.5 mg/kg q HS[1]	Main use in neuropathic and sickle cell pain situations. Can cause fatal dysrhythmia in overdose.[1] Promotes suicidal tendency[1]
Gabapentin	PO 100 mg bid or tid titrated up to 3,600 mg/24 hours[1]	Main indication is neurologic pain[1]
Quetiapine, risperidone, chlorpromazine, haloperidol	Quetiapine: 6.25 or 12.5 mg PO qd (hs); in acute agitation with pain repeat q6 hr; increase up to 25 mg/dose if needed.[1] Risperidone: Useful for PDD spectrum or tic disorder and chronic pain; 0.25–1 mg (in 0.25 mg increments) q d or bid[1]	Can cause extrapyramidal symptoms; lowers seizure threshold in increasing doses[1]
Fluoxetine	PO 10-20 mg q d in the morning[2]	Indications are anxiety disorders with arousal amplifying pain. Also used in PDD in very low doses[2]
Sucrose solution via pacifier or gloved finger (all PO)[2]	Preterm infants (gestational age): 28 weeks: 0.2 mL swabbed into mouth; 28–32 weeks: 0.2–2 mL, depending on suck/swallow; More than 32 weeks: 2 mL term infants: 1.5–2 mL over 2 minutes[1]	Wait for 2 minutes before starting procedure; analgesia may last up to 8 minutes.[1] Consider one more dose if needed

(PO, per oral; IV, intravenous; PR, per rectal; NSAIDs, nonsteroidal anti-inflammatory drugs; PDD, pervasive development disorder).

Chapter 46: Pain Management and Sedation

Situations Requiring Pain Management and Sedation in Children

- Systemic diseases or organ involvement:
  - Infections, rheumatic or rheumatoid diseases, renal or intestinal colic, malignancy
- Procedural pain—IV access (central, peripheral), bone marrow (BM) aspiration, wound suturing, lumbar puncture and biopsy (Refer Chapter 8 for pain management and sedation in rapid sequence ventilation), CT, and MRI
- Anxiety or panic disorders in hospital environment or due to disease process
- Trauma care
- Oral or anal or rectal or genital mucosal ulcer pain.

TREATMENT MODALITIES

- Nonpharmacological
- Pharmacological.

Nonpharmacological

- Psychological and physical techniques like relaxation, distraction by music, dance, video, television
- Pet therapy
- Acupuncture
- Local heat application
- Massage
- Yoga practice.

Key role is by the pediatrician involving the child, nurse and parents.

Pharmacological

- Topical application—for IV access, lumbar puncture (LP), other needle procedures, painful mouth or genital ulcers (aphthous, viral infections), choice agents are lidocaine cream 5% or *EMLAP* (a topical *e*utectic *m*ixture of *l*idocaine *a*nd *p*rilocaine).[1]
- Local infiltration—0.25–0.5% lidocaine infiltration up to a maximum safe dose of 5 mg/kg; recommended for wound suturing, LP, bone marrow aspiration, pleural, pericardial and ascites tap, biopsy, etc.
- Systemic analgesia—*routes are to be oral or IV or PR or nasal but never intramuscular (IM).*
  - Procedure-related pain—optional use; drugs preferred are: IV pentazocine HCl + promethazine HCl (1 mg/kg/dose, each can be repeated 4 hourly).

Flowchart 46.1: Stepwise addition of drugs depending on the severity of pain as per the WHO criteria.

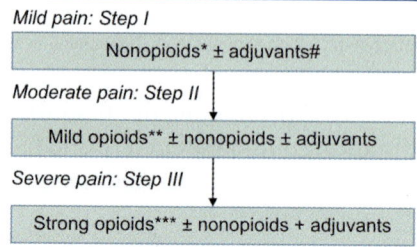

*Paracetamol, ibuprofen, celecoxib or IV ketorolac. Sucrose solution—oral.
**Codeine 0.5–1 mg/kg/dose q 4–6 hourly.
***Morphine (O) 0.3 mg/kg/dose q 4 hours, IV 0.05 mg/kg/dose q 4 hours, methadone (O) 0.2 mg/kg/dose q 8 hours, IV 0.1 mg/kg q 8 hours.
#Diazepam (O) 0.2–0.3 mg/kg/dose,[3] tricyclic antidepressants—amitriptyline 0.1–0.2 mg/kg at bedtime.

- For CT/MRI—chloral hydrate (O, P/R) 30 minutes before the procedure. If unsuccessful, a combination of IV ketamine (0.5–2 mg/kg) with IV midazolam (0.05–0.15 mg/kg) is advised, may be repeated.[4]
- Disease or treatment-related pain—stepwise addition of drugs depending on the severity of pain as per the WHO criteria (Flowchart 46.1).

SPECIAL SITUATIONS

- Deafferentation pain—carbamazepine (O).
- Central nervous system invasion—dexamethasone (IV/O).
- Muscle spasm—benzodiazepines.
- Bone pain—corticosteroids.
- Colicky pain—atropine, hyoscyamine.

CONCLUSION

Pain in children is under-recognized and undertreated; should be assessed by pain rating scale and analgesic therapy be given as per the WHO guidelines.

REFERENCES

1. https://archieve.org/stream/nelson20/1102djvu.txt (internet 15-Apr-2017).
2. Zeltzer LK, Krane EJ. Pediatric Pain Management. In: Kliegman RM, Stanton BMD, St. Geme J, Schor NF (Eds). Nelson Textbook of Pediatrics. US: Elsevier; 2011.
3. Carlton KK Lee. Drug Dosages. The Harriet Lane Handbook. US: Elsevier; 2002.
4. Gal P, Reed MD. Medications. In: Kliegman R, Behrman R, Jenson H, Stanton B (Eds). Nelson Textbook of Pediatrics. US: Saunders; 2007.

Chapter **47**

Brain Death and Legal Aspects

Manju George Elenjickal, S Sushamabai

ABSTRACT

Brain death is the irreversible cessation of all cortical and brain stem functions. The three parameters to be satisfied for brain death are irreversible coma with a known cause, apnea and absence of brainstem reflexes. The ancillary investigations: electroencephalogram (EEG) and cerebral blood flow (CBF) study though not a must may be occasionally required in selected situations for confirmation. The pediatrician's role is to diagnose brain death clinically; complete the documentation and counsel the bereaved parents, subsequent care of the body and appropriate communications if organ donation is planned or helping the parents to decide withdrawing supportive care to the brain-dead child.

INTRODUCTION

Brain death is the irreversible cessation of all functions of the entire brain, including the brainstem and is the legal death presently accepted. Cessation of heartbeat and interruption of blood circulation are not legal declaration of death. The diagnosis of brain death is made essentially by repeated clinical examination but at times EEG and cerebral blood flow (CBF) studies may be required.

Components of Clinical Brain Death

The components of clinical brain death diagnosis are:
- *Irreversible coma:* It should be due to a known cause. Coma is complete unresponsiveness even to noxious stimuli—can be assessed by AVPU (Alert, responds to Voice, responds to Pain, Unresponsive) scale. The presence of spinal cord reflexes is not against brain death.

Note: The cause of coma should be diagnosed by detailed history and relevant investigations to rule out reversible conditions.

- *Absence of brainstem reflexes:* Pupillary light reflex (midbrain), doll's eye reflex or oculocephalic reflex (midbrain, pons), corneal reflex (pons), oculovestibular reflex (midbrain, pons), gag and cough reflex (done by introducing a suction catheter through the endotracheal tube to the carina to stimulate cough—indicates involvement of medulla).
- *Apnea*: It is the absence of respiratory effort to an adequate response and is confirmed by *apnea test*, the procedure being:
    - Ensure stable vitals, correct metabolic derangement if any, stop drugs producing apnea, maintain body temperature; should be done by the same physician; preoxygenate the patient with 100% oxygen for 10 minutes; adjust the ventilation to achieve pCO_2—40 mm Hg; assess the baseline blood gas values; stop mechanical ventilation; maintain 100% oxygen through a T-piece attached to endotracheal (ET) tube or via a resuscitation bag; monitor vitals and blood oxygen saturation (SpO_2); obtain blood gas after 10 minutes and then every 5 minutes; brain death is considered if no respiratory effort with pCO_2 more than or equal to 60 mm Hg or more than or equal to 20 mm Hg above baseline.

Note: Apnea test, as it may destabilize the patient, is performed only if the first two criteria of brain death are satisfied.

The pediatrician's responsibilities in brain death are:
- Confirmation of brain death.
- Decision for discontinuation of medical support.
- Continuing medical support for organ donation if planned.
- Support, help and counseling the family for decision making.

Two examinations (by different treating physicians) including apnea testing, separated by an observation period (24 hours for neonates from 37 weeks of gestation to term infants 30 days old and 12 hours for infants and children more than 30 days of age) are needed. An observation period of 24–48 hours prior to initiation of brain death assessment is recommended following cardiopulmonary resuscitation (CPR) or severe acute brain injury.

ANCILLARY STUDIES

- EEG should reveal electrocerebral silence for 30 minutes. Disadvantages are artifacts in tracing and the presence of suppressing levels of drugs given to the patient giving erroneous impression.
- Cerebral blood flow studies—absence of the radionuclide agent in the brain is supportive of brain death.

Documentation should be complete and should reveal:
- Etiology and irreversibility of coma.
- Absence of confounding factors: Hypothermia, hypotension, hypoxia, significant metabolic derangement, significant levels of drugs that depress the brain.
- Absence of motor response to noxious stimulation.
- Absence of brainstem reflexes: Pupillary light reflex, oculocephalic reflex, corneal reflex; cough and gag reflex.
- Absence of respiratory effort in response to an adequate stimulus; blood gas reports at the beginning and at the end of the apnea test should be documented.

SUBSEQUENT CARE

- Inform the family about the meaning of brain death and also the details about the total dependence on mechanical gadgets like ventilator.
- Continue supportive care till decisions are made by the family about potential organ donation and comes to terms with the diagnosis, this may take hours to days.
- Do not attempt to force the parents into early decisions about further care and the withdrawal of support.
- Once the family is prepared, supportive care may be withdrawn so that the child will experience natural death.

Organ Donation

- The correct time to refer families for organ donation is when the diagnosis of brain death is done.
- Provide appropriate care for the organs to be transplanted to maintain optimal organ perfusion by increasing the rate of IV fluid infusion, provide nutritional support, minimize the use of vasopressors, and use antibiotics.
- Proceed for the legal steps to organ donation.

CONCLUSION

Brain death should be certified by two examinations separated by age, appropriate time interval, by two different doctors, and if needed by apnea test.

Section 7

ENDOCRINE AND METABOLIC EMERGENCIES

Chapter 48

Diabetic Ketoacidosis

S Sushamabai

ABSTRACT

Diabetic ketoacidosis (DKA) is the commonest potentially fatal endocrine emergency encountered in pediatrics. The diagnostic criteria are blood glucose more than or equal to 200 mg/dL, metabolic acidosis (blood pH <7.35) and ketosis (blood ketones ≥3 mmol/L, urine ketones >2+). The classical presentation is a known diabetic child on inadequate insulin presenting with abdominal pain, vomiting and dehydration. Clinical severity grading is mild, moderate and severe. The priorities are correction of fluid and electrolyte balance, detection and management of infections, and insulin therapy. Systematic human monitoring and capillary blood glucose estimation are crucial to detect cerebral edema and speed up recovery. The features of cerebral edema and its management are also included.

INTRODUCTION

Diabetic ketoacidosis (DKA) is the most common endocrine emergency in pediatrics and is a life-threatening complication of childhood diabetes.

CLINICAL PRESENTATION

- Suspect DKA in any child who is critically ill, comatose, has repeated vomiting, unaccountable dehydration, labored breathing, dyspnea or acute abdominal symptoms.
- In a child with established diabetes presenting with any intercurrent illness always exclude coexisting DKA.

DIAGNOSTIC CRITERIA

All should be satisfied:
- Blood glucose more than or equal to 200 mg/dL (11.1 mol/L).
- Metabolic acidosis: Venous blood pH less than 7.35.
- Ketosis: Blood ketones more than or equal to 3 mmol/L, urine ketones >2+

Table 48.1: Severity grading of DKA in children.

Parameter	Mild	Moderate	Severe*
Symptoms Signs	Vague Fatigue	Drowsy but arousable Some dehydration Kussmaul breathing	Deepening coma Severe dehydration circulatory/respiratory/renal failure
Venous pH	>7.25–7.35	7.15–7.25	<7.15
Care area	Emergency room	High-dependency unit.	Pediatric ICU

*Note: Severe hypernatremia (corrected Na >150 mEq/L) also is severe DKA.

Patient Approach

Proceed to severity grading as in Table 48.1.

Simplified approach in 13 steps in letters A to M is detailed below:

0–20 min: Parallel history and stabilization.
Airway—clear the secretions.
Breathing—give 100% O_2; keep resuscitation set ready; intubate if respiratory compromise.
Circulation—assess central and peripheral pulsations, blood pressure (BP), capillary refill time (CRFT); start normal saline (NS) 20 mL/kg in 20–60 minutes if in shock or severe dehydration. In mild DKA intravenous (IV) fluids may not be required. Put indwelling catheter if comatose; secure two IV access.
Dextrose—estimate capillary blood glucose (CBG) by glucometer; recheck CBG by venous blood sugar at least 12 hourly.
Electrolytes—send blood for serum sodium, potassium, calcium, phosphorus (S. Na, K, Ca, P) along with renal function test (RFT), venous blood gas (VBG), liver function test (LFT), S. amylase, lipase, HbA1c and C-peptide; keep separate IV access for frequent blood sample collection.

20–30 minutes: Fluid and electrolyte therapy.
Fluid calculation—simplified *Milwaukee protocol*
Volume required: 4 L/m²/day [body surface area (BSA)];—BSA calculate as:

Wt in kg	BSA as m²
1–5	(0.05 × kg) + 0.05
6–10	(0.04 × kg) + 0.1
11–20	(0.03 × kg) + 0.2
>20	(0.02 × kg) + 0.4

$$\text{Rate of infusion for next 23 hours} = \frac{\text{Calculated fluid- 1st hour bolus}}{23} = \text{mL/hour}$$

Type of fluid after 1st hour bolus is ½ NS.

30–40 minutes: **G**lucose administration.
- When blood glucose (BG) reaches 300 mg/dL change ½ NS to 5% dextrose (D) ½ NS 1:1 ratio. Rate of fall of BG ideally should be 50–100 mg/hr.

40–50 minutes: **H**ypokalemia correction.
- Add potassium to IV fluids up to 40 mEq/L (20 mEq of K acetate and K phosphate each) after the child has voided urine or if severe hypokalemia as evidenced by ECG changes (flat T-waves, appearance of U waves, widening of QRS) or if low value of S. K in lab report.

50–60 minutes: **I**nsulin infusion.
- Start early 1st hour as continuous infusion @ 0.1 U/kg/hr till BG reaches less than 300 mg/dL.
- Add 10% D to ½ NS when BG reaches 200 mg/dL; thereafter reduce the insulin infusion rate to 0.05–0.02 U/kg/hr.
- Switch to subcutaneous (s/c) insulin 1 U/kg/day, divided 6 hourly when the child becomes alert, venous pH more than 7.30, no evidence of dehydration and no vomiting. Give 1st dose of s/c insulin along with first food.
- Continue IV insulin infusion for 30 minutes more.

Preparation of insulin infusion: Dissolve 50 units of regular insulin in 50 mL NS so that 1 mL provides 1 unit insulin. Infuse @ 0.1 mL/kg/hr using infusion pump. For the 1st dose 25 mL extra infusion has to be prepared to flush the tubing.

Joined infusion: Using a Y-tube connection joined infusion of insulin and IV fluids can be set up to reduce the number of IV access in difficult situations where infusion pump is not available. Single dose of IM insulin prior to transportation also is advised in such areas.

Beyond 60 minutes:
Ketoacid correction (bicarbonate therapy)—indications are:
- Venous pH less than 6.9.
- Circulatory or renal failure.

Dose 1 mEq/kg of sodium bicarbonate in equal dilution as infusion in 1 hour.
Laboratory report evaluation and correction:
- Assess corrected sodium as:

$$\frac{\text{Measured Na} + 1.6 \times (\text{measured glucose in mg/dL} - 100)}{100}$$

- If the value is more than 150 mEq/L prolong the rehydration time 12 hours more to avoid cerebral edema.
- Consider additional investigations as computed tomography (CT) or magnetic resonance imaging (MRI), lumbar puncture (LP), chest X-ray (CXR), blood or urine or other body fluid culture as per clinical picture after stabilization. The common associated infections in DKA are pneumonia, urinary tract infection (UTI), cellulitis, meningitis and moniliasis of external genitalia.
- Start empirical antibiotic therapy (ceftriaxone ± vancomycin ± amikacin) for associated infections within the first hour.

Monitoring: Maintain a flow chart revealing:
- Hourly vitals, Glasgow Coma Scale (GCS), pupil size, capillary glucose, electrocardiograph (ECG) changes, insulin dose, input and output (I/O) chart until blood glucose (BG) is 250 mg/dL.
- 6-hourly VBG, serum electrolytes (SE), urine sugar, acetone (ideally with each void).
- Others as per clinical indication daily.

Problems Encountered

Cerebral Edema

- Occurs 4–12 hours after starting treatment while the patient reveals improvement clinically and biochemically.
- Clinical features are headache, irritability and rapid fall in GCS, dilated or unequal pupils, papilledema, bradycardia, irregular shallow respiration and seizures.
- The clinician should be vigilant about this complication while the patient reveals improvement with treatment.

Treatment

- 30° head end elevation.
- Intravenously 20% mannitol 2 mL/kg in 5 minutes may be repeated.
- Prolong the rehydration period for 12–24 hours more.
- Hyperventilation if needed.

Recovery Phase

Features are:
- Alert
- Stable vitals
- No vomiting
- Blood pH more than 7.30
- Serum Na 135–145 mEq/L
- Blood glucose (BG) less than 200 mg/dL.

Management

- Shift to recovery ward.
- Start insulin replacement therapy.
- Medical nutrition therapy (MNT).
- Diabetes education and care.
- Long term follow-up.

CONCLUSION

Diabetic ketoacidosis is the most common fatal endocrine emergency in children but with vigilant monitoring and systematized therapy the patient can be saved.

FURTHER READING

1. Bajpai A. Type I diabetes mellitus in children and adolescents in India. In: Clinical practice guidelines (Ed). Diabetic Ketoacidosis. Lucknow: ISPAE; 2011.

Chapter 49

Acute Adrenocortical Insufficiency

S Sushamabai

ABSTRACT

Acute adrenocortical insufficiency (AACI) is a life-threatening endocrine emergency in children. It is due to low serum cortisol of congenital or acquired causes. Clinical presentation can be recurrent vomiting, failure to thrive (FTT) with/without ambiguous genitalia and unexplainable dehydration in young infants, congenital adrenal hyperplasia being the most common cause at this age; autoimmune disease and infections are the causes in older children. Hyponatremia, hyperkalemia, hypoglycemia, and metabolic acidosis support the diagnosis. Treatment is fluid and electrolyte administration and intravenous (IV) hydrocortisone.

INTRODUCTION

Acute adrenocortical insufficiency (AACI) is a life-threatening endocrine emergency due to low serum cortisol most often associated with aldosterone deficiency. Suspect AACI in:
- Newborn babies presenting with recurrent vomiting, shock, unexplainable dehydration, failure to thrive with or without ambiguous genitalia.
- Older children having lethargy, recurrent vomiting, anorexia, weight loss or poor weight gain, hypotension, hypoglycemia, dehydration, shock.

ETIOLOGY

- *Newborns:* Birth injuries leading to adrenal hemorrhage, congenital adrenal hyperplasia (CAH), septicemia, disseminated intravascular coagulation (DIC).
- *Infants and children:* Sepsis, meningococcemia, severe dengue illness with bleeding, child abuse, Addison disease, long-term steroid therapy, drug-induced (etomidate).

DIFFERENTIAL DIAGNOSIS

- Diarrhea with dehydration.
- Septic shock.
- Renal tubular acidosis.
- Poisoning.
- Inborn errors of metabolism.

Patient Approach

- Admit in pediatric intensive care unit (PICU) if the child is in shock; stabilize Airway, Breathing and circulation (ABC); assess blood glucose; correct hypoglycemia if present.
- Send blood for venous blood gas (VBG), Na, K, Cl, HCO_3, random blood sugar (RBS), Ca, P, renal function test (RFT), cortisol (adrenocorticotropic hormone [ACTH], aldosterone, 17-hydroxyprogesterone [17-OHP] and plasma renin additionally if CAH is suspected).
- The metabolic derangements supporting the diagnosis of adrenal insufficiency are hyponatremia, hyperkalemia, hypoglycemia and metabolic acidosis.
- The hormonal derangements diagnostic of AACI are low levels of plasma cortisol and aldosterone. High 17-OHP and plasma renin are supportive of CAH.

Note: Metabolic acidosis need not be prominent in newborns and young infants due to defective ketoacid metabolism; in older children hyperkalemia is a late feature.

- ACTH stimulation test with cosyntropin—collect the first blood sample for basal value of cortisol, administer cosyntropin 0.250 mg as rapid intravenous (IV), collect 2 more samples 30 and 60 minutes after the test injection. This test is advised if the cortisol value is low but there is strong clinical suspicion of adrenal insufficiency.
- Evaluate ECG to detect hyperkalemia characterized by tent shaped T-waves of more than 5 divisions.
- Start IV 5% dextrose in normal saline 20–60 mL/kg in 20–60 minutes. Repeat up to three boluses till hypoglycemia, hyponatremia and hypotension are corrected. Continue maintenance fluid therapy with 5% dextrose normal saline (DNS) till the dehydration and dyselectrolytemia are corrected. Treat hyperkalemia (Chapter 53).
- Intravenous hydrocortisone—10 mg (infant), 25 mg (toddler), 50 mg (child), 100 mg (adolescent) as bolus followed by same dose divided 6 hourly for 24–48 hours, then half the dose for 24 hours. Switch over to oral maintenance dose (10–20 mg/m^2/day divided 2–3 times daily) assessing

Flowchart 49.1: Algorithm of acute adrenocortical insufficiency management.

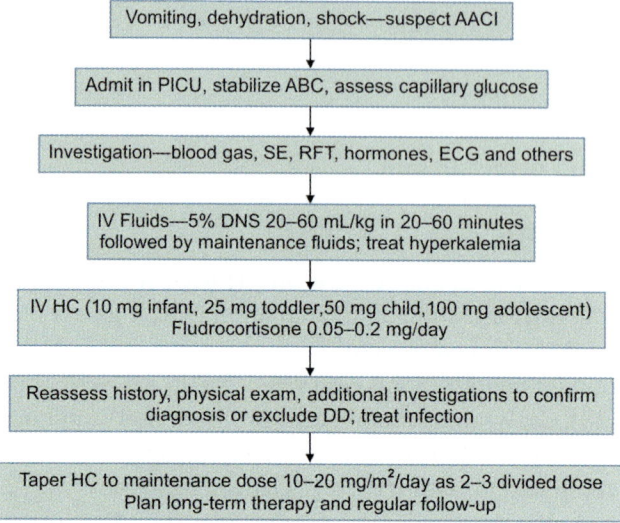

(AACI, acute adrenocortical insufficiency; PICU, pediatric intensive care unit; ABC, airway, breathing and circulation; RFT, renal function test; ECG, electrocardiograph; IV, intravenous; DNS, dextrose normal saline; DD, differential diagnosis; SE, serum electrolytes)

clinical response. Prednisolone in ¼ dose of hydrocortisone in 2 divided doses is an alternative.
- Add fludrocortisone 0.05–0.2 mg/day in 2 divided doses if mineralocorticoid deficiency is suspected.
- Reassess the history and clinical examination. Plan further investigations as per clinical diagnosis. Ultrasonography or magnetic resonance imaging (USG/MRI) abdomen to assess the adrenal size as well as to rule out renal tubular acidosis is a must.
- Maintenance dose of hydrocortisone has to be increased 2–3-fold in periods of stress like infection, vomiting.
- Replacement therapy during surgery should be the full dose as in AACI.
- Plan proper long-term follow-up program which include:
  – Growth monitoring and blood pressure (BP) once in 3 months.
  – Serum electrolytes, blood sugar and 17-OHP estimation every 6 months.
- Surgical consultation for ambiguous genitalia and reconstructive surgery for sex determination should be done at the earliest in CAH.

Algorithm of AACI management has been shown in Flowchart 49.1.

CONCLUSION

Acute adrenocortical insufficiency is a fatal endocrine emergency but timely diagnosis and treatment with IV fluids and hydrocortisone will save life.

Chapter 50

Puberty Menorrhagia

S Sushamabai

ABSTRACT

Puberty menorrhagia is abnormal menstrual bleed in adolescents. It can be heavy regular bleed or intermenstrual bleeding. The most common etiology is immaturity of the hypothalamic-pituitary axis; congenital or acquired coagulopathies, uterine or vaginal tumors or malignancies, hemangiomas and pelvic infection are other causes. Critically ill patients with severe anemia should be cared in ICU, stabilized and urgent whole blood or packed red blood cell (PRBC) should be given. Intravenous (IV) estrogen for 24–48 hours along with progestin is the specific hormone therapy to stop bleeding. Investigations are complete blood count (CBC) with coagulation profile and transabdominal pelvic ultrasonography (USG) abdomen to exclude utero-ovarian mass. Local vaginal examination should be done in all. Follow-up treatment with combined oral contraceptive (COC) pills is advised thereafter. Cyclical therapy with COC pills is needed in those with mild and moderate anemia with active bleeding. Those with coagulopathies require long-term menstrual suppression. Patients in whom hormone therapy is to be avoided oral tranexamic acid is the drug advised.

INTRODUCTION

Puberty menorrhagia is uterine bleeding of excessive amount or of increased duration, occurring regularly in adolescents. The preferred term at present is *abnormal uterine bleeding (AUB)*—indicating menstrual bleed abnormal in regularity, volume, frequency or duration. The type can be specified as heavy regular bleed or inter menstrual bleeding.

ETIOLOGY

- Ovulation dysfunction termed as dysfunctional uterine bleeding (DUB)—anovulation due to immaturity of the hypothalamic-pituitary-ovarian axis in first-two years of menarche.

- Uterine problems—fibroid, cervical polyp, malignancy, intrauterine devices, hemangioma, pelvic infection, ectopic pregnancy, retained products of conception.
- Vaginal causes—injury (sexual abuse), foreign body inside vagina, cancer.
- Systemic diseases—coagulopathies (congenital or acquired), leukemia, chronic liver disease. The commonest ones are von-Willebrand disease (VWD) and platelet function disorders.
- Drug-induced—intake of contraceptives, anticoagulants, etomidate, others.

Patient Approach

- Initial quick assessment by brief history and physical examination. Assess the quantity and duration of bleeding. Enquire fever, abdominal pain, amenorrhea, past or family history of bleeding disorders, history of injury and ecchymosis or drug intake.
- Assess vital parameters, severity of anemia; organomegaly, abdominal tenderness, utero ovarian mass, vaginal foreign body or injury.
- Admit in PICU if severe anemia [hemoglobin (Hb) <8 g/dL] or postural hypotension or syncope or unstable vitals. Stabilize Airway, Breathing and Circulation (ABC) with bolus normal saline (NS) and O_2. Send blood for CBC, peripheral smear for abnormal cells and platelet morphology, bleeding time (BT), clotting time (CT), prothrombin time (PT), activated partial thromboplastin time (APTT), blood grouping, typing, cross matching. Start whole blood or packed RBC transfusion 10–20 mL/kg in 2–4 hours.
- Detailed history and physical examination after stabilization:
  - Menstrual history—age of onset, pattern.
  - Severity assessment of bleeding—frequent number of pads changed, passing of clots larger than 1 inch, bleeding more than 7 days—all indicate severe bleeding.
  - Family history (mother, sisters) of menstrual irregularities and gynecological problems.
  - Confidential history of (H/O) sexual activity, drug intake.

Physical Examination

- Vitals, growth parameters, body mass index (BMI), sexual maturity rating (SMR), signs of androgen excess (hirsutism, severe acne).
- External genitalia for injury, foul-smelling discharge, ulcers, foreign body;
- Transabdominal pelvic ultrasonography (USG) to detect uterine or ovarian mass and anatomical abnormalities.
- Arrange for pelvic examination if needed.

- Additional investigations as liver function test (LFT), renal function test (RFT), thyroid function test (TFT), coagulation factor assay and platelet function studies as per suspected etiology.

Specific Therapy

Mild anemia—Hb more than 10 g/dL:
- Reassurance, close follow-up, menstrual charting.
- Iron supplementation as per the degree of anemia.
- If active bleeding add *COC* pills containing estrogen and progestin:
  - One pill BD till bleeding stops, then one daily for 3 weeks.
  - After withdrawal bleeding stops, start one pill daily for 3 weeks.
  - Repeat for 3 cycles.

Moderate anemia—Hb 8–10 g/dL:
- No need for hospital admission if stable.
- COC pill 1 q 6 hourly for 4–7 days, then taper to once daily dosing and stop in 2 weeks.
- After withdrawal bleeding has stopped, start COC pill one daily for 3 weeks.
- Repeat for 3–6 cycles.

Severe anemia—Hb less than 8 g/dL:
- Hospitalize—urgent investigations for coagulopathy and malignancies.
- Airway, Breathing and Circulation stabilization, blood or PRBC transfusion.
- Combined oral contraceptive-2 pills twice daily for 5–7 days; if severe vomiting administer IV conjugated estrogens 25 mg q 6 hourly, along with progestin for 24–48 hours.
- Continue with COC pills as for moderate anemia.
- After bleeding is controlled taper COC pill to once daily for 3 weeks.
- After withdrawal bleeding has stopped, start COC pill one daily for 3 weeks.
- Repeat cycle for 3–6 months.

Patients who want to avoid hormone therapy:
- Oral tranexamic acid 1.3 g TDS for 5 days.
- It has increased risk of thrombosis when combined with hormone therapy.

Long-term menstrual suppression—may be required for those with bleeding diathesis:
- Oral medroxyprogesterone acetate (MPA) on continuous daily basis *OR*
- Continuous COC pill *OR*

Flowchart 50.1: Algorithm of management of abnormal uterine bleeding.

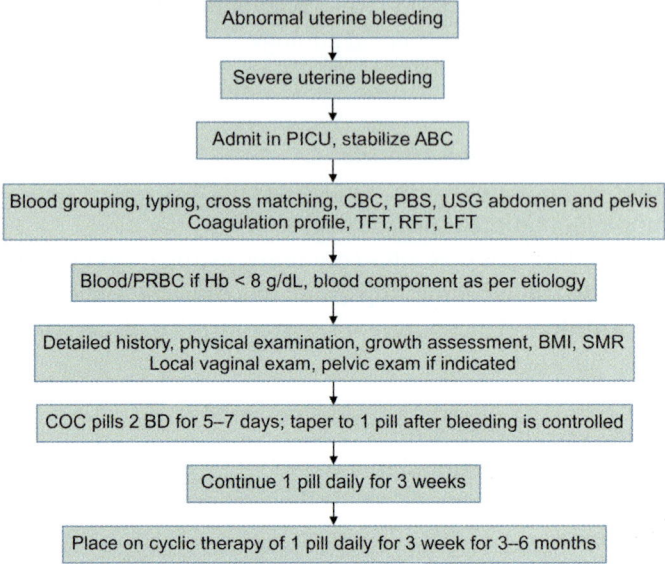

(PICU, pediatric intensive care unit; ABC, airway, breathing and circulation; CBC, complete blood count; PBS, peripheral blood smear; USG, ultrasonography; TFT, thyroid function test; RFT, renal function test; LFT, liver function test; PRBC, packed red blood cell; BMI, body mass index; SMR, sexual maturity rating; COC, combined oral contraceptive)

- Depo-medroxy progesterone acetate (DMPA) 150 mg intramuscular (IM) once in every 3 month.

Algorithm of management of abnormal uterine bleeding is shown in Flowchart 50.1.

CONCLUSION

Puberty menorrhagia should be investigated to exclude nonhormonal causes and should be treated with estrogen progestin combination.

Chapter 51

Diabetes Insipidus

S Sushamabai

ABSTRACT

Diabetes insipidus (DI) is the clinical situation of polyuria and polydipsia due to vasopressin deficiency or insensitivity of the kidneys to vasopressin. It can present as a medical emergency in young infants, postoperative patients, following trauma, meningitis, encephalitis, leukemia, lymphoma etc. in vasopressin deficiency. Nephrogenic DI can be genetic or acquired. The diagnostic criteria are polyuria more than 2 L/m²/24 hr; serum osmolality more than 300 mOsm/L and urine osmolality less than 300 mOsm/L. Diabetes mellitus and chronic renal failure are the main differential diagnoses. The details of vasopressin administration, fluid therapy and the drug therapy in central and nephrogenic DI are discussed.

INTRODUCTION

Diabetes insipidus (DI) is the clinical situation of polyuria and polydipsia due to vasopressin deficiency (central DI) or insensitivity of the kidneys to vasopressin (nephrogenic DI).

DIAGNOSTIC CRITERIA

- Polyuria more than 2 L/m²/24 hours
- Serum osmolality more than 300 mOsm/L
- Urine osmolality less than 300 mOsm/L.

Box 51.1 reveals the differential diagnosis of DI.

Box 51.1: Differential diagnosis of DI.

Central
- Genetic
  - Acquired
  - Trauma, neurosurgery
  - Congenital malformations of pituitary gland

Contd...

Contd...

- Neoplasms involving pituitary
- Infections (meningococcemia, TB)
- Autoimmune
- Drug-induced—phenytoin
- Infiltrates—leukemia, histiocytosis

Nephrogenic diabetes insipidus
- Genetic
- Acquired
  - Renal anomalies, chronic renal failure (CRF)
  - Hypocalcemia
  - Drug-induced

Primary polydipsia

Diabetes mellitus

CLINICAL PRESENTATION AND MANAGEMENT

- Suspect DI in post-traumatic or neurosurgery patients with polyuria, dehydration, shock and hypernatremia.
- Children or infants with failure to thrive, unexplained fever, dehydration, primary and secondary enuresis, polyuria, polydipsia.

Patient Approach

Sick child—exclude osmotic diuresis (mannitol, hyperglycemia, radioactive contrast material) and polyuria due to fluid administration (serum osmolality >300 mOsm/L).

Note: Sick children can have stress hyperglycemia or secondary to steroid administration.

- Not sick child—proceed systematically with detailed history, physical examination and investigations to assess the etiology.
- Assess the degree of dehydration, growth parameters for failure to thrive (FTT), pallor, lymphadenopathy, hepatosplenomegaly, visual function and central nervous system (CNS).

Investigations

- Urine—albumin, sugar, specific gravity, osmolality, culture
- Serum osmolality, Na, K, Ca
- Renal function test (RFT)
- Others as per suspected etiology.

The diagnostic features of DI are serum osmolality more than 300 mOsm/kg with urine osmolality less than 300 mOsm/kg and hypernatremia.

Management

Acute Central Diabetes Insipidus

- Treat shock
- Subsequent fluid management for maintenance requirement—3 L/m²/day till urine output is 2–4 mL/kg/hr. Monitor S. Na, K and glucose.
- Aqueous vasopressin (pitressin)—indicated in acute central DI following neurosurgery (dose 1.5 mU/kg/hr) along with fluid restriction to 1 L/m²/24 hr. Monitor urine output, urine specific gravity and S. Na. Taper and stop when urine output stabilizes to 2–4 mL/kg/hr.

Permanent Central Diabetes Insipidus

- 1-deamino-8-D-arginine-vasopressin (DDAVP) oral tablets 25–300 µg q 8–12 hr. Intra nasal spray 10 µg/0.1 mL. Use with caution in children as it may cause severe hyponatremia.
- Treat the etiology.

Monitoring the acutely ill child:
- Hourly intake output chart, vitals, hydration status.
- 6 hourly S. Na, K, glucose, osmolality till steady.
- Urine Na (U. Na), specific gravity and osmolality as indicated.

Nephrogenic Diabetes Insipidus

- Treat the etiology—hypocalcemia, hyperkalemia, offending drugs, renal anomalies.
- Congenital nephrogenic DI:
  - Hydrochlorothiazide 2–3 mg/kg/day alone or with amiloride 20 mg/1.73 m²/day decreases polyuria.
  - High-dose vasopressin with indomethacin is advised in children with genetic defects in V2 receptor revealing reduced affinity for vasopressin.
- High calorie low-sodium diet.
- Fluid intake 3 L/m²/day.

CONCLUSION

Diabetes insipidus due to vasopressin deficiency presents with polyuria and polydipsia; can be diagnosed by serum and urine osmolarity and should be treated with IV vasopressin in postoperative patients.

Chapter 52

Thyroid Crisis

S Sushamabai

ABSTRACT

Thyroid crisis or thyroid storm is an occasional endocrine emergency encountered in children. The features are delirium, restlessness, tachycardia and heart failure. Diagnosis is confirmed by thyroid function studies revealing high triiodothyronine (T3), thyroxine (T4) and low thyroid-stimulating hormone (TSH). Early diagnosis and intensive treatment including Airway, Breathing and Circulation (ABC) stabilization, fluid and electrolyte therapy and infection control are needed. The specific therapy for hyperthyroidism is propylthiouracil, potassium iodide, propranolol and steroids.

INTRODUCTION

Thyroid crisis or thyroid storm is a rare endocrine emergency of hyperthyroidism in children. Clinical features are acute onset of:
- Hyperthermia
- Restlessness and delirium
- Severe tachycardia
- Heart failure.

It may rapidly progress to delirium, coma and death unless treated at the earliest.

PATHOGENESIS

Due to the potentiating action of catecholamines by the thyroid hormones in high level.

Precipitating Events

Infection, trauma, radioactive iodine therapy and surgery.

DIFFERENTIAL DIAGNOSIS AND MANAGEMENT

- Viral myocarditis
- Scorpion envenomation.

Patient Approach

General

- Admit in pediatric intensive care unit (PICU); administer oxygen; proceed to parallel history and physical examination.
- Stabilize ABC; assess blood glucose, correct the abnormality.
- Send blood for T_3, T_4 and free T_3, free T_4, TSH, Serum Electrolytes (SE), glucose, complete blood count (CBC), renal function test (RFT) and liver function test (LFT).
- The supportive lab findings are elevated T_3, T_4 and free T_3, T_4 and low TSH.
- Assess electrocardiogram (ECG) for tachycardia and arrhythmias; proceed to corrective measures.
- IV fluids—correction of shock followed by maintenance fluid therapy.
- Restrict fluids to 2/3 maintenance if in cardiac failure.
- Digitalization if needed.
- Correction of electrolyte imbalance.
- Treat fever with paracetamol or cooling blanket; avoid aspirin.
- Sedation with phenobarbitone for restlessness.
- Administer multivitamins.

Specific Therapy

- Propyl thiouracil 400 mg q 8 hours PO; administer through NG tube if vomiting.
- Saturated solution of potassium iodide 3 drops q 8 hours.
- Propranolol 1 mg/kg IV q 6 hours till heart rate slows down (avoid in cardiac failure or asthma).
- Prednisone 20 mg q 12 hours till stable.
- Supportive therapy:
  - Treat infection or other precipitating factors.

CONCLUSION

In children presenting with delirium, restlessness, tachycardia, and cardiac failure, consider the possibility of thyroid storm which can be effectively treated with propylthiouracil, steroids, potassium iodide, and propranolol.

Chapter 53

Disorders of Electrolyte Metabolism

S Sushamabai

ABSTRACT

Chapter deals with the deficiency and excess of five important electrolytes, namely, sodium, potassium, calcium, magnesium, and phosphorus. The life-threatening effects of the imbalance of these electrolytes are seizures, coma, paralysis, and cardiac arrhythmias. The diagnostic criteria, pathogenesis, investigations, and systematic management of these dyselectrolytemias are dealt with.

HYPERNATREMIA

Definition

Serum sodium (serum Na) concentration more than 145 mEq/L.

Causes

- Water loss:
  - Diarrhea, vomiting, nasogastric aspiration
  - Diuretics (mannitol), osmotic cathartics (lactulose)
  - Babies under radiant warmers
  - Excessive sweating
  - Burns
  - Diabetes mellitus and insipidus
  - Acute tubular necrosis, chronic renal failure
- Excess sodium intake:
  - Improper formula, oral rehydration salt (ORS)
  - Sodium bicarbonate therapy (oral/parenteral)
  - Intentional salt intake (child abuse)
  - Iatrogenic—oral or intravenous (IV) fluids.

Clinical Presentation

- Irritability, restlessness, weakness, lethargy, thirst, fever, seizures, and coma.

- Signs of dehydration may be masked—"Doughy feel of skin pinch of abdomen".
- Clinical features of underlying illness will be superimposed.

Pathophysiology

Acute and severe hypernatremia causes osmotic shift of water from neurons leading to shrinkage of the brain, tearing of the blood vessels, and intracranial hemorrhage.

Complications

Brain hemorrhage—can be subarachnoid, subdural or parenchymal.

Patient Approach

- Suspect hypernatremia in children with diarrhea, vomiting, irritability, convulsions, coma, renal disease or any serious illness.
- Admit in pediatric intensive care unit (PICU); stabilize airway, breathing, and circulation (ABC); parallel history and physical examination to assess the etiology and severity.
- Send blood for serum electrolytes, renal function test (RFT), and random blood sugar.
- Treat shock with normal saline (NS) 10–20 mL/kg in 20–60 minutes till it is corrected.
- Control seizures—Ideal drug is fosphenytoin.
- Plan further investigations as per etiology.
- Estimate the fluid deficit for hypernatremia (deficit = 4 mL/kg/each mEq of Na >145 mEq/L).
- Calculate hourly fluid requirement as—maintenance + deficit/48 hours.
- Type of fluid is 1/4–1/2 NS in 5% dextrose, add KCl 20 mEq/L (in children without dehydration, initial bolus NS is not needed).
- Assess the time for correction of hypernatremia based on initial sodium concentration as:
    - 145–157 mEq/L = 24 hours
    - 158–170 mEq/L = 48 hours
    - 171–183 mEq/L = 72 hours
    - 184–196 mEq/L = 84 hours
- Monitor serum Na 4–6 hourly
- Adjust the sodium content of the fluid based on subsequent serum sodium levels; rate of fall of serum Na should be 10–12 mEq/L/24 hr
- Consider dialysis if serum Na is more than 180 mEq/L
- Treat the etiology.

Flowchart 53.1: Management of hypernatremia.

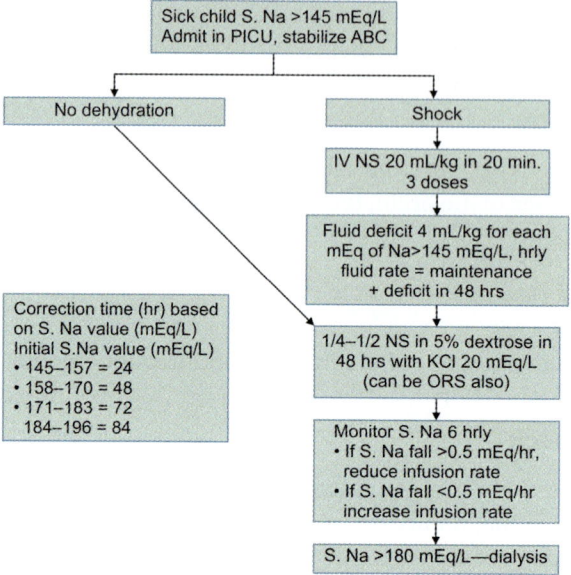

(ABC, airway, breathing, and circulation; IV, intravenous; NS, normal saline; ORS, oral rehydration solution; PICU, pediatric intensive care unit; S. Na, serum sodium)

Children not sick and tolerating oral feeds can be managed with ORS, normal food and low salt fluid or drinking water (Flowchart 53.1).

HYPONATREMIA

Definition

Serum Na less than 135 mEq/L.

Hyponatremia is a common electrolyte abnormality seen in critically ill children, can occur with normal, low or high amounts of total body sodium. Clinical presentation and management depends on:
- Acute (<48 hr) or chronic (>48 hr).

Etiology

- *Hypovolemic* (total body sodium << total body water):
  - Extra renal loss (urine Na <10 mEq/L)—diarrhea, vomiting, sweating, fistulas, drains, third space loss, and cerebral salt wasting.
  - Renal loss (urine Na >20 mEq/L)—diuretic therapy, osmotic diuresis (mannitol), renal tubular acidosis, and adrenal insufficiency.

- *Eu/normovolemic* (total body water > total body Na, urine Na >10 mEq/L)
  - Central nervous system—infections (meningitis, encephalitis), trauma, tumors, and syndrome of inappropriate antidiuretic hormone.
  - Respiratory—asthma, pneumonia.
  - Drug-induced—vincristine, cyclophosphamide.
  - Postoperative.
- *Hypervolemic* (total body water >> body Na, urine Na <10 mEq/L)
  - Chorionic villus sampling—congestive cardiac failure
  - Hepatic—chronic or acute liver failure
  - Renal—nephrotic syndrome and renal failure.

Clinical Presentation

- *Mild hyponatremia (Serum Na 120–130 mEq/L)*
  - Headache, vomiting, lethargy, confusion
  - Depressed deep tendon reflexes
  - Can be in apparent.
- *Severe hyponatremia (Serum. Na <120 mEq/L)*
  - Coma, seizures, features of brainstem herniation, apnea, cardiac arrhythmias, shock, and central diabetes insipidus *(Note—symptoms can occur with rapid fall of S. Na to 125 mEq/L).*

Pathophysiology

- Hyposmolality due to hyponatremia produces influx of water intracellularly leading to cerebral edema, raised intracranial pressure, brain ischemia, and herniation.
- Extrusion of intracellular electrolytes and organic osmolytes (such as glutamate and aspartate which are excitatory amino acids) can produce seizures without obvious cerebral edema.

Patient Approach

- Suspect hyponatremia in any child with dehydration, critical illness, seizures, and coma
- Admit in PICU; stabilize ABC; assess blood glucose; send blood for serum. Na, K, venous blood gas (VBG), serum osmolality, urine Na, urine osmolality, RFT and others as per suspected etiology.
- While stabilizing the child assess, the duration of hyponatremia as acute or chronic and the body fluid volume (as normo-, hypo- or hypervolemic) by brief history and physical examination; in most situations it will be possible.
- Treat hypotension first irrespective of the serum sodium level with IV bolus NS 20 mL/kg in 20–60 minutes up to three doses as per need.
- Proceed to detailed history and physical examination.

Further Correction

- *Acute and symptomatic hyponatremia:*
  - Rapid correction with 3% saline—4–6 mL/kg in 1–2 hours (1 mL/kg of 3% saline increases serum. Na 1 mEq/L).
  - Stop 3% saline infusion once the child is symptom free or acute rise in serum. Na of 10 mEq/L is noted in first 5 hours.
  - Correct the remaining deficit over 24–48 hours; the quantity of sodium deficit is calculated by the following formula:

  $$\text{mEq of Na} = (Cd - Ca) \times Fd \times \text{body weight in kg}$$

  [Cd is the desired concentration = 135 mEq/L, Ca is the actual sodium concentration, Fd is the fractional distribution of Na in the body = 0.6]
  - The rate of correction is 0.6–1 mEq/L/hr till S. Na is 125 mEq/L and then at a slower rate.
  - The type of fluid is 5% dextrose with 0.45% NS. Add KCl 20 mEq/L if there is hypokalemia.

Note—rapid correction can lead to central pontine myelinolysis and permanent damage.

- *Chronic hyponatremia:*
  - Correct the deficit over 48–72 hours (calculation as above)—rate of correction being 0.5 mEq/L/hr.
- *Asymptomatic hyponatremia:*
  - World Health Organization ORS 245 in maintenance dose till correction is complete.
- *Hypervolemic hyponatremia:*
  - Restrict sodium and water intake two-thirds to one-half of the maintenance requirement.
- *Syndrome of inappropriate antidiuretic hormone:*
  - Fluid restriction two-thirds of maintenance requirement.
- *Treat the underlying cause:*
  - Addison disease—IV hydrocortisone
  - Renal failure—dialysis
  - Drug induced—stop, reduce or change the drug
  - Hypoalbuminemia—IV 25% albumin infusion (0.5–1 g/kg) slow infusion in 2 hours followed by IV furosemide 1–2 mg/kg.

Monitoring

- Clinical: Hourly vitals, Glasgow Coma Scale, pupils, SpO_2, input/output chart
- Laboratory: Serum Na 4–6 hourly—others as per situation.

Sodium content of various preparations:
- 1 mL 3% saline = 0.5 mEq
- 1 mL NS = 0.15 mEq
- 1 mL low Osm ORS = 0.075 mEq
- 1 g common salt = 17 mEq.

HYPERKALEMIA

Hyperkalemia indicates high serum potassium (Serum K); age-wise values being:
- Less than 2 months: More than 7 mmol/L
- More than 2–12 months: More than 6 mmol/L
- More than 12 months: More than 5 mmol/L

Hyperkalemia is a life-threatening emergency and should be controlled immediately.

Causes

- *Pseudohyperkalemia:*
    - Squeezed or hemolyzed sample
    - Sample from the limb infused with potassium-rich fluid
    - Thrombocytosis and leukocytosis.
- *True hyperkalemia:*
    - Increased intake (oral, IV fluid, packed cell transfusion)
    - Renal failure, renal tubular acidosis type IV
    - Drug-induced—angiotensin-converting enzyme (ACE) inhibitors, diuretics, and nonsteroidal anti-inflammatory drugs
    - Adrenal insufficiency—congenital or acquired
    - Acidosis
    - Massive hemolysis
    - Tumor lysis syndrome
    - Periodic paralysis.

Clinical Presentation

- Nausea, vomiting, paresthesia, twitching, and fatigue
- Suspect hyperkalemia in a critically ill child, especially if any of the above factors are associated
- Cardiac arrhythmias.

Patient Approach

- Admit in PICU; stabilize ABC
- Immediate electrocardiogram (ECG) to assess the severity (Table 53.1)

Table 53.1: ECG changes in hyperkalemia.

Abnormality	Serum K (mmol/L)
Tented T waves (>10 mm)	5.5–6.5
Prolonged PR interval Flat P waves QRS widening	>6.5–8
Absent P waves Bundle branch blocks Sine waves	>8

- Send blood samples for serum K (assess plasma K if accurate value is needed), blood gas analysis, blood sugar, RFT, others as per indication.

Correction of Hyperkalemia

- Discontinue potassium containing fluids and drugs inducing hyperkalemia
- Stabilize myocardial membrane to prevent fatal arrhythmia:
  - Intravenous 10% calcium gluconate 0.5 mL/kg in 5–10 minutes (immediate action, infuse in 30 minutes if on digoxin, discontinue if bradycardia develops)
- Enhance cellular uptake of potassium:
  - Nebulized salbutamol 0.5–1 mL in 3 mL NS in 20 minutes (rapid action, lasts for 2 hours)
  - Intravenous sodium bicarbonate 1 mEq/kg in 5% dextrose in 5–10 minutes (immediate action)
  - Intravenous regular insulin 0.1 U/kg with 50% glucose solution 1 mL/kg over 1 hour (onset of action by 30 minutes)
- Eliminate body potassium (especially in renal failure):
  - Sodium polystyrene sulfonate (Kayexalate) oral or per rectum (PR) 1 g/kg up to a maximum of 15 g/dose in 20% sorbitol; repeat every 2 hours; onset of action in 1 hour; lowers serum K 1 mEq/L
  - Intravenous furosemide 1 mg/kg
  - Thiazide diuretics (if renal function is normal) 2 mg/kg in 2 divided doses daily
  - Hemodialysis
- Specific therapy for the etiology (e.g. steroids, mineralocorticoids in Addison disease) (Flowchart 53.2).

Flowchart 53.2: Management of hyperkalemia.

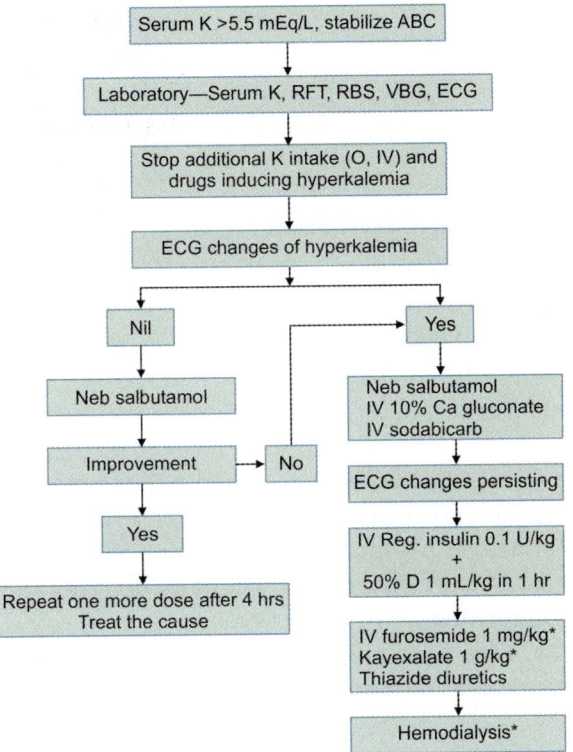

*In renal failure.
(ABC, airway, breathing, and circulation, ECG, electrocardiogram; IV, intravenous; RBS, random blood sugar; RFT, renal function test)

HYPOKALEMIA

Hypokalemia is defined as serum K less than 3.5 mEq/L. The condition is common in children, but perceived less and is potentially fatal if not corrected promptly.

Causes

- Gastrointestinal loss—diarrhea, vomiting, nasogastric aspiration, and laxative use
- Poor intake—severe acute malnutrition and improper parenteral fluid therapy
- Renal loss—renal tubular acidosis, Cushing syndrome, congenital adrenal hyperplasia, high renin conditions, and syndromes (Bartter, Gitelman, Liddle)

- Drug-induced—diuretics, insulin, salbutamol, and steroids
- Hypomagnesemia.

Clinical Presentation

Muscle weakness, hypotonia, neck flop, paralysis, ileus, and cardiac arrhythmias.

Patient Approach (Flowchart 53.3)

- Suspect hypokalemia in critically ill children, those with contributory factors and in cardiac arrhythmias.
- Admit in PICU; stabilize ABC; document blood pressure; the value will be helpful to assess the etiology.
- Send blood for serum K, serum Na, serum magnesium (S. Mg), VBG, and RFT.
- Assess the severity by ECG changes (T wave flattening, ST depression, U wave appearance, arrhythmias in the order of severity).
- Decide treatment as per the severity, cause, renal status, and duration of hypokalemia. Usually the etiology will be evident from the history and physical examination.
- Consider 24 hours urine potassium (U_K) estimation if the etiology is not clear (spot U_K creatinine ratio also is reliable).

Treatment

- Stop all ongoing loss (diuretic therapy) and correct hypomagnesemia.
- Immediate correction of dehydration by bolus NS.

Flowchart 53.3: Diagnostic approach to hypokalemia.

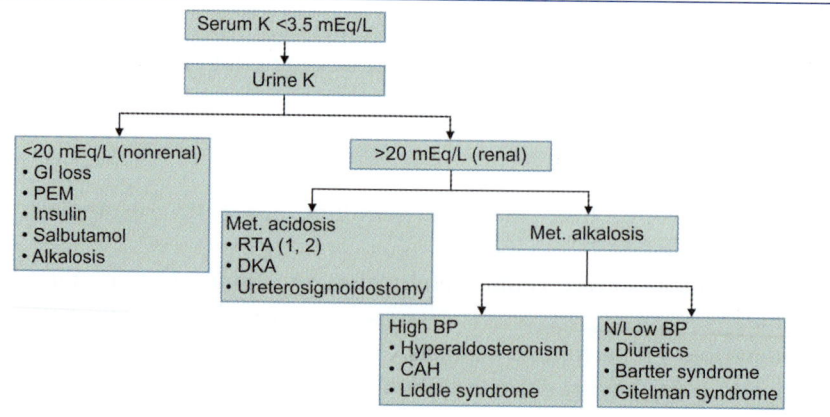

(BP, blood pressure; CAH, congenital adrenal hyperplasia; DKA, diabetic ketoacidosis; GI, gastrointestinal; PEM, protein–energy malnutrition; RTA, renal tubular acidosis)

- Acidosis should be corrected only after bringing serum K up to 2.8 mEq/L
- Correction of hypokalemia:
    - Mild form (Serum K 2.5–3.5 mEq/L): Oral potassium chloride solution (15 mL = 20 mEq) 2–4 mEq/kg/day, maximum 240 mEq/day divided q6 hours. Dilution and sweetening is needed as the solution is bitter. If intolerant to oral preparation consider IV infusion as written for severe form.
    - Severe form (Serum K <2.5 mEq/L or clinically cardiac arrhythmia): Requires IV replacement. Increase the concentration of potassium in the IV fluid up to 40 mEq/L (use potassium chloride, acetate or phosphate as per underlying clinical situation). Infuse at 0.5 mEq/kg/hr. ECG monitoring is recommended
    - Disease-specific therapy:
        - Lifelong potassium supplementation in renal tubular acidosis.
        - ACE inhibitors in Bartter and Gitelman syndromes.
        - Triamterene in Liddle syndrome.
- Correction of hypomagnesemia.

HYPERCALCEMIA

Hypercalcemia is defined as serum calcium (S. Ca) more than 11 mg/dL. Even mild persistent elevation requires detailed investigations since Ca metabolism is tightly controlled by the body.

Causes

- Hyperparathyroidism
- Vitamin D intoxication
- Malignancies—leukemia, lymphoma, neuroblastoma
- Granulomatous disease—sarcoidosis, tuberculosis
- Thyrotoxicosis
- Prolonged immobilization
- Intake of thiazide diuretics.

Clinical Presentation

- Weakness, fatigue, and irritability
- Anorexia, nausea, and abdominal pain
- Acute pancreatitis
- Renal calculi, polyuria, and polydipsia
- Cardiac arrhythmias.

Investigations

- Serum calcium more than 11 mg/dL
- Serum phosphorus will be less than 3 mg/dL
- Normal alkaline phosphatase
- Elevated parathyroid hormone (PTH) in hyperparathyroidism
- Other investigations as per suspected etiology.

Treatment

- Stop vitamin D and Ca supplementation and diuretic therapy.
- Promote urinary Ca excretion—administer IV NS to produce urine output 3–5 mL/kg/hr; monitor potassium.
- Intravenous furosemide to increase urine output; watch for other electrolyte imbalance when furosemide is given.
- Peritoneal or hemodialysis in renal failure.
- Treatment of underlying cause.
- The safety of bisphosphonates in children is not well-established.

HYPOCALCEMIA

Hypocalcemia is defined as serum Ca less than 8 mg/dL or ionized calcium less than 4 mg/dL.

Normal serum Ca is 8.8–10.8 mg/dL.

Causes

- Vitamin D deficiency
- Disorders of vitamin D metabolism
- Hypoparathyroidism
- Protein–energy malnutrition
- Hypomagnesemia
- Renal failure
- Renal tubular acidosis
- Acute pancreatitis
- Metabolic alkalosis
- Tumor lysis syndrome.

Clinical Presentation

- Seizures, irritability, and muscle cramps
- Laryngospasm
- Tetany
- Growth retardation.

Patient Approach

Symptomatic

- Admit in PICU; stabilize ABC.
- Send blood for sugar, Ca, Mg, Na, K, and VBG estimation.
- Electrocardiogram evaluation for QTc which will be increased (depends on the severity and etiology—N <0.45).
- Intravenous 10% calcium gluconate 1–2 mL/kg (elemental Ca 9.3 mg/mL) slowly, monitoring the heart rate; repeat 6 hourly for 24–48 hours *Caution—intravenous calcium gluconate, if extravasated, can produce severe tissue necrosis.*
- Continue treatment with oral calcium 40–80 mg/kg/day of elemental calcium (calcium carbonate yields 40% elemental calcium) till the etiology is corrected.
- Correction of Mg deficiency, acidosis or alkalosis, if detected.
- Vitamin D supplementation in deficiency, liver or renal diseases; use the appropriate preparation.

HYPERMAGNESEMIA

Definition

Plasma magnesium (Mg) more than 2.5 mg/dL. Symptomatic hypermagnesemia occurs with values more than 4.5 mg/dL, a rarely encountered pediatric emergency.

Causes

- Increased intake—antacids, laxatives, enema, acute asthma on IV magnesium sulfate therapy
- Transplacental transfer in neonates if high maternal levels of Mg
- Chronic renal failure
- Tumor lysis syndrome.

Pathophysiology

High Mg inhibits acetyl choline release, the effects being exaggerated by aminoglycoside antibiotics.

Clinical Presentation

- Flushing, lethargy, poor suck, hypotonia, and hyporeflexia
- Nausea and vomiting
- Resistant hypocalcemia
- Hypotension, cardiac arrhythmias, and respiratory muscle weakness.

Investigations
- Plasma Mg, serum Ca, and RFT
- Electrocardiogram—prolonged PR, QRST intervals.

Diagnosis
- Clinical presentation, history suggestive of increased intake, and renal failure
- Laboratory confirmation.

Treatment
- Stop excess Mg intake (oral, enema, IV, intramuscular)
- Hydration (oral, IV) to produce diuresis
- Loop diuretic—furosemide 1-2 mg/kg q12 hourly
- Hemodialysis in renal failure
- Cardiac arrhythmia or respiratory muscle paralysis, renal failure—intravenous calcium gluconate 100 mg/kg equally diluted slowly
- Respiratory and cardiac support.

HYPOMAGNESEMIA

Hypomagnesemia is serum Mg below 1.5 mEq/L (*N* value—1.5-2.3 mg/dL). Symptomatic hypomagnesemia occurs if the value is less than 1.2 mEq/L. Severe hypomagnesemia is serum Mg 0.2-0.8 mg/dL. Though a common clinical situation, it is rarely recognized.

Causes
- Gastrointestinal losses—diarrhea, vomiting, nasogastric suction, and chronic malabsorption
- Renal—chronic use of thiazide diuretics, mannitol therapy, recovery phase of acute tubular necrosis, Gitelman and Bartter syndromes, familial hypomagnesemia-hypercalciuria nephrocalcinosis
- Protein-energy malnutrition refeeding phase
- Intrauterine growth retardation
- Infants of diabetic mothers
- Diabetic ketoacidosis
- Pancreatitis.

Clinical Presentation

Clinical features are secondary to hypocalcemia (by impairing the release of PTH) and hypokalemia as follows:
- Tetany, seizures, and signs of latent tetany
- Hypotonia, ileus, neck flop, and cardiac arrhythmias
- Suspect in refractory hypocalcemia and hypokalemia.

Investigations

- Serum magnesium, other electrolytes as per suspected etiology
- Renal function test
- Urine Mg 24 hours sample or spot urine Mg creatinine ratio.

Treatment

- Severe hypomagnesemia—intravenous Mg sulfate 25–50 mg/kg (0.05–0.1 mL/kg of 50% solution or 2.5–5 mg/kg of elemental Mg) as slow infusion, repeated q6 hourly for two to three doses. Consider lower doses in renal insufficiency.
- Long-term therapy—Oral Mg gluconate provides 5.4 mg of elemental Mg/100 mg preparation. Sustained release oral preparations or intramuscular injections are alternatives but should be used with caution in renal insufficiency.

HYPERPHOSPHATEMIA

Definition

Increase in plasma phosphorus (P) above the normal range for age as shown below:

Age	Phosphorus (mg/dL)
0–5 days	4.8–8.2
1–3 years	3.8–6.5
4–11 years	3.7–5.6
12–15 years	2.9–5.4
16–19 years	2.7–4.7

Causes

- Chronic renal failure
- Excessive intake (cow's milk, medicinal)
- Phosphate retention enemas and laxatives
- Vitamin D intoxication
- Hypoparathyroidism
- Tumor lysis syndrome
- Rhabdomyolysis
- Acute hemolysis
- Hyperthyroidism.

Clinical Features

- Features of hypocalcemia
- Systemic calcification—renal, pulmonary, and conjunctival

Laboratory Evaluation

- Blood urea and serum creatinine
- Serum electrolytes and uric acid
- Others as per suspected etiology.

Treatment

- Mild form with normal renal function:
    - Restrict dietary phosphate (milk, egg, meat, and fish), intravenous fluids to enhance renal function.
- Severe form:
    - Oral phosphorus binder—calcium carbonate along with food
    - Dialysis especially in renal failure
- Chronic hyperphosphatemia:
    - Diet restriction and phosphorus binders
- Treat the etiology.

HYPOPHOSPHATEMIA

Definition

Plasma phosphorus below the normal range for age (refer to "Hyperphosphatemia" section of this chapter).

Causes

- Vitamin D deficiency
- Rickets (hypophosphatemic, Fanconi syndrome)
- Protein-energy malnutrition
- Refeeding syndrome
- Sepsis
- Metabolic acidosis
- Respiratory alkalosis
- Drug-induced—diuretics, glucocorticoids, antacids, and phosphate binders
- Insulin infusion
- Premature infants
- Hungry bone syndrome
- Dialysis
- Total parenteral nutrition.

Clinical Features

Can be acute or chronic; severe hypophosphatemia (<1.5 mg/dL) can be life-threatening; features are as follows:
- Rickets in chronic cases

- Rhabdomyolysis (if severe acute)
- Neurologic—proximal muscle weakness, atrophy, tremors, ataxia, seizures, delirium, and coma
- Respiratory—acute respiratory failure and ventilator dependence
- Cardiac arrhythmias.

Diagnosis

From history, physical examination, and investigations.

Investigations

- Serum calcium, P, alkaline phosphatase, 25 OH D, PTH
- Others as per etiology revealed by clinical assessment.

Treatment

- Mild chronic depletion—oral phosphate in divided doses; treat the etiology
- Severe—intravenous Na/K phosphate depending on plasma K level—dose 0.8–1.6 mmol/kg over 6 hours followed by 2–3 mmol/kg/day in divided doses:
    - Increase the intake of dietary phosphate (dairy products, meat, fish)
    - Discontinue phosphate binding agents
    - Disease-specific therapy.

CONCLUSION

In all critically ill children, serum electrolyte estimation and appropriate correction is mandatory.

Chapter 54

Hyperammonemia

S Sushamabai

ABSTRACT

Hyperammonemia (plasma ammonia >300 mmol/L) is a fatal metabolic emergency. The causes can be inborn errors of metabolism (IEM) or acquired liver failure of acute or chronic nature. Pathogenesis is development of brain edema and encephalopathy. The condition has to be suspected in children with recurrent vomiting, seizures, and progressive liver disease. The clinical features are similar to liver failure—varying degrees of altered sensorium, seizures, bulging fontanel, papilledema, jaundice, and hepatomegaly. The treatment is as for hepatic encephalopathy along with elimination of ammonia by administering sodium benzoate, sodium phenyl acetate, and arginine hydrochloride. Megavitamin therapy is empirically advised in IEM. Peritoneal or hemodialysis (preferable) for hyperammonemia should be considered if medical therapy fails. L-carnitine is beneficial in carnitine deficiency disorders and is needed in children getting benzoate therapy.

INTRODUCTION

Hyperammonemia is a fatal metabolic emergency due to increased plasma ammonia (>300 μmol/L) of diverse etiology. The situation is not uncommon in children but is rarely recognized and managed appropriately.

CAUSES

- Inborn errors of metabolism—urea cycle disorders, organic acidemias, lysinuric protein intolerance, hyperornithinemia–hyperammonemia–homocitrullinuria syndrome, transient hyperammonemia of the new born, and hyperinsulinemic hyperammonemia
- Acute or chronic liver failure (drug-induced or congenital or acquired liver diseases)
- Sepsis.

PATHOPHYSIOLOGY

- Ammonia is the toxic end product of amino acid catabolism which is normally converted to urea by liver and is excreted through urine.
- Excess ammonia is converted to osmotically active glutamine by the astrocytes in the brain leading to brain edema and encephalopathy.
- In metabolic disorders and sepsis, excess ammonia accumulates whereas in liver diseases, degradation to urea and excretion do not occur.
- The clinical manifestations of hyperammonemia are due to brain edema associated with the underlying etiology.

CLINICAL PRESENTATION

- Vomiting, poor feeding, lethargy, tachypnea, convulsions, and deepening coma
- Recurrent episodes of encephalitis.
- Signs of raised increased intracranial pressure (ICP)—bulging fontanel, dilated pupils (in the new born period and infancy), and papilledema (older age group).
- Evidence of underlying diseases—jaundice, hepatomegaly, bleeding tendency, and features of sepsis.
- Features of hyperammonemia in early infancy are usually due to inborn errors of metabolism
- In a previously diagnosed child, symptoms can be precipitated if treatment is irregular, after high protein intake or infections.

PATIENT APPROACH

- Initial stabilization (airway, breathing, and circulation) and therapy for brain edema depending on the severity of the situation (Chapter 33).
- After stabilization proceed to detailed history. Unexplained sibling death, seizures, mental retardation, recurrent encephalopathy, Reye-like syndrome, recurrent vomiting, and food intolerance in blood relatives may indicate inborn errors of metabolism.
- Physical examination—assess for failure to thrive, developmental delay, abnormal odors (body, urine), dysmorphism, jaundice, hepatosplenomegaly, and neurological abnormality.

LABORATORY EVALUATION

- Urine—routine, culture, neurometabolic screening (NMS) which includes reducing sugars (glucose, galactose, and fructose), ketone bodies,

dinitrophenylhydrazine for keto acids, $FeCl_3$ test, cetyltrimethylammonium bromide for mucopolysaccharides, and acetone.
- Blood—complete hemogram, culture, serum glutamic pyruvic transaminase, glucose, renal function test, venous blood gas, plasma ammonia (ideally fasting), pyruvate, and lactate.
- Ultrasonography (USG) abdomen to evaluate the liver and other abdominal organs.
- Cerebrospinal fluid—cell count, biochemistry including lactate, culture.
- Others as per indication.

Note—plasma ammonia is to be estimated immediately after collection. It is mandatory for each laboratory to have standardized value.

DIAGNOSIS

From the history, physical examination and screening investigations for liver disease and sepsis.

DIFFERENTIAL DIAGNOSIS

- Sepsis
- Meningitis
- Chemical or drug poisoning
- Hepatic or renal failure
- Recurrent encephalitis of other etiology.

Remember—a child having compensated hyperammonemia, encephalopathy can be precipitated by superadded infection, vomiting, or high-protein diet.

Proceed as per Table 54.1 for the diagnosis by interpreting plasma NH_3, pH, pCO_2, and urine NMS.

Table 54.1: Laboratory interpretation in hyperammonemia.

Disease	Plasma NH_3	pH, pCO_2	Urine NMS	Plan
Urea cycle disorder	High/N	Met. alkalosis	Normal	Further inv
Organic acidemias	N/High	Anion gap acidosis	$FeCl_3$+ Ketosis+ DNPH+	Further inv
Amino acidopathy	N	Normal	DNPH+	Further inv
Galactosemia	N	Normal	Reducing Sugar+	Further inv

(DNPH, dinitrophenylhydrazine; NMS, neurometabolic screening)

TREATMENT

- Nil oral till diagnosis of hyperammonemia is confirmed and the sensorium has started improving.
- Gastric decompression and intravenous (IV) ranitidine.
- Correction of dehydration by bolus normal saline (NS). Maintenance fluid—1/2 NS with 10% dextrose to prevent protein catabolism (add lipids 1–2 g/kg/24 hr + proteins 0.25 g/kg/24 hr as per availability).
- Vitamin K or fresh frozen plasma as per requirement.
- Correction of acidosis—intravenous sodium bicarbonate/peritoneal/hemodialysis.
- Treat the precipitating event—fever control and sepsis.
- Control of seizures (lorazepam, fosphenytoin), and raised ICP (mannitol, 3% saline).
- Empirical megavitamin therapy—thiamine 100–500 mg, riboflavin 100–500 mg, biotin 5–20 mg, pyridoxine 40 mg, vitamin B12 1 mg/day as per suspected metabolic disorder.
- Elimination of body ammonia:
    - Fluids and electrolytes as described.
    - Remove the excess ammonia by priming dose as described in Table 54.2
    - Continue infusion (benzoate and acetate 250–500 mg/kg/24 hr each + arginine 200–600 mg/kg/24 hr) added to the daily IV fluid
    - If IV preparations are not available, oral sodium benzoate and acetate in same dose can be used q 6 hourly.
    - Consider peritoneal or hemodialysis if no improvement.
- Carnitine 50–100 mg/kg/24 hr div q 12 hourly for children having carnitine deficiency or on benzoate therapy.
- Switch over to oral feeds (protein 0.5–1 g/kg/day) and drugs (benzoate and acetate 250–500 mg/kg/day div q 6 hourly).

Arrange follow-up evaluation and detailed investigations. Protein-restricted diet (0.5–1 g/kg/day) or appropriate readymade protein diet for

Table 54.2: Elimination of body ammonia.	
Sodium benzoate	250 mg/kg
Sodium phenyl acetate	250–500 mg/kg
Arginine hydrochloride	200–600 mg/kg*

To be added to 10% glucose as 20 mL/kg infusion in 1–2 hours.
Sodium content of the preparation should be calculated in the daily intake.
*Avoid in organic acidemia and arginase deficiency.

the metabolic disorder is to be adhered lifelong. Most children gradually recover and can be maintained on protein-restricted calorie-sufficient vitamin-enriched diet.

CONCLUSION

Hyperammonemia is an occasional fatal emergency encountered in children, can be due to IEM or liver disease; is to be treated as for hepatic encephalopathy along with sodium benzoate and acetate and arginine hydrochloride.

Chapter **55**

Approach to Inborn Errors of Metabolism

S Sushamabai

ABSTRACT

Inborn errors of metabolism (IEM) are inherited disorders of metabolism causing altered protein synthesis. They can present as trivial to lethal illness. The common age group is newborn to infancy. The clinical features are lethargy, poor feeding, vomiting, convulsions, failure to thrive (FTT), recurrent encephalopathy, unexplained organomegaly, developmental delay or regression, mental retardation, muscle weakness and cardiomyopathy. This chapter deals with the systematic approach, laboratory evaluation and treatment. Supportive therapy for fluid and electrolyte maintenance, seizure control, treatment of hyperammonemia and megavitamin therapy are included.

INTRODUCTION

Inborn errors of metabolism (IEM) or inherited disorders of metabolism are single-gene mutation disorders causing altered protein synthesis and manifest as varying spectrum of diseases of trivial to lethal nature. These proteins can be enzymes, receptors, transport vehicles, membranes or structural elements. The mutations can produce structural (qualitative) or quantitative defect. Clinical manifestations are due to:
- End-product deficiency (essential metabolite)
- Accumulation of intermediate toxic metabolite
- Accumulated metabolites of alternate pathways.

CLINICAL PRESENTATION

- Common age group is newborn period to infancy
- The affected infant is normal at birth; becomes symptomatic within days to months (this point rules out birth injuries, intrauterine insults or infections, chromosomal abnormalities or other genetic diseases)
- The common symptoms are:
  - *Newborns:*
    - Lethargy, poor feeding, vomiting, and jaundice

- Convulsions not responding to intravenous (IV) glucose or calcium
- Coma.

Note—consider IEM as a possibility in neonates with suspected sepsis without any conclusive evidence.
- *Older age group*—additional manifestations are:
  - Failure to thrive, unusual odor of body or urine, abnormal urine color
  - Developmental delay or regression
  - Recurrent seizures
  - Mental retardation or growth retardation
  - Features of renal failure or renal stones
  - Liver failure or gall stones
  - Unexplained organomegaly
  - Muscle weakness or cardiomyopathy
  - Recurrent encephalopathy or Reye-like syndrome.

PATIENT APPROACH

- Suspect the possibility of IEM in a sick neonate, or any child with the above symptoms.
- Admit in pediatric intensive care unit if sick; stabilize airway, breathing, and circulation (ABC); correct dehydration and hypoglycemia; proceed to detailed evaluation after stabilization.
- Enquire past history of recurrent episodes of seizures or the features mentioned above, treatment given, outcome, investigations done and their reports.
- Family history consanguinity, abortion, sibling deaths due to undiagnosed illness, mental retardation, seizures, and developmental delay or regression.
- Physical examination for:
  - Abnormal body or urine odor, body color (albinism, jaundice), and hair changes
  - Failure to thrive, micro or macrocephaly, cataract, developmental delay, spasticity, and hypotonia.

LABORATORY EVALUATION

- *See* Table 54.1 for investigations.
- Additional investigations for urea cycle disorders, organic acidemias and amino acidopathy as per diagnosis made by the clinical details and screening investigation results.

TREATMENT

- Supportive therapy—ABC stabilization, correction of hypoglycemia
- Fluid and electrolyte balance
- Treatment of hyperammonemia (refer to Chapter 54)
- Seizure control
- Control of fever and sepsis
- Special diets as per diagnosis (if available); otherwise, protein-restricted calorie adequate and vitamin-rich diet should be advised (refer to Chapter 54)
- Peritoneal or hemodialysis to remove the accumulated noxious compounds
- Activation of alternate pathways to reduce the noxious compounds, e.g. sodium benzoate and phenyl acetate as in hyperammonemia
- Administration of deficient metabolites:
    - Carnitine—50 mg/kg/day as IV infusion in carnitine deficiency followed by oral preparation
    - Thiamine—100–500 mg/day in pyruvate dehydrogenase deficiency and maple syrup urine disease
    - Biotin—5–20 mg/day in biotinidase deficiency and propionic acidemia
    - Riboflavin—200–300 mg/day in glutaric aciduria type 1
    - Vitamin B12—1–2 mg/day in methyl malonic acidemia
    - Vitamin B6—200–1,000 mg/day in classic homocystinuria
- Plan for definite therapy—bone marrow or liver transplantation.

CONCLUSION

In infants and children presenting with lethargy, poor feeding, vomiting, seizures, FTT, recurrent encephalopathy, organomegaly and developmental delay or regression, IEM should be considered as differential diagnosis and appropriate management should be implemented at the earliest.

Heat Stroke

Manju George Elenjickal, S Sushamabai

ABSTRACT

Heat stroke is hyperthermia exceeding 40°C oral temperatures with altered sensorium leading to high mortality and is a preventable emergency. The situation is occasionally encountered in adolescents in sports activity and in child laborers. The body should be immediately cooled at the site itself. Immediate stabilization, fluid and electrolyte therapy, early dobutamine administration, seizure control, and management of metabolic complications are the treatment in the hospital. Cardiac arrhythmias and liver and renal failure are the serious complications encountered. This health hazard should be prevented by health education to avoid excess heat exposure and adequate fluid intake.

INTRODUCTION

Heat stroke is defined as hyperthermia exceeding 40°C oral temperature with altered sensorium with or without anhidrosis. It is a medical emergency with 50% mortality which is preventable.

CLINICAL PRESENTATION

It is of two types: (1) Exertional and (2) Nonexertional or classic.

Exertional Heat Stroke

- Affects young individuals during extreme physical exertion in a hot environment like children playing outdoor, child labor, and athletes.
- Features—hyperthermia, diaphoresis, and delirium.
- Preceding symptoms—nausea, vomiting, abdominal pain, muscle cramps, diarrhea, head ache, dizziness, weakness, dyspnea, and syncope.
- Complications—disseminated intravascular coagulation, acute renal failure, liver failure, rhabdomyolysis, and lactic acidosis.

Nonexertional Heat Stroke or Classic

- Affects older individuals in epidemic form during heat waves (periods of prolonged elevations in ambient temperature). Direct exposure to sunlight is not a prerequisite.
- Features—hyperthermia, altered sensorium, and anhidrosis.
- Predisposing factors—chronic preexisting diseases like congestive heart failure, diabetes, and renal or liver disease.
- Drug intake—diuretics, beta-blockers, vasodilators, antihistamines, and anticholinergics.
- Skin disorders with poor sweating—ectodermal dysplasia, scleroderma, and congenital absence of sweat glands.

Note—in both groups patients may present as emergency—coma, convulsions, and shock.

DIFFERENTIAL DIAGNOSIS

Conditions with high fever, tachypnea, and hypotension such as septic shock, severe pneumonia, meningitis, intracranial bleeding, other types of internal bleeding.

PATIENT APPROACH

- Have an index of suspicion of the possibility of heatstroke in children and adolescents subjected to child labor, vigorous exercise in hot environment, and those with other risk factors as mentioned earlier.
- Admit in pediatric intensive care unit; stabilize airway, breathing, and circulation; intubate if comatose; treat shock with normal saline/Ringer's lactate 20–30 mL/kg in 1 hour.
- Detailed history and physical examination to exclude the differential diagnosis.
- Once heat stroke is suspected, start cooling the body from the site where the patient is picked up. Immersion in cold water, transport in AC ambulance, removal of restrictive clothing, promotion of evaporative heat loss by intermittently spraying tepid water over the patient, blowing a fan, and applying ice packs over axilla and groin are various methods to bring down the body temperature.
- Massage vigorously the skin especially torso and neck to promote the return of cool peripheral blood to overheated brain and viscera.
- Continuous monitoring of core temperature, nasogastric aspiration to assess gastrointestinal bleeding and indwelling Foley catheter to assess urine output and renal status.

INVESTIGATIONS

Complete blood count, platelet count, urinalysis, random blood sugar, renal function tests (RFT), liver function test, creatine phosphokinase, chest X-ray, electrocardiography, serum electrolyte (Na, K, Ca, P), blood gas, echocardiography, cerebrospinal fluid studies, ultrasonography abdomen, CT or MRI brain as per clinical findings of organ impairment and possible differential diagnosis.

SUBSEQUENT MANAGEMENT

- Fluid and electrolyte administration to correct shock, hypoglycemia, and dyselectrolytemia.
- Monitor body temperature to bring it down to 39°C in 1 hour. Active measures for cooling can be stopped at this point.
- Continue supportive measures with monitoring till stable for 24 hours.

MONITORING

- Hourly vitals, SpO_2, Glasgow coma scale, watch for seizures
- 3 hourly gastric aspirate to detect internal bleeding
- 6 hourly input/output chart to assess renal status
- Urinalysis and RFT daily
- Evaluate for features of hepatic failure daily
- Others as per situation.

COMPLICATIONS

- Seizures—control with diazepam/lorazepam/barbiturates. Avoid phenytoin. If refractory, paralyze and ventilate.
- Shock—fluid resuscitation, dobutamine if fluid refractory.
- Cardiac arrhythmias, ischemia—fluid and electrolyte balance and specific therapy.
- Hepatic failure—avoid paracetamol and supportive therapy.
- Renal failure—due to rhabdomyolysis; liberal fluid resuscitation to maintain urine output 3 mL/kg/hr, urine alkalinization, and mannitol. Dialysis in resistant cases.
- Metabolic—problems encountered are hypoglycemia, hyperkalemia, hypophosphatemia, and hypocalcemia (latter three are due to muscle necrosis). Detect and treat.
- Compartmental syndrome due to muscle necrosis—surgical intervention, if needed.

PREVENTION

- Avoid excessive exposure to sun heat; proper fluid intake when the ambient temperature is high.
- Athletes should be given proper health education about the amount and type of fluid intake.
- Children with risk factors should be well-informed about the situation and adequate fluid intake should be advised.

CONCLUSION

Heat stroke is a preventable medical emergency especially encountered in adolescents in sports activity and in child laborers and should be treated aggressively.

Chapter 57

Severe Acute Malnutrition

S Sushamabai

ABSTRACT

Severe acute malnutrition (SAM) is a complex metabolic emergency due to reduced calorie and protein in the diet; delay in correction may lead to death or disability. The chapter deals with the diagnostic criteria and management as per World Health Organization (WHO) recommendations. The patient approach should be as immediate stabilization in the initial 2–7 days followed by subsequent rehabilitation which may spread for months. Initial stabilization is to correct hypoglycemia, hypothermia, dehydration, dyselectrolytemia, infections, micronutrient deficiency, and initiation of feeding with F-75 formula. Subsequent rehabilitation deals with continuation of feeding, catch-up growth, sensory stimulation, and follow-up program.

INTRODUCTION

Severe acute malnutrition is a complex metabolic emergency of protein energy undernutrition resulting in death if not treated appropriately in time. The diagnostic criteria (defined by WHO and United Nations International Children's Emergency Fund) are any one of the following:
- Weight for height less than 3 standard deviations of median WHO reference
- Visible severe wasting
- Presence of bipedal pitting edema
- Mid-upper arm circumference less than 11.5 cm (not applicable in infants <6 months age).

CAUSES

- Defective food intake—poverty, ignorance, food deprivation, broken families, diseases like cleft palate, gastrointestinal anomalies, and chronic diseases.

- Defective nutrient absorption or assimilation—malabsorption syndromes, chronic diarrhea, and inborn errors of metabolism (IEM)
- Increased demand—prematurity, low birth weight, chronic infections [like tuberculosis (TB) and human immunodeficiency virus (HIV)], hypercatabolic diseases like diabetes mellitus and insipidus, renal tubular acidosis, and chronic systemic diseases (congenital heart disease, congestive heart failure, chronic lung disease, and chronic renal failure).

Note—those with defective food supply are primary SAM whereas those subsequent to underlying diseases are secondary SAM.

CLINICAL PRESENTATION

- Children with SAM are usually brought for the complaints of superadded infections which may be fever, acute or chronic diarrhea, pneumonia, pyoderma, and sepsis or meningitis
- Edema
- Symptoms of metabolic imbalance like seizures due to hypoglycemia or other electrolyte imbalance
- Rarely the primary complaint is poor food intake, lack of weight gain or weight loss.

DIFFERENTIAL DIAGNOSIS

- Nonedematous SAM—IEM, acquired immunodeficiency syndrome
- Edematous SAM—nephrotic syndrome, chronic liver failure, congestive cardiac failure, and protein-losing enteropathies.

INVESTIGATIONS

- For all—complete blood count, peripheral blood smear for malarial parasite and to assess the type of anemia
- Urine routine and culture
- Stool microscopy, pH, sugar
- Serum proteins—total, albumin, globulin
- Blood culture
- Mantoux test
- Chest skiagram to detect TB/pneumonia and to assess the heart
- HIV serology
- Renal function tests, liver function test, serum electrolytes, and blood glucose (BG)
- Others as per clinical indication.

PATIENT APPROACH

Patient approach is in two phases: (1) Initial stabilization and (2) subsequent rehabilitation.

Initial Stabilization

Initial stabilization (2–7 days)—detection and management of complications:
- *Hypoglycemia*—blood glucose less than 54 mg/dL or less than 3 mmol/L
  - Measure BG on admission. If not measured, assume hypoglycemia and treat.
  - If symptomatic (seizures, coma, lethargy, shock, hypothermia), give intravenous (IV) 10% dextrose 5 mL/kg followed by 10% dextrose 50 mL oral or through nasogastric (NG) tube.
  - Estimate BG level every 30 minutes till stable. Start F-75 feeds after the completion of dextrose feeds, every 2 hourly including night feeds.
  - For those with asymptomatic hypoglycemia start oral 10% glucose feeds and then change to F-75 feeds as above.

Note—hypoglycemia, hypothermia and infection occur as triad; hence detect and treat the others.
- *Hypothermia*—rectal temperature less than 35.5°C/95.5°F.
  - Cover with warm clothes including head. Keep the room warm. Use radiant warmer or spotlight above the child. Promote bedding in and skin-to-skin contact with the mother
- *Dehydration:*
  - Difficult to estimate in children with SAM; assume that those with watery diarrhea have some dehydration.
  - Signs of dehydration are thirst, hypothermia, rapid weak pulse, delayed CRFT (>3s) and dry mucosa.
  - Skin pinch is unreliable in wasted and edematous child.

Severe dehydration with shock—IV Ringer Lactate with 5% dextrose or normal saline with 5% dextrose 15 mL/kg in 1 hour to a maximum of two boluses (monitor for signs of over hydration/cardiac decompensation).
- Follow-up therapy with oral rehydration therapy with oral rehydration "solution" (ORS- 245)—5–10 mL/kg/hr orally or by NG tube.

Some dehydration—ORS 245—5–10 mL/kg every 30 minutes for first 2 hours, then 5–10 mL/kg/hr for next 4–10 hours. Replace ongoing loss with 5–10 mL/kg/hr/each watery stool.
- Continue breast feeding.

- Initiate F-75 feeds 2 hours after rehydration alternating with ORS till rehydration is complete.
- *Dyselectrolytemia:*
    - *Hypokalemia*—clinical features of severe hypokalemia are flaccid weakness of abdominal, skeletal, and respiratory muscles. Electrocardiography (ECG) features are ST depression, T wave inversion, and appearance of U waves. IV potassium infusion is indicated if serum potassium (S.K) is less than 2 mEq/L or ECG changes with serum K less than 3.5 mEq/L. Infusion rate can be as 40 mEq/L of IV fluid or as 0.3–0.5 mEq/kg/hr. Continue oral potassium chloride 3–4 mEq/kg/day for 2 weeks more (syrup KCl 15 mL = 20 mEq).
    - *Hypomagnesemia*—always coexistent. Clinical features (seizures, tetany, neck floppiness, cardiac arrhythmias, persistent diarrhea) may not be perceived. All SAM children should be given intramuscular (IM) magnesium sulfate (50%) 0.3 mL/kg up to a maximum of 2 mL on day 1 of treatment; thereafter replace with oral magnesium 0.8–1.2 mEq/kg/day till there is complete recovery.
- *Infections:*
    - Classical signs of infection as fever and tachycardia may not be present; hypothermia and hypoglycemia herald sepsis.
    - Assume serious infection in all SAM children at admission.
    - Start empirical antibiotic therapy (ampi + genta/third generation cephalosporins) after sending cultures. Switch over to appropriate antibiotics as per culture report.
- *Micronutrient deficiency—will be always present:*
    - Treat with twice the recommended dietary allowance
    - Vitamin A: Day 1
        - Less than 6 months: 50,000 U
        - 6 months–1 year: 100,000 U
        - More than 1 year: 200,000 U
    - Vitamin D: If rickets—Stoss therapy (3–600,000 U as single dose per os on day 1)
    - Vitamin K: Day 1—2.5 mg IM
    - Thiamine, Riboflavin, Niacin—0.5 mg, 0.6 mg, 6.6 mg/1,000 kcal, respectively
    - Folic acid:
        - Day 1: 5 mg
        - Day 2 onward: 1 mg/day
    - Zinc: Day 1 onward—2 mg/kg/day
    - Cu: Day 1 onward—0.2–0.3 mg/kg/day
    - Iron: Day 7 onward—3 mg/kg/day.

Table 57.1: Starter formula for F-75 diet (75 kcal/100 mL milk).

Cow's milk	30 mL
Sugar	1.5 teaspoon
Oil	0.5 teaspoon
Water to make up	100 mL

Table 57.2: Formula for F-100 diet (100 kcal/100 mL milk).

Cow's milk	95 mL
Sugar	1 teaspoon
Oil	0.5 teaspoon
Water to make up	100 mL

Table 57.3: Starter Formula for Lactose Free F-75 Diet (75 kcal/100mL).

Cow's milk	30 mL
Sugar	1 teaspoon
Oil	0.5 teaspoon
Powdered puffed rice	1 teaspoon
Water to make up	100 mL

Severe anemia—hemoglobin <4 g/dL—WBT 10 mL/kg in 3 hr or packed red blood cell 5–7 mL/kg in 2 hours.

- *Initiate feeding:*
    - As early as possible—oral/NG tube.
    - Total fluids—130 mL/kg/day (100 mL/kg if edema).
    - Total calories—150–200 mL/kg/day.
    - Start as small, frequent (2 hourly) feeds including night hours.
    - Continue breastfeeding.
    - Starter formula—F-75 (75 kcal/100 mL, milk based) can be prepared as described in Table 57.1.
    - Start with 80 kcal/kg/day; gradually increase to 100 kcal/kg/day by increasing 10 mL successively until some amount is left uneaten.
    - Start F-100 diet (100 kcal/100 mL) once F-75 is tolerated; can be prepared as described in Table 57.2.
    - Substitute low lactose/lactose free diet if lactose intolerance with diarrhea; can be prepared as shown in Table 57.3 (F-75 diet).

Note—ready-to-use therapeutic food (RUTF) can be replaced for the above high calorie, high protein diet if available.

Subsequent Rehabilitation

- *Catch-up growth:*
    - As the appetite improves, encourage food intake to reach 150–200 kcal/kg/day and proteins 4–6 g/kg/day
    - Switch over to appropriate home diet
    - Continue breast feeding.
- *Sensory stimulation:*
    - Provide-stimulating environment
    - Instruct mother to impart tender loving care
    - Structured play therapy for 15–30 min/day
    - Promote physical activity as soon as the child improves.
- *Prepare for follow-up:*
    - Parameters of recovery are
        - Disappearance of edema
        - At least 15% weight gain or
        - Weight for height is 90% of median
    - Alert, active, eating a diet of 120 kcal/kg/day
    - On exclusive oral feeding
    - Consistent weight gain of 5 g/kg/day
    - Free from infection
    - Immunization is updated
    - Caretaker is reliable for home care.

CONCLUSION

Severe acute malnutrition is a fatal medical emergency involving multiple metabolic derangements and should be detected and rectified to prevent death due to under nutrition.

FURTHER READING

1. Dalwai S, Choudhury P, Bavdekar SB, et al. Consensus statement of the Indian Academy of Pediatrics on integrated management of severe acute malnutrition. Indian Pediatr. 2013;50:399-404.

Chapter 58

Intravenous Fluid Therapy

S Sushamabai

ABSTRACT

Intravenous (IV) fluid therapy is often lifesaving in the emergency department. Therapy is to be categorized as maintenance, replacement of the ongoing loss, and deficit present. Maintenance requirement is calculated according to Holliday and Segar formula. The fluid should be isotonic either normal saline (NS) or 1/2 NS with 5% dextrose along with KCl. Replacement therapy fluid depends on the type and quantity of fluid lost from the body. It has to be replaced volume by volume 1 to 6 hourly. Deficit therapy is the therapy for dehydration. The fluid should be either Ringer's lactate (RL) or NS. The volume to be administered should be calculated by history and examination to assess the degree of dehydration and the type of dyselectrolytemia. Proper monitoring is mandatory to prevent complications of IV fluid therapy.

INTRODUCTION

Intravenous fluid therapy is often required in pediatric practice mostly in emergency care areas and for perioperative care as a lifesaving treatment.

INDICATIONS

- Stabilization of the critically ill child
- Severe dehydration due to any cause
- Shock
- As a supportive therapy for reduced fluid acceptability
- Excessive ongoing fluid loss with insufficient oral replacement as in vomiting, diarrhea, gastric aspiration, diabetes, burns, renal tubular acidosis, dengue shock syndrome, etc.
- Children awaiting surgery or procedures to prevent dehydration, dyselectrolytemia and ketoacidosis
- Children on ventilator support, in coma and having inborn errors of metabolism
- For electrolyte therapy in children with specific dyselectrolytemia.

ROUTES OF ADMINISTRATION

- Peripheral veins—most commonly used
- Scalp veins—newborns and young babies
- Central veins—ventilated patients and for administering medicines through central veins.

In emergency situations, if venous access is not obtained, intraosseous route can be utilized.

COMPONENTS OF IV FLUID THERAPY

- Maintenance fluid
- Replacement fluid
- Deficit fluid.

Maintenance Fluid Therapy

- Indicates the normal requirement for a child without any disease-causing fluid and electrolyte imbalance but who cannot be fed orally.
- Calculated by Holliday and Segar formula based on the body weight of the patient as shown below:

Weight in kg	Fluid/day (mL)
0–10	100 mL/kg
11–20	1,000 mL + 50 mL/kg for each kg >10 kg
>20	1,500 mL + 20 mL/kg for each kg >20 kg

Note: Maximum requirement/day is 2,400 mL. For overweight children calculation should be for the 50th percentile weight of the child's height.

Type of Fluid

- Should be isotonic to plasma. The choice fluids are NS or 1/2 NS with added 5% dextrose and KCl 20 mEq/L.
- The selection should be based on the clinical situation and body requirement for Na and K

Note: The fluid requirement has to be increased or decreased depending on the clinical situation.

Rate of Infusion

The rate of infusion according to different body weights is described on next page.

Body weight in kg	Fluids/hr
0–10	4 mL/kg
>10–20	40 mL + 2 mL kg/hr × (wt–10 kg)
>20	60 mL + 1 mL/kg/hr × (wt–20 kg)*

Note: The maximum fluid rate is 100 mL/hr.

Replacement Fluid Therapy

- Indicates therapy of the ongoing abnormal fluid loss from the body.
- Can be gastrointestinal (vomiting, gastric aspirate, diarrhea), renal (polyuria), third space loss or chest tube drain.
- Child has to be placed on maintenance therapy.
- Losses are to be added to the maintenance requirement every 1–6 hours as mL/mL loss.
- The fluid composition advised is:
  - Gastric aspirate/vomiting—NS + 10 mEq/L KCl
  - Diarrhea—5% dextrose 1/2 NS + 30 mEq/L NaHCO$_3$ + 20 mEq/L KCl
  - Polyuria:
    - Measure urine output + urine Na
    - Replace mL/mL with the fluid based on measured serum electrolytes
  - Third space loss/chest tube output—NS/RL as mL/mL loss.

Deficit Therapy

- Indicates the therapy for dehydration.
- Quantity depends on the degree of dehydration (some/severe) and the cause of dehydration.
- The degree of dehydration is to be assessed by history regarding the quantity of fluid loss, the cause of dehydration, the amount and the type of fluid given at home, urine output of the patient and by assessing the clinical signs of dehydration.
- If signs of dehydration are present, restore the intravascular volume with NS/RL 20 mL/kg in 20–60 minutes. Repeat the amount up to a total of 100 mL/kg or till signs of dehydration disappear.
- Calculate the total requirement for 24 hours.
- Deduct the deficit therapy already administered from 24 hours fluid needed. Administer the remaining volume in next 24 hours as 5% dextrose NS + 20 mEq/L KCl.
- Assess the ongoing loss. Give correction as described in replacement therapy.

COMPLICATIONS OF IV FLUID THERAPY

- Overhydration
- Dehydration
- Dyselectrolytemia
- Anaphylaxis
- Venous thrombophlebitis
- Febrile reactions
- Defective food intake
- Deficiency diseases after prolonged IV fluid administration.

CONCLUSION

Intravenous fluid therapy is life-saving, should be appropriately calculated and administered regarding the volume, composition, and the rate of infusion.

Section 8

RENAL SYSTEM

Chapter 59

Acute Kidney Injury

S Sushamabai

ABSTRACT

Acute kidney injury (AKI) is the revised terminology for acute renal failure and is defined as sudden deterioration in renal function resulting in accumulation of nitrogenous waste products in the body and electrolyte imbalance due to renal function impairment. The most common type is prerenal failure due to diarrhea or other types of fluid loss. In intrinsic renal failure, acute poststreptococcal glomerulonephritis, nephrotoxic drug intake, and snake envenomation are the leading causes. Postrenal causes are surgical problems. The clinical features of AKI are reduced urine output, edema, altered sensorium, convulsions, vomiting, anemia, and growth retardation. Severity staging of AKI can be done by AKI network (AKIN) or pediatric risk, injury, failure, loss and end stage renal disease (RIFLE) criteria. History, physical examination, and simple laboratory investigations are sufficient to differentiate between prerenal, intrinsic renal and postrenal causes. Volume replacement and diuretic therapy with furosemide and low-dose mannitol are effective in correcting prerenal failure as well as to prevent most cases of intrinsic renal failure. Indications for dialysis and types of dialysis recommended are also described.

INTRODUCTION

Acute kidney injury, formerly termed as acute renal failure (ARF), is the sudden deterioration in fluid and electrolyte homeostasis and retention of nitrogenous waste products in the body due to rapid decline in renal function.

DIAGNOSTIC CRITERIA

The term AKI has replaced ARF because of the lack of clear definition for ARF. Patients are diagnosed to have AKI if there is reduction in renal function within 48 hours. Staging of AKI based on AKIN criteria can be simplified as shown in Table 59.1.

Pediatric RIFLE criterion that includes risk, injury, failure, loss and end stage renal disease, is based on glomerular filtration rate and categorizes severity by rise in serum creatinine:
- *Stage I: More than 150%*

Table 59.1: Staging of acute kidney injury.

Stage	Serum creatinine criteria	Urine output criteria
1	Increase in S. Cr ≥ 0.3 mg/dL or 1.5–2 folds from baseline	<0.5 mL/kg/hr for > 6 hr
2	Increase in S. Cr > 2–3 fold	<0.5 mL/kg/hr for >12 hr
3	Increase in S. Cr > 3 fold or ≥ 4 mg/dL with acute increase of ≥ 0.5 mg/dL	<0.3 mL/kg/hr for > 24 hr or anuria for >12 hr

Note: Only one criterion (creatinine/urine output) needs to be fulfilled to qualify for a stage. Patients on renal replacement therapy are considered in Stage 3 or above.
(S. Cr, Serum creatinine)

- *Stage II: More than 200%*
- *Stage III: More than 300%.*

COMMON CAUSES

- *Prerenal:*
  - Hypovolemia (dehydration, blood loss, diuretics)
  - Third space loss (sepsis, nephrotic syndrome)
  - Heart failure
  - Perinatal asphyxia
  - Hypoalbuminemia
- *Intrinsic renal:*
  - Glomerular nephritis of various causes
  - Prolonged prerenal insult
  - Sepsis—leading to multiple organ dysfunction syndrome
  - Drug-induced (nonsteroidal anti-inflammatory drugs, aminoglycosides)
  - Hemolytic uremic syndrome
  - Acute tubular necrosis (snake/wasp envenomation)
  - Tumor lysis syndrome
  - Renal vein thrombosis.
- *Postrenal:*
  - Obstructive uropathies (congenital, stones)
  - Urolithiasis
  - Hemorrhagic cystitis
  - Neurogenic bladder.

PATIENT APPROACH

- Detailed history—suggestive of fluid loss (diarrhea/vomiting/starvation/polyuria), drug intake, poor urine stream, high colored urine, periorbital edema, skin rashes, cardiac symptoms, past and family history of renal disease should be obtained.

- Seizures, edema, vomiting, and altered sensorium can be the presenting features of AKI.
- Detailed physical examinations for signs of dehydration, edema, altered sensorium, skin rashes, bleeding, hyper/hypotension, and abdominal masses are helpful to detect the underlying etiology.
- Look for features of chronic renal disease like anemia, growth retardation, hypertension, and acidotic breathing.
- Place bladder catheter to assess urine output and also to detect posterior urethral valve.

INVESTIGATIONS

Should be prompt:
- Urinalysis—protein, sugar, microscopy, osmolality, sodium, culture and sensitivity.
- Blood—hemoglobin (Hb), total and differential count, platelet count, reticulocyte count, peripheral smear study, hematocrit, renal function test (RFT), liver function test, serum Na, K, Ca, P, blood pH, C3 complement, lactic dehydrogenase (LDH), antistreptolysin O, and antinuclear antibody.
- Chest X-ray and abdominal ultrasonography.
- Others including renal biopsy as per clinical diagnosis.

MANAGEMENT

Depends on the type and etiology of renal failure.

Prerenal failure (indices—urine specific gravity >1.020, urine Na <20, urine osmolality >500 mOsm/kg, Fe Na <1)

Hypovolemic—due to diarrhea, vomiting, gastric aspirate, burns, blood loss, dengue shock syndrome
- Start fluid challenge—normal saline (NS) 20 mL/kg as intravenous (IV) bolus in 20–60 minutes as per volume status. Repeat two more boluses monitoring for features of hypervolemia (respiratory distress, edema, lung crackles, and raised central venous pressure). Fluid replacement in hypovolemic renal failure will be followed by diuresis of 2–4 mL/kg by 2 hours.
- If oliguria persists 2 hours after fluid replacement, administer loop diuretic—furosemide 2–4 mg/kg IV or IV bumetanide 0.1 mg/kg. Add mannitol 0.5 mg/kg as single IV dose especially in hemo- or myoglobinuria.
- Continuous infusion with low-dose dopamine (2–3 µg/kg/min) can be tried.

- If no response to diuretic challenge, stop diuretics; consider fluid restriction.
- *Congestive cardiac failure*: Assess the hydration status and do the correction; use inotropes to improve cardiac output.
- *Third-space loss*: Administer colloids or plasma 10 mL/kg in 2 hours in addition to fluid correction.
- *Hypovolemia due to hemorrhage and after fluid bolus*: Consider blood transfusion 10–20 mL/kg in 2–4 hours.
- Once dehydration is corrected, continue appropriate fluid therapy (IV/oral) till the cause is corrected.
- Manage the complications as in intrinsic renal failure.

Intrinsic renal failure (Indices—urine specific gravity <1.010, urine Na >40 mEq/L, urine osmolality <350, Fe Na >2%)

Fluid Management

- Maintain intake output chart.
- Prevent fluid overload by restricting intake to 400 mL/m^2/day as 5% dextrose (oral replacement should be salt-free fluid) plus the amount equal to previous days urine output as 1/2 NS.
- Replace blood or gastrointestinal loss as equal amounts of blood/NS, respectively.
- For children with excess fluid overload, consider further fluid restriction.
- In respiratory distress due to pulmonary edema, administer oxygen and furosemide (2–4 mg/kg IV); consider dialysis.

Electrolyte Management

- Monitor serum Na, K, HCO$_3$, Ca, and P.
- Treat metabolic acidosis if bicarbonate is less than 8 mEq/l till pH <7.15 or if hyperkalemia. Give sodium bicarbonate IV (1 mEq/kg) till the value is 12 mEq/L followed by oral solution.
- Provide medical therapy for other electrolyte disorders (Chapter 53). The common problems encountered are hyperkalemia, hyponatremia, hypocalcemia, and hyperphosphatemia.

Others

- *Edema*: Restrict salt and water; administer diuretics.
- *Hypertension*: Isradipine (0.05–0.15 mg/kg/dose) for rapid reduction in blood pressure; for sustained effect amlodipine, propranolol or labetalol are recommended.
- *Seizures*: Control with benzodiazepines.

- *Anemia*: Usually mild (Hb 9–10 g/dL). Give fresh washed red blood cell transfusion (5–10 mL/kg) in 2 hours if Hb is less than 7 g/dL. In hypervolemic patients, transfusion should be slow in 4–6 hours.
- *Nutrition*: Diet should be high calorie (90–120 cal/kg/day as per age), protein restricted (0.8–1.2 g/kg/day), salt restricted, and fluid balanced. Consider total parenteral nutrition if oral intake is inappropriate. Restrict sodium, potassium, and phosphorus.
- *Infections*: Observe strict asepsis, recognize infections promptly and treat. Avoid nephrotoxic antibiotics. Dose adjustment depends on creatinine clearance. For aminoglycosides like amikacin, dose adjustment can be done by increasing the *interval method* by multiplying the usual interval by serum creatinine value.

COMPLICATIONS

- Volume overload with hypertension leading to left ventricular failure or encephalopathy
- Persistent electrolyte imbalance
- Metabolic acidosis unresponsive to medical therapy
- Neurologic symptoms—altered sensorium, seizures
- Calcium, phosphorus imbalance with tetany.

INDICATIONS FOR DIALYSIS

- Anuria or oliguria
- Refractory volume overload evidenced by refractory hypertension or pulmonary edema
- Persistent hyperkalemia, hypocalcemic tetany, and metabolic acidosis
- Increasing blood urea nitrogen more than 100–150 mg/dL
- Snake envenomation
- Drug poisoning—phenobarbitone
- Inborn errors of metabolism—hyperammonemia
- Inability to provide adequate nutrition.

TYPES OF DIALYSIS

- *Peritoneal dialysis*: Therapy of choice in sick and unstable neonates and infants.
- *Intermittent hemodialysis*: Advised in patients with stable hemodynamic status. The procedure lasts for 3–4 hours, three to seven times in a week.
- *Continuous renal replacement therapy*: Indicated in patients with unstable hemodynamic status, sepsis and multiorgan failure.

FOLLOW-UP

- All children with AKI need regular follow-up; those with prerenal AKI and rapid recovery, first follow-up can be after 2 weeks, thereafter every 3 months for a period of 1 year is ideal.
- During follow-up, assess for anemia, growth retardation, edema, and status of the associated illness.
- Urine for albumin and microscopy and RFT are a must at each visit; others as per the etiology of AKI and the clinical status.

OUTCOME

- Depends on the underlying cause.
- Most patients with AKI due to renal limited conditions recover completely if timely appropriate treatment is given.
- Acute kidney injury with multiorgan failure carries high mortality rate; medical management for chronic renal insufficiency for variable periods will be required in a good number of such patients with parenchymal damage.
- In those with AKI and obstructive uropathies, prognosis depends on the nature of obstruction and the surgical correction made or possible.

CONCLUSION

Acute kidney injury should be properly classified and treated as per clinical picture and investigations.

Chapter 60

Renal Tubular Acidosis

S Sushamabai

ABSTRACT

Renal tubular acidosis (RTA) is an emergency of diverse etiology; common presentation is in infants as non-anion gap metabolic acidosis and dyselectrolytemia. The clinical types are distal (type 1, hypokalemic), proximal (type II, hypokalemic), combined (type III), and hypoaldosteronism (type IV, hyperkalemic). The common clinical presentations are failure to thrive (FTT), poor weight gain, recurrent vomiting, unaccountable dehydration, rickets, jaundice, and developmental delay. The differential diagnosis and investigations are detailed. Stepwise approach to treatment includes correction of dehydration followed by correction of hypokalemia and acidemia intravenously. Oral sodium bicarbonate should be started as the child improves and should be maintained lifelong. Children with hypokalemia require potassium citrate orally lifelong. Periodic follow-up for growth monitoring, metabolic equilibrium, and renal status and timely correction are advised. Vitamin D and calcium (Ca) should be administered if there is development of rickets.

INTRODUCTION

Renal tubular acidosis includes diverse group of diseases inherited as well as acquired characterized by normal anion gap metabolic acidosis with normal glomerular filtration rate.

DIAGNOSTIC CRITERIA

- Non-anion gap metabolic acidosis. Anion gap is calculated as [Serum Na − (Cl + HCO_3)]. Normal value is 8–12 mEq/L. Value less than 12 mEq/L is suggestive of normal anion gap.

Note: Other causes of acidosis should be ruled out by history, physical examination, and relevant investigations.

CLINICAL TYPES

- Proximal—type II (less common, hypokalemic)
- Distal—type I (more common, hypokalemic)
- Hyperkalemic—type IV (hypoaldosteronism/pseudohypoaldosteronism)
- Combined—type III (combined proximal and distal).

PATHOPHYSIOLOGY

- *Distal RTA—most common form:*
    - Can be sporadic, inherited, or acquired.
    - The primary problem is defective secretion of hydrogen ion causing severe metabolic acidosis with the urine pH always >5.5, loss of sodium bicarbonate at the distal tubule, increased chloride absorption, and hyperchloremia.
    - Hypokalemia is always present due to the increased urinary secretion of potassium instead of H^+.
    - Hypercalciuria is usual leading to nephrocalcinosis and nephrolithiasis.
    - Hypocitraturia and bone disease are common.
- *Proximal RTA:*
    - Can be sporadic, inherited, or acquired.
    - Renal tubular acidosis may be rarely isolated but mostly a component of generalized proximal tubular dysfunction as in Fanconi syndrome.
    - The primary problem is defective proximal tubular reabsorption of bicarbonate producing marked bicarbonaturia, urine pH being <5.5 since distal tubular acidification is intact.
    - In Fanconi syndrome, varying degrees of proteinuria, glycosuria, uricosuria, aminoaciduria, phosphaturia, and increased urinary Na and K may occur.
- *Hyperkalemic RTA—can be due to:*
    - Hypoaldosteronism—impaired aldosterone production seen in Addison disease, congenital adrenal hyperplasia (CAH), or as isolated abnormality.
    - Pseudohypoaldosteronism—impaired renal responsiveness to aldosterone seen in acute pyelonephritis and acute or chronic urine retention.
    - Clinical features are due to impaired H^+ ion and K secretion.
    - Can be part of Addison disease, CAH or obstructive uropathy.
    - Very rarely inherited isolated forms can occur.
    - Laboratory features are hyperchloremic non-anion gap metabolic acidosis with hyperkalemia.

CLINICAL PRESENTATION

Usually presents in infancy as:
- Failure to thrive and growth retardation
- Recurrent episodes of vomiting, polyuria, and fever
- Unaccountable dehydration and acidotic breathing
- Polyuria and excessive thirst
- Gross motor delay and hypotonia
- Episodic weakness
- Rickets and bone pains
- Features of underlying disease like jaundice, hepatomegaly, cataract, anemia, obstructive uropathy, CAH, and pigmentation.

PATIENT APPROACH

- Suspect RTA in any infant or child with FTT or growth retardation, recurrent vomiting, dehydration, acidotic breathing, motor delay, hypotonia, and episodic weakness.
- Admit in pediatric intensive care unit and stabilize airway, breathing, and circulation if severe dehydration or acidosis.
- Send blood for sugar, Na, K, Cl, HCO_3, Ca, P, renal function test, and for arterial blood gas/venous blood gas analysis.
- Ultrasonography abdomen to exclude nephrocalcinosis or obstructive uropathy.

Note: In diarrhea or diseases with dehydration, the diagnostic investigations should be done or repeated after correcting the metabolic impairment.

DIFFERENTIAL DIAGNOSIS

- Diarrhea with dehydration
- Recurrent vomiting of medical or surgical causes leading to dehydration
- Congenital adrenal hyperplasia
- Protein energy malnutrition
- Diabetic ketoacidosis
- Inborn errors of metabolism
- Septic shock.

DETAILED INVESTIGATIONS

- *To differentiate the type of RTA—Urinalysis*: Ideally collect the first morning sample for pH and anion gap (urine Na + urine K – urine Cl)
    - *Proximal RTA*—Urine pH <5.5, acidemic blood, negative urine anion gap
    - *Distal RTA*—Urine pH >6, acidemic blood, positive urine anion gap

- *To diagnose the etiology*: Urine culture, albumin, amino acids, sugar, phosphate, urine Ca/creatinine (Cr) ratio and microscopy, and other investigations as per clinical assessment.

SUBSEQUENT MANAGEMENT

- Correction of dehydration—normal saline 10–20 mL/kg in 20–60 minutes.
- Correction of hypokalemia: Add potassium chloride to the intravenous (IV) drip up to 20–40 mEq/L (IV KCl 1 mL = 2 mEq). Can be given as oral potassium citrate solution (1 mL contains 2 mEq of potassium and bicarbonate) as clinical improvement starts, and the child tolerates oral medicines.
- Correction of acidosis—sodium bicarbonate 5–20 mEq/kg/day as continuous IV infusion added to the running fluid or as oral in divided doses till blood bicarbonate is in the acceptable range = 15 mEq/L (10% IV sodium bicarbonate 1 mL = 0.9 mEq; oral sodium bicarbonate 325 mg one tablet = 4 mEq).
- Correction of underlying problems:
  - Phosphate and vitamin D supplementation additionally in Fanconi syndrome
  - Fludrocortisone 0.1–0.15 mg/day in type IV RTA.

Discharge Criteria

- Correction of dehydration and acidosis clinically, near normal electrolyte values.
- Accepting feeds and reveals weight gain.

FOLLOW-UP AND LONG-TERM THERAPY

- All children with RTA should be kept under periodic follow-up (once in 3 months) to monitor hydration, clinical acidosis, growth and development, and treatment compliance.
- Renal function test, serum electrolytes, and blood gas should be evaluated twice yearly and appropriate correction should be done.
- Ultrasonography abdomen yearly to detect nephrocalcinosis or progressive renal damage.
- Urine Ca/Cr ratio which should be maintained at 0.2.
- Vitamin D and Ca deficit should be corrected.

CONCLUSION

Renal tubular acidosis is non-anion gap metabolic acidosis usually due to inherent defects in bicarbonate homeostasis requiring lifetime sodium bicarbonate therapy.

Chapter 61

Hematuria

S Sushamabai

ABSTRACT

Hematuria is the presence of more than or equal to 5 RBCs/µL of urine, usually pathological, rarely can be innocent. Other causes of red urine should be excluded by history. The common causes of hematuria are infections, trauma, viral hemorrhagic fevers, urolithiasis, and poststreptococcal glomerulonephritis (PSGN). Differentiating features between glomerular, tubular, and lower urinary tract hematuria, initial stabilization, subsequent management, and further follow-up are discussed. The initial stabilization depends on the severity of hematuria and subsequent approach is as per underlying etiology.

INTRODUCTION

Hematuria is defined as the presence of at least 5 RBCs/µL of urine. *Significant hematuria* is >50 RBCs/µL of urine.

PATIENT APPROACH

History—Consider other causes for red urine as:
- Hemoglobinuria and myoglobinuria
- Drug intake—rifampicin, pyridium, nitrofurantoin, and metronidazole
- Vegetables and fruits—beetroot, blackberry, rhubarb
- Food coloring
- Metabolites—urates, porphyrin, tyrosinosis, and homogentisic acid.

Assess the Degree of Hematuria—Gross or Trivial

Common causes of gross hematuria:
- Urinary tract infections—bacteria, adenovirus
- Urolithiasis
- Trauma—accidental, battered child

- Coagulopathy:
  - Congenital (hemophilias, platelet function disorders)
  - Acquired [immune thrombocytopenic purpura (ITP), hemolytic-uremic syndrome, disseminated intravascular coagulation (DIC)]
- Glomerular diseases:
  - Postinfectious glomerulonephritis
  - Henoch–Schönlein purpura (HSP) nephritis
  - Immunoglobulin A nephropathy
  - Alport syndrome
  - Systemic lupus erythematosus
- Hemorrhagic fevers—dengue and others
- Sickle cell disease
- Tumors and malignancies.

Have a quick assessment of the child for the severity of bleeding.
- Assess the sensorium, vitals, degree of pallor.
- Altered sensorium (irritability/coma) herald hypotension in hemorrhagic fevers or hypertensive encephalopathy in glomerulonephritis.
- Tachycardia and pallor indicate gross amount of blood loss and the urgency for blood transfusion.
- Admit in pediatric intensive care unit if massive hematuria, febrile, altered sensorium, hypo/hypertension, spontaneous bleeding in other body parts, severe abdominal pain, and history or evidence of trauma.
- Stabilize airway, breathing, and circulation; start bolus normal saline if in shock.
- Administer analgesic and antispasmoic for renal colic. Avoid nonsteroidal anti-inflammatory drugs.
- Send blood for hemoglobin, total leukocyte count, differential leukocyte count, PLC, PBS, reticulocyte count, coagulation profile, grouping, typing and cross matching, serum electrolytes (Na, K, Ca, P, Cl), renal function test, liver function test.
- Urgent ultrasonography abdomen to detect urolithiasis, tumors, trauma, renal anomalies, and liver disease.
- Evaluate urine for color, proteins, sugar, microscopy (RBC morphology), culture, and sensitivity.
- Differentiate the hematuria according to the site of origin as:
  - Glomerular—cola/tea-colored urine, proteinuria more than 100 mg/dL, deformed RBCs, RBC casts
  - Tubular—presence of white blood cells, tubular epithelial cell casts, normal-shaped RBCs
  - Lower urinary tract—bright red/pink colored urine, gross and/or terminal hematuria, blood clots, and normal-shaped RBCs.

Detailed History and Physical Examination

- Recent history of pyoderma/tonsillitis, presence of edema, oliguria—PSGN.
- Severe abdominal pain is characteristic of renal calculi; can occur in HSP due to intestinal edema and/or gangrene.
- Dysuria is characteristic of lower urinary tract infection (UTI); flank pain indicates acute pyelonephritis.
- Enquire about the past history of UTI/other urinary problems.
- Family history of renal diseases, kidney transplantation, and bleeding diathesis.
- Bleeding from skin and/or mucosa may suggest ITP, coagulopathy, and DIC.
- Palpable purpura and arthritis are features of HSP.
- Palpable abdominal mass can indicate renal or other malignant tumors or renal anomalies.

Plan further investigations and management accordingly. Children with asymptomatic microscopic hematuria for more than 1 year (persistent) should be subjected to renal biopsy for histopathological diagnosis.

CONCLUSION

Hematuria usually heralds serious urinary or systemic diseases and should be evaluated thoroughly.

Chapter 62

Acute Pyelonephritis

S Sushamabai

ABSTRACT

Acute pyelonephritis is an infectious emergency of renal parenchyma and pelvis especially in young infants. The typical clinical presentation is high fever, abdominal pain, vomiting, and renal angle tenderness. The condition should be suspected in children presenting with febrile seizures, sepsis, recurrent abdominal pain/diarrhea, and fever of unknown origin. Prompt stabilization, early urine culture with properly collected sample, empirical antibiotic therapy, and US imaging of the abdomen to detect surgical problems are the initial priorities. The ideal empirical antibiotic is ceftriaxone. Subsequent management and imaging studies, follow-up and long-term chemoprophylaxis are also discussed.

INTRODUCTION

Acute pyelonephritis is a serious form of urinary tract infection in children mostly occurring in infants less than 1 year. The term indicates bacterial infection of the renal parenchyma and pelvis though to some extent rest of the urinary tract also is affected. The common organisms are *Escherichia coli*, *Klebsiella*, and *Proteus* groups.

CLINICAL PRESENTATION

- Classical symptoms are high fever (>102.2°F), abdominal or flank pain, vomiting. In infants less than 2 years age, fever without focus may be the only clinical manifestation.
- Suspect acute pyelonephritis in infants with febrile seizures, fever with abdominal pain/diarrhea/jaundice/features of sepsis/irritability/abdominal distension.
- Newborns can present with weight loss, poor feeding, irritability, and jaundice.
- Dysuria, frequency, and dribbling are features of lower urinary tract infection and can be present if the lower urinary tract also is affected. Fever usually indicates pyelonephritis.

- The pathognomonic clinical sign is renal angle tenderness. Supportive findings are signs of dehydration, ileus, and shock.

PATIENT APPROACH
- Admit in pediatric intensive care unit if the patient is in septic shock, has seizures, jaundice, repeated vomiting/poor drinking, ileus, dehydration or less than 1 month age.
- Stabilize airway, breathing, and circulation; send samples for urine and blood cultures, urine albumin and microscopy, complete blood count, PBS, renal function test (RFT), liver function test and serum electrolytes. Polymorphonuclear leukocytosis in blood is characteristic of acute pyelonephritis.
- Ideal sample for urine culture is the midstream specimen obtained after cleaning the introitus in girls and retracted prepuce in boys.
- If the child is not toilet trained or prepuce cannot be retracted or unconscious, catheterized or suprapubic aspirate urine sample should be collected at the earliest so as to start empirical antibiotic therapy.
- Urine collection bag sample revealing bacterial growth may be due to skin contamination and not reliable.
- Prompt plating of the sample is a must to avoid overgrowth of contaminants.
- Urinary tract infection can be considered if a single pathogen colony count is obtained in:
  - Midstream sample more than or equal to 100,000/mL *or*
  - Suprapubic/catheterized sample more than or equal to 50,000 or more than or equal to 10,000/mL in a symptomatic child
- Ultrasonography abdomen should be done at the earliest to exclude perinephric/renal abscess, anomalies of the urinary tract, and liver or biliary problems.
- High levels of C-reactive protein and procalcitonin are characteristic of acute pyelonephritis.
- Start empirical antibiotic therapy (after the cultures are sent) as shown below:
  - Intravenous ceftriaxone 50–75 mg/kg/day or
  - Intravenous cefotaxime 100 mg/kg/24 hr div (divided) q 8 hr or
  - Intravenous ampicillin 100 mg/kg/24 hr div q 6 hr with gentamicin 3–5 mg/kg/24 hr in 1–3 div doses. Assess renal function test before starting aminoglycoside therapy
- Antibiotics should be changed as per culture and sensitivity report.
- Failure to respond within 48 hours of appropriate antibiotics, poor urine stream, abdominal mass, non-*Escherichia coli* pathogen, urosepsis, and elevated serum creatinine are red flag signs for imaging studies.

SUBSEQUENT MANAGEMENT

- Surgical intervention should be considered if there is renal/perirenal abscess or evidence of urinary obstruction.
- Continue supportive therapy till the vitals are stable. Intravenous (IV) maintenance fluids need to be continued for 24 hours more after the child is tolerating oral fluids and medicines.
- Intravenous antibiotics should be given for a minimum period of 48 hours. Total duration of antibiotic therapy is 7–14 days depending on the associated complications.
- A voiding cystourethrogram is recommended for all patients less than 3 years age:
  - With atypical features
  - Abnormal USG findings
  - Recurrent UTI
- Dimercaptosuccinic acid scan is advised:
  - After 4–6 months of treatment in all patients more than 3 years to detect renal scarring
  - All patients less than 3 years of age with abnormal voiding cystourethrogram (VCUG)
- Imaging studies need be repeated if there are abnormalities.
- Repeat urine culture is advised 1 week after stopping antibiotics to ensure clearance of infection.
- Factors contributing to recurrent UTI should be assessed. They are constipation, pinworm infestation, adherent labia, adherent prepuce, improper voiding habits and improper cleaning habits. Appropriate fluid intake, treatment of constipation, 3 hourly voiding habits and proper cleaning of the perineum should be advised. Other problems are to be corrected.
- Antimicrobial prophylaxis is advised for children with recurrent UTI having underlying problems like severe vesicoureteral reflux, urinary calculi, obstructive uropathy, and neuropathic bladder. The recommended agents are trimethoprim–sulfamethoxazole and nitrofurantoin in 30% of the normal therapeutic doses as single dose daily till the abnormalities are corrected surgically or by self-remission. Amoxicillin and cephalexin are alternatives but more prone for drug resistance.
- Administration of probiotics is found to be beneficial so as to replace the urogenital pathologic flora.

OUTCOME

- Timely diagnosis and prompt appropriate management results in full recovery unless there are underlying renal anomalies.
- Delay in diagnosis, improper/inadequate treatment, and follow-up can lead to hypertension and progressive renal damage.
- The prognosis of patients with underlying renal problem depends on the type of anomaly, the treatment provided and the follow-up care.

CONCLUSION

Acute pyelonephritis is a severe infection of the kidneys and can lead to severe sepsis especially in young infants and should be evaluated in febrile children.

Section 9

GASTROINTESTINAL SYSTEM

Chapter 63

Fulminant Hepatic Failure

Carol Sara Cherian, S Sushamabai

ABSTRACT

Fulminant hepatic failure or acute liver cell failure (ALF) is a clinical syndrome of rapid and severe impairment of liver cell function ending in death. Most children recover with timely intensive supportive therapy. The diagnostic criteria are hepatic coagulopathy [international normalized ratio (INR) >1.5] not corrected by vitamin K with clinical hepatic encephalopathy or INR more than 2 regardless of hepatic encephalopathy with biochemical evidence of acute liver injury of less than 8-week duration. The etiology can be viral infections, toxic liver damage or autoimmune diseases. Clinical assessment for prognostication of encephalopathy is included. Stepwise management includes fluid and electrolyte maintenance, prevention of hypoglycemia, bowel sterilization, prevention and treatment of bleeding, broad spectrum antibiotic therapy to control infections, and management of seizures. N-acetyl cysteine therapy is beneficial and is discussed in detail. Those with poor prognostic predictors should be considered for liver transplantation.

DEFINITION

Fulminant hepatic failure or acute liver failure[1] is a clinical syndrome of rapid and severe impairment of liver cell function without liver cell necrosis.

The diagnostic parameters are:
- Biochemical evidence of acute liver injury (<8-week duration)
- No evidence of chronic liver disease
- Hepatic coagulopathy[2] [prothrombin time (PT) >15 s/INR >1.5] not corrected by vitamin K with clinical hepatic encephalopathy *or*
- Prothrombin time more than 20 seconds or INR more than 2 regardless of the presence of clinical hepatic encephalopathy.

Note: Hepatic encephalopathy is not a must to diagnose acute liver failure (ALF). INR should be measured 8 hours after parenteral vitamin K.

SYMPTOMS

Increasing jaundice, fever, lethargy, anorexia, persistent vomiting, abdominal pain, altered sensorium, seizures, and bleeding.

SIGNS

Change in sleep rhythm, varying degrees of coma, extensor responses, brisk deep tendon reflexes, decerebrate/decorticate spasms, fetor hepaticus, asterixis, jaundice ± hepatomegaly or rapidly shrinking liver, and bleeding tendency.

COMMON CAUSES

- Infections—viral hepatitis, bacterial sepsis, leptospirosis, and malaria
- Drugs and toxins—paracetamol, antituberculosis (TB) drugs, valproic acid, mushrooms, and anesthesia overdose
- Metabolic—Reye syndrome, tyrosinemia, Wilson disease, galactosemia, others
- Shock.

PATHOPHYSIOLOGY

Liver cell damage can be produced by:
- Direct toxic effect and/or ischemic/immune-mediated destruction following the insults.
- Subsequent to this, there is impairment of synthetic, excretory, detoxifying and metabolic liver functions resulting in multisystem dysfunction.
- Hepatic encephalopathy is due to high serum levels of ammonia, amines and false neurotransmitters which are not cleared by the damaged liver.

DIFFERENTIAL DIAGNOSIS

Meningitis, encephalitis, septic shock, severe malaria, and typhoid fever with toxemia.

PATIENT APPROACH

Goals of therapy are:
- Diagnose the etiology and treat
- Provide liver support to prevent ongoing damage
- Detect the associated complications and treat.

Step I—Parallel History, Quick Assessment, Stabilization, Investigations

- Admit in pediatric intensive care unit.
- Brief history; assess the vitals, oxygen saturation (SpO_2), Glasgow coma scale (GCS), capillary blood glucose.
- Stabilize airway, breathing, and circulation; correct hypoglycemia.
- Bladder catheterization and indwelling catheter to measure urine output till the child is conscious to void.
- Nasogastric aspiration and stomach wash with normal saline; no oral feeds till improvement.
- Proceed to mechanical ventilation if in advanced coma (stage 3 or 4).
- Send blood for complete blood count, PBS for MP, culture including fungal agents, coagulation profile, liver function test (LFT), renal function test (RFT), serum electrolytes (SE), plasma ammonia, venous blood gas (VBG), viral markers, leptospira antibody and Wilson's disease workup. Prolonged PT, elevated serum glutamic pyruvic transaminase, and blood ammonia support the diagnosis of fulminant hepatic failure.
- Toxicology screening if suspected.
- Cerebrospinal fluid studies are mandatory to exclude meningitis if there is no absolute contraindication for lumbar puncture.
- Keep blood sample for grouping, typing and crossmatching.
- Send urine for routine examination and culture; consider toxic and metabolic screening if suspected.
- Assess blood loss—arrange for blood transfusion if actively bleeding or Hb less than 7 g/dL; administer whole blood 15–20 mL/kg in 4 hours.
- For children in deep coma—secure two IV accesses—one for repeated blood sampling and the other for administration of drugs and fluids.
- Arrange for urgent bedside ultrasonography abdomen to detect the liver size and preexisting abnormality and to assess the status of the gallbladder.
- Chest X-ray is should be done to exclude associated pneumonia.
- Proceed to detailed history and physical examination after stabilization.

Step II—Assess the Severity of Encephalopathy

Staging of hepatic encephalopathy is described in Table 63.1.

Post-stabilization therapy:
- Correction of dehydration and hypoglycemia.
- Maintenance fluid—2/3 of normal + gastric aspirate loss. Type of fluid—10% dextrose with 1/2 normal saline and KCl 40 mEq/L + multivitamins + minerals (Ca, Mg, P).

Table 63.1: Clinical staging of hepatic encephalopathy.

Parameter	Staging			
	I	II	III	IV
Symptoms	Lethargy, reversal of day and night sleep	Drowsiness, mood swings, disorientation	Stupor but arousable, confused, incoherent speech	Coma
Signs	Trouble in drawing figures, performing mental tasks	Asterixis, fetor hepaticus, incontinence	Asterixis, hyperreflexia, rigidity, extensor reflexes	Areflexia, flaccidity, no asterixis
EEG	Normal	Generalized slowing, q waves	Markedly abnormal, triphasic waves	Markedly abnormal bilateral slowing, d waves, electric-cortical silence

(EEG, electroencephalography)

- Intravenous vitamin K 0.2 mg/kg/day (max 10 mg/day) till recovery.
- Intravenous ranitidine as prophylaxis to prevent gastrointestinal (GI) bleeds—1–5 mg/kg/day divided (div) q 8 hourly.
- Intravenous pantoprazole at double dose if gut bleeding—2 mg/kg bolus followed by 0.2 mg/kg/hr as infusion for 72 hr or till bleeding stops; continue with oral dose till recovery (stop ranitidine if pantoprazole is introduced).
- Lactulose retention enema 1:3 dilution in water q 6 hourly.
- Oral lactulose 0.5–1 mL/kg q 2–4 hr to produce 2–3 loose stools/day.
- Oral neomycin 50–100 mg/kg/day div q 8 hourly.
- Intravenous antibiotics—cefotaxime + amikacin + cloxacillin if infection; antifungal therapy if indicated.
- Intravenous N-acetyl cysteine—150 mg/kg in 15–60 minutes diluted in 5% dextrose or NS; maintenance 12.5 mg/kg/hr for 4 hours, then 6.25 mg/kg/hr till recovery as indicated by INR less than 1.5.
- Specific therapy for etiology—N-acetyl cysteine (acetaminophen poisoning), acyclovir (herpes simplex virus infection), penicillin (amanita poisoning), lamivudine or entecavir (hepatitis B virus chronic infection), prednisone (autoimmune hepatitis), and pleconaril (enteroviral infection).
- Consider the need for liver transplantation in stage 3 or 4 coma; other advanced forms of liver supportive therapy should be used as bridge therapy as per facility.

- Oral feeds can be started as the sensorium and the liver function laboratory parameters reveal improvement:
  - Start with simple sugars followed by fruit juices
  - Gradual introduction of family diet
  - Restrict protein in the diet to 0.5 g/day in the initial days.

Step IV—Monitoring

- *Clinical:*
  - Hourly heart rate, respiratory rate, blood pressure, SpO_2, GCS, pupils, deep tendon reflex, and plantar response
  - 4-hourly temperature, input/output chart, encephalopathy grading, GI bleed quantity
  - Daily liver span and sepsis evaluation.
- *Laboratory:*
  - 4-hourly random blood sugar
  - 12-hourly S.Na, K, C a, P
  - Daily platelet count, prothrombin time, hemoglobin, blood urea, serum creatinine, and venous blood gas
  - Once in 3 days LFT, plasma NH_3.

Step V—Management of Complications

- *Cerebral edema:* Most common cause of death; anticipate/suspect if:
  - Sudden deterioration of sensorium (GCS-score decreasing)
  - Bradycardia, apnea, pupillary changes, and papilledema
  - Posturing and seizures.
- *Treatment:*
  - Head end elevation 30–45°, minimize suction, and noxious stimuli.
  - Treat fever, seizures, electroencephalographic recording to detect nonconvulsive seizures, treat accordingly.
  - Reduce fluid volume to two-thirds of maintenance requirement.
  - Treat hypoglycemia, hypoxemia, hypotension, dyselectrolytemia (Na, Ca, P).
  - Treatment of brain edema—IV mannitol (20%) 5 mL/kg bolus followed by 2 mL/kg q 6 hr × four doses or 3% saline if the patient is in shock.
  - Early intubation, mechanical ventilation in grade III/IV encephalopathy.
- *Coagulopathy:*
  - Fresh frozen plasma/platelets/cryoprecipitate as per need
  - Recombinant factor VII_a in refractory cases.
- *Convulsions:*
  - Intravenous phenytoin/phenobarbitone 15 mg/kg loading dose followed by 5 mg/kg/day div q 12 hr.
- *Sedation—Lorazepam/Fentanyl*

Refer respective chapters for respiratory failure, shock, renal failure, and dyselectrolytemia.

Poor prognostic predictors:
- Age less than 1 year
- Encephalopathy stage IV
- International normalized ratio more than 4
- Need for dialysis
- Plasma ammonia more than 200 µmol/L.

Arrange for liver transplantation in such children.

CONCLUSION

Fulminant hepatic failure is rapid and severe impairment of liver cell function in a previously normal liver and should be evaluated and aggressive treatment should be given in children with acute liver disease.

REFERENCES

1. Bernal W, Auzinger G, Dhawan A, et al. Acute liver failure. Lancet. 2010;376:196-201.
2. Srivastava A, Yacbha SK, Poddar U. Predictors of outcome in children with acute viral hepatitis and coagulopathy. J Viral Hepat. 2012;19:e194-201.

Chapter 64

Reye Syndrome

S Sushamabai

ABSTRACT

Reye syndrome (RS) is acute and fatal hepatic encephalopathy due to transient mitochondrial dysfunction of the liver induced by viral infections, toxins and drugs. Clinical features are repeated vomiting, seizures, coma and hepatomegaly. Raised serum glutamic pyruvic transaminase (SGPT)/serum glutamic oxaloacetic transaminase (SGOT) and plasma ammonia along with prolonged prothrombin time (PT) are supportive of diagnosis. Clinical staging system can be used for prognostication. Supportive therapy for encephalopathy is the only treatment.

INTRODUCTION

Reye syndrome is acute encephalopathy and fatty degeneration of the liver due to transient severe mitochondrial dysfunction of the liver.

ETIOLOGY

- Viral infections—influenza, varicella precipitated by aspirin or antiemetic intake
- Toxins—aflatoxins
- Drug-induced—valproic acid, cyanide, nimesulide
- Inborn errors of metabolism—suspect when repeated episodes occur.

PATHOGENESIS

- Mitochondrial dysfunction of the liver results in hypoglycemia, hyperammonemia, dyselectrolytemia, and subsequent encephalopathy.

Table 64.1: Clinical staging of Reye syndrome.

Symptoms	Signs	Stage	Prognosis
Vomiting, lethargy	Hepatomegaly	I	Good
Delirium, confusion	Hyperventilation, hyperreflexia	II	Good
Light coma, seizures±	Decorticate rigidity	III	Guarded
Deep coma, seizures	Fixed pupils, decerebrate rigidity	IV	Grave
Deep coma, decerebrate posturing	Fixed pupils, loss of DTR, flaccidity	V	Grave

(DTR, deep tendon reflexes)

CLINICAL FEATURES

- Repeated episodes of vomiting (may be preceded by a mild prodromal illness)
- Lethargy, coma, and seizures
- Hepatomegaly.

Clinical severity grading can be assessed as in Table 64.1.

DIFFERENTIAL DIAGNOSIS

- Accidental drug ingestion
- Meningitis
- Encephalitis
- Head injury
- Intracranial space-occupying lesion (ICSOL)
- Storage diseases with metabolic encephalopathy.

INVESTIGATIONS

- Ultrasonography abdomen to assess the nature of hepatomegaly
- Complete blood count, urine routine and acetone
- Liver function test—normal serum bilirubin with raised SGPT and SGOT, high plasma ammonia, and prolonged PT support the diagnosis of RS
- Random blood sugar—reveals nonketotic hypoglycemia
- Venous blood gas and serum electrolytes
- Renal function test—elevated blood urea and serum creatinine
- Cerebrospinal fluid studies to rule out meningitis
- Computed tomography or magnetic resonance imaging brain if ICSOL suspected.

TREATMENT

- Admit in pediatric intensive care unit; stabilize airway, breathing and circulation; assess and correct blood glucose level
- Intravenous (IV) fluids—2/3 maintenance requirement containing 10% dextrose with 40 mEq/L potassium, in 1/2 normal saline to maintain the serum Na between 140 mEq/L and 145 mEq/L; adjust the fluid volume to maintain urine output 1–2 mL/kg/hr
- Vitamin K 5 mg IV, repeat daily till PT is less than 1.2
- Anticonvulsant therapy—fosphenytoin + Phenobarbitone (Ch 35)
- Treatment of cerebral edema-fever and seizure control, head-end elevation 30°, IV mannitol/3% saline, intubation, hyperventilation
- Bowel sterilization—nasogastric tube aspiration, ampicillin, lactulose (as in acute liver failure)
- Fresh frozen plasma 10 mL/kg in 1–2 hours
- Intravenous ranitidine 3–5 mg/kg/day divided q 8 hourly.

SUBSEQUENT MANAGEMENT

As the signs of recovery start, the child can be gradually switched over to oral feeds as in hepatic encephalopathy and other medicines can be tapered.

OUTCOME

- Good with early diagnosis and intensive supportive therapy
- Recurrent episodes indicate the possibility of inborn errors of metabolism and have to be investigated accordingly.

CONCLUSION

Children presenting with repeated vomiting, seizures, coma, hepatomegaly, and raised SGPT, should be evaluated for Reye syndrome and aggressively treated.

Chapter 65

Acute Diarrhea and Dehydration

Carol Sara Cherian, S Sushamabai

ABSTRACT

Diarrhea is frequent passing of watery loose stools leading to loss of fluids and electrolytes from the body. The illness can produce death due to dehydration, dyselectrolytemia, and severe undernutrition. The World Health Organization (WHO) definition for diarrhea is passing of loose watery stools more than three times/day. The leading cause of diarrhea is viral infection. The patient assessment is essentially clinical by ask, look, and feel steps. The dehydration can be no, some, or severe degrees and the therapy plans are A, B, and C, respectively. In plan A and B fluid replacement is by ORS and in plan C, dehydration is corrected with intravenous (IV) Ringer lactate or normal saline. Zinc is essential for recovery; vitamin A and folic acid therapy are beneficial if there is deficiency. Drug therapy as per WHO protocol is outlined. Diet therapy in acute and persistent diarrhea is also included.

INTRODUCTION

Diarrhea as per WHO definition is more than three episodes of watery stools in 24 hours. Different types of diarrhea are:
- *Acute diarrheal disease (ADD)*—sudden onset of loose stools lasting less than 14 days
- *Persistent diarrhea*—acute onset diarrhea of infectious etiology lasting more than 14 days leading to undernutrition
- *Dysentery*—bloody diarrhea of infectious etiology
- *Chronic diarrhea*—insidious onset diarrhea lasting more than 14 days and is of noninfectious etiology.

ACUTE DIARRHEAL DISEASE

Etiology

- *Infectious:*
  - *Viral*—rotavirus (most common), calicivirus, adenovirus, coronavirus, cytomegalovirus, and picornavirus

- *Bacterial*—*Escherichia coli, Shigella, Vibrio cholerae, Salmonella, Campylobacter, Yersinia*
- *Parasitic*—*Giardia lamblia, Entamoeba histolytica,* malaria, and *Cryptosporidium parvum.*
- *Noninfectious*: Drugs, toxins, food induced, pesticides (organophosphates), and heavy metals (mercury, copper, arsenic, tin, fluoride).

Pathophysiology

- Direct invasion of intestinal mucosa by pathogens or by toxin action producing loss of fluids and electrolytes (Na, Cl, HCO_3, K).
- Hypoglycemia due to vomiting, purging, and poor intake.
- Net effects are dehydration, dyselectrolytemia, shock, and renal failure.
- Repeated episodes cause protein-energy malnutrition (PEM).

Clinical Presentation

- Vomiting, watery stools with/without fever, and abdominal cramps.
- Features of complications—excessive thirst, altered sensorium, convulsions, reduced urine output, and abdominal distension.
- Features of associated illness—pneumonia, meningitis, osteomyelitis, urinary tract infection (UTI), and PEM.

Patient Approach

- *Ask*: Duration, frequency, and volume of diarrheal stools, vomiting, associated blood in stools, fluids given (type and quantity), frequency of urine output, thirst, and other symptoms (high fever, convulsions, dysuria, cough, dyspnea, indicating associated serious infections).
- *Look*: Altered sensorium, sunken eyes, dry mucosa, rapid breathing, and abdominal distension.
- *Feel*: AF tension, rapid/feeble/thready pulse, CRFT, blood pressure, skin pinch return, and cold extremities.
- *Assess*: The degree of dehydration (Table 65.1).
- *Act*: Admit in pediatric intensive care unit or high-dependency unit if in severe dehydration or reveal associated problems as sepsis, pneumonia, meningitis, features of dyselectrolytemia, convulsions, shock, organ failure, and severe PEM.
    - Stabilize airway, breathing, and circulation (ABC); assess capillary glucose; correct hypoglycemia if detected.
    - Investigations:
        - Most patients of ADD without underlying problems do not require any investigation.

Table 65.1: Assessment of dehydration.

Signs	No dehydration	Some dehydration	Severe dehydration
Sensorium*	Normal	Irritable	Lethargy/coma
Thirst*	Drinks normally	Drinks eagerly	Unable to drink
Skinfold*	Instant recoil	Recoil in <2 s	Recoil in >2 s
Eyes	Normal	Slightly sunken	Deeply sunken
Tears	Present	Decreased	Absent
Mouth and tongue	Moist	Dry	Parched
CRFT	Normal <3 s	Prolonged >3 s	Prolonged >3 s
Extremities	Warm	Cold	Cold, mottled, cyanotic
Urine output	Normal	Decreased	Minimal
Treatment plan	A	B	C

*Key signs of dehydration.
Diagnose dehydration—If 1 key sign + 2 or more other signs or 2 key signs

Table 65.2: Fluid therapy—Plan C.

Age	Initial fluid, duration	Subsequent fluid, duration
<1 year	30 mL/kg in 1 hr	70 mL/kg in 5 hr
>1 year	30 mL/kg in 1/2 hr	70 mL/kg in 2.5 hr

Type of fluid—Ideal RL, alternate NS. (RL, Ringers lactate; NS, normal saline)
Note: Repeat the initial volume if the child continues to have feeble/nonpalpable radial pulse.

- If severe dehydration or associated problems consider blood gas, renal function test (RFT), serum electrolytes (SE), blood glucose (BG), complete blood count, prothrombin time, stool, and urine microscopy and culture, chest X-ray (CXR), blood culture, cerebrospinal fluid studies, etc.
- *Start fluid resuscitation—Plan C (Table 65.2) for severe dehydration:*
    - *Monitoring*—assess for the disappearance of clinical signs of dehydration after each bolus and for the appearance of signs of over hydration.
    - *Consider additional therapy* for associated disease, zinc, probiotics, vitamin A, and folic acid for control of diarrhea.
    - *Start oral fluids and feeds* once the signs of dehydration start disappearing. Continue with plan B therapy, if there are features of some dehydration and with plan A, if no dehydration.
- *Some dehydration—Plan B therapy:*
    - Manage in oral rehydration therapy area with ORS (245) 75 mL/kg in 4 hours. Give breastfeeds in-between; if not breastfed, give 100–200 mL milk/feed with plain water in-between.

Chapter 65: Acute Diarrhea and Dehydration

- Method—cup and spoon (nasogastric tube administration can be tried if acceptability is poor). Stop ORS when the child is active, playful, has no diarrhea or dehydration.
- If vomiting, wait for 10 minutes. Then give one teaspoon (5 mL) ORS every 2-3 minutes.
- ORS is inappropriate in severe dehydration, for initial fluid therapy and in paralytic ileus.
- ORS may be ineffective in children with a high stool purge rate (>5 mL/kg/hr), repeated vomiting (>3/hr), glucose malabsorption, and with incorrect preparation.
- Monitor the amount of ORS given, number of stools passed, for signs of overhydration or persistence of dehydration. Give ORS 10 mL/kg/stool in 1 hour, in sips for each stool loss in between.
- Reassess after 4 hours. Classify dehydration, select appropriate plan of treatment. Begin feeding; demonstrate to mother how to prepare ORS and the method of administration. If no dehydration, send home with two packets of ORS. Follow instructions as given in Plan A.
- *No dehydration—Plan A therapy:*
  - Manage at home. Follow three rules:
    - Give more fluids 5-10 mL/kg/stool in 1 hour. Fluids can be ORS 245/ORS equivalents, for example, Kanji water with salt added to taste, salted yoghurt drink, vegetable or chicken soup.
    - Give enough food—continue breastfeeding for babies less than 6 months age; for more than 6 months age, add homemade foods at least six times/day along with breastfeeds.
    - Advise to bring the child back to hospital if diarrhea persists beyond 3 days, many watery stools or blood in stools, vomiting, poor eating/drinking, increased thirst, fever or decreased urine output.

Drug Therapy in Diarrhea

- Elemental zinc:
  - 10 mg/day × 2 weeks in babies less than 6 months age
  - 20 mg/day × 2 weeks in those above 6 months age
- Probiotics—*Lactobacillus, bifidobacterium*
- Vitamin A, folic acid—as in PEM (Chapter 57)
- Indications for antibiotics:
  - Systemic infections (select appropriately)
  - Bacterial dysentery (shigellosis)
    - Intravenous ceftriaxone 50-100 mg/kg/day × 5 days if sick
    - PO cefixime 10 mg/kg/day, divided q 12 hr or ciprofloxacin 20-30 mg/kg/day, divided q 12 hr (in less sick children) × 3 days

- Cholera:
  - Children more than 7 years—tetracycline 12.5 mg/kg 4 times daily × 3 days/doxycycline 6 mg/kg single dose.
  - Children less than 7 years—erythromycin 12.5 mg/kg/dose q 6 hr × 3 days *or* azithromycin 20 mg/kg single dose.
  - Amebic dysentery—metronidazole 10 mg/kg/dose q 8 hr × 7 days followed by paromomycin 25–35 mg/kg/day divided q 8 hr × 7 days *or* diloxanide furoate 20 mg/kg/day in 3 divided doses × 7 days.
  - Giardiasis—metronidazole 5 mg/kg/dose q 8 hr × 7 days *or* furazolidone *or* albendazole.

Prevention—Educate regarding:
- Safe drinking water and clean eating habits
- Rotavirus vaccine is effective in preventing diarrhea due to rotavirus infection.

PERSISTENT DIARRHEA

Etiopathogenesis

- Undernutrition subsequent to diarrhea impairs the repair of intestinal epithelium producing malabsorption. A vicious cycle of increasing malabsorption and nutritional deterioration occurs.
- Inadequate food intake associated with diarrhea aggravates malnutrition.
- Persistent infection by organisms like *E. coli* (enteroaggregative and enteroadherent types) and cryptosporidium add to the problem.
- Cow's milk protein allergy, lactose, and other carbohydrate intolerance can occur.
- Repeated antibiotic administration producing pathogenic bacterial or fungal overgrowth in the intestine.

Clinical Presentation

- Prolonged diarrhea with frequent loose stools
- Progressive weight loss leading to overt malnutrition
- Associated infections—tuberculosis, UTI, pneumonia, sepsis, and cellulitis
- Features of micronutrient deficiency—anemia, vitamin A, B complex, and D deficiency
- Gaseous distension of abdomen, explosive stools, and perianal excoriation due to lactose intolerance.

Indications for Hospitalization

- Age less than 4 months and not breast fed
- Severe dehydration
- Associated severe malnutrition
- Presence of systemic infection.

Patient Approach

- Stabilize ABC; assess BG; correct hypoglycemia.
- Correction of dehydration—IV or oral rehydration as per clinical assessment
- Consider investigations—blood and urine culture, CXR, stool (microscopy, phototherapy, sugar, occult blood), SE, RFT, liver function test, and Mantoux test
- Continue breastfeeding:
  - Reduce lactose load in the diet by adding cooked rice or banana powder in babies more than 3 months age
  - Greater than 4-month age babies if stool pH is <5.5 and reducing substances more than or equal to 1%, advise the following:
    - Milk-based low-lactose diet (*diet A*—milk + rice + sugar + oil + water) (Table 57.3) *or*
    - Lactose-free diet (*diet B*—egg white + rice + sugar + oil + water)
- Treatment of PEM (Chapter 57)
- Broad-spectrum antibiotics (cefotaxime + amikacin) for infections
- Additional vitamins and minerals (vitamin A, zinc, folic acid) as for severe acute malnutrition (Chapter 57)
- Parameters for discharge:
  - Recovery from diarrhea
  - Improved appetite
  - Weight gain:
  - A regular follow-up to assess growth and detect the recurrence of diarrhea
- Persistence of diarrhea and poor weight gain:
  - Consider reinvestigation
  - Change to monosaccharide-based diet (diet C-comminuted chicken/egg white + glucose + oil)
- Continued diarrhea and dehydration—reinvestigate to exclude intractable diarrhea of infancy. Consider IV hyperalimentation followed by slow enteral alimentation.

CONCLUSION

Children with diarrhea should be clinically evaluated for dehydration and ORS therapy be started to prevent dehydration and IV fluids to treat severe dehydration.

FURTHER READING

1. Bhatnagar S, Lodha R, Choudhury P, et al. IAP guidelines 2006 on management acute diarrhea. Indian Pediatr. 2007;44:380.
2. Lopez AL. Cholera. In: Kliegman R, Stanton B, St Geme J, Schor N, Behrman R (Eds). Nelson Textbook of Pediatrics, 19th edition. US: Elsevier/Saunders; 2011. pp. 965-8.
3. World Health Organization. (2005). The treatment of diarrhoea. [online] WHO website. Available from http://www.who.int/maternal_child_adolescent/documents/9241593180/en/ [Accessed September 2018].

Chapter 66

Gastrointestinal Bleeding

Carol Sara Cherian, S Sushamabai

ABSTRACT

Gastrointestinal (GI) bleeding (GIB) is a common emergency in children and may end up in death which can be prevented by timely treatment. Bleeding can occur from upper or lower GI tract (GIT) due to local or systemic causes. Upper GIB (UGIB) due to local causes is the most common and is mostly mucosal or nonvariceal, presents with hematemesis. Lower GI bleed presents as melena or hematochezia. Assessment and immediate stabilization should proceed parallel. All patients with lower GI bleed should be investigated for upper GI bleed also. The roles of proton pump inhibitors in upper GI mucosal bleed and vasopressin, as well as early endoscopic ligation in variceal bleed, are discussed. The additional investigations in lower GI bleed are stool examination, colonoscopy, biopsy, and more advanced radiological investigations.

INTRODUCTION

Gastrointestinal bleeding is a common emergency in children and may become occasionally fatal. Timely diagnosis and intervention can prevent death. Bleeding can be from upper or lower GIT.

UPPER GASTROINTESTINAL BLEEDING

Upper gastrointestinal bleeding—indicates bleeding from a site proximal to the ligament of Treitz (at the level of duodenojejunal flexure).

Common Causes of UGIB beyond Neonatal Period

- *Local bleeding:*
  - *Nonvariceal (most common):*
    - Mallory–Weiss tears
    - Drug-induced erosions [nonsteroidal antiinflammatory drugs (NSAIDs), steroids]
    - Stress ulcers

- Esophagitis
- Foreign body impaction
- Trauma
- Caustic ingestion
- Duodenal and peptic ulcers
- Polyps, tumors, and vascular malformations
- *Variceal*—less common, usually massive
- *Generalized bleeding:*
  - Hemorrhagic fevers (dengue and others)
  - Disseminated intravascular coagulation and sepsis
  - Hereditary bleeding disorders (hemophilia)
  - Henoch–Schönlein vasculitis
  - Snake envenomation
  - Poisoning—arsenic, Cu, plant seeds (*Abrus precatorius*)
  - Liver failure
  - Renal failure.

Clinical Presentation

- Vomiting of frank blood or coffee-colored material ranging from trivial to large amounts; may contain clots. Blood when exposed to gastric or intestinal juices quickly darkens to coffee color.
- Nausea, vomiting, or diarrhea can precede large amounts of hematemesis.
- Features of hypovolemic shock as pallor, tachycardia, low blood pressure, and altered sensorium occur if the hematemesis is massive.
- Suspect massive occult bleeding (>30% of blood volume for the body weight) if the patient has features of hypovolemic shock with minimal hematemesis.
- Associated symptoms and signs of underlying cause may be evident.
- Features of hepatic coma may appear in patients with liver disease and hematemesis due to the breakdown products of intraluminal blood and elevated serum bilirubin.
- Consider hemoptysis or swallowed blood from epistaxis and gum bleeds as alternate possibilities that are to be excluded by history and examination. In hemoptysis, respiratory symptoms and signs will be present.

Patient Approach

Depends on the amount of blood vomited or lost and the underlying etiology; verify by history and by guaiac test of gastric fluid to confirm true bleeding.

Step I—Assess the Severity and Stabilize

Massive hematemesis
- Admit the patient in PICU; assess vitals; stabilize airway, breathing, and circulation; suck the airway; administer O_2 5–10 L/min. Pallor, tachycardia, narrow pulse pressure, and orthostatic or overt hypotension indicate massive blood loss. Proceed to intubation and mechanical ventilation if there is airway compromise.
- Secure two intravenous (IV) lines; start IV normal saline (NS) 20 mL in 10–20 minutes, repeat two more boluses till signs of shock disappear.
- Collect blood for complete blood count, coagulation profile, grouping and cross matching, random blood sugar, serum electrolytes, renal function test, liver function test, and culture; also urine routine and culture (Box 66.1).
- Nasogastric (NG) aspiration (use an age-appropriate large bore NG tube) for gastric decompression, to confirm hematemesis and to assess the quantity of blood loss.
- Indwelling catheter to assess urine output; maintain a strict intake-output chart including gastric aspirate.
- Urgent ultrasonography (USG) abdomen to evaluate the liver, patency of portal vein and to detect esophageal varices.
- Bedside Doppler studies for portal venous flow direction urgently.
- Vitamin K 5 mg IV single dose, correction of coagulopathy by fresh frozen plasma and/or platelet transfusion as needed (Chapter 79).

Box 66.1: Diagnostic workup of LGIB.

For all (UGIB and LGIB)
- CBC, PBS, coagulation profile, grouping, typing, cross matching, SE, RBS, RFT, LFT
- Blood and urine culture, sensitivity
- USG abdomen and upper GI endoscopy

Colitis presentation
- Stool microscopy, occult blood, culture and sensitivity, assay for clostridium difficile toxin
- Colonoscopy with biopsy for histology, culture, immunohistochemistry

Noncolitis presentation
- Colonoscopy and biopsy or polypectomy
- ^{99m}Tc pertechnetate scan for Meckel's diverticulum/intestinal duplication
- Triple-phase CT angiography and selective cannulation of mesenteric vessel for embolization in aneurysmal bleed
- Capsule endoscopy is useful to evaluate the small intestine
- Tagged RBC scan is helpful to locate the site of bleeding when it is obscure
- Preoperative endoscopy in significant ongoing bleeding from unknown site

(CBC, complete blood count; CT, computed tomography; GI, gastrointestinal; LFT, liver function test; LGIB, lower gastrointestinal bleeding; PBS, peripheral blood smear; RBC, red blood cell; RBS, random blood sugar; RFT, renal function test; SE, serum electrolytes; UGIB, upper gastrointestinal bleeding; USG, ultrasonography)

- Proton pump inhibitor—IV pantoprazole 2 mg/kg/dose as loading dose followed by 0.2 mg/kg/hr infusion for 72 hours; once stabilized, change to double dose orally for 2 weeks.
- Whole blood transfusion 20 mL/kg in 2–4 hours if the child continues to be in shock in spite of fluid boluses.
- Packed cell transfusion to bring up hemoglobin to 8 g/dL.
- Antibiotics—third-generation cephalosporin for 7 days, if any associated infection especially in children with variceal bleeding.

Step II—Detailed History and Subsequent Management

- Nil oral till active bleeding stops as assessed by gastric aspirate and endoscopy.
- Parenteral fluid therapy—correction of dehydration followed by maintenance fluid as D5 1/2 NS with KCl 20–40 mEq/L; replace gastric aspirate loss as NS volume by volume to the maintenance requirement.
- Gastroenterology consultation for endoscopy within 24 hours to visualize the bleeding area (variceal/nonvariceal).
- For variceal bleeding, add vasopressin (0.33 U/kg over 20 minutes as bolus followed by continuous infusion of the same dose on an hourly basis) or octreotide IV infusion 1–5 µg/kg/hr
- Endoscopic sclerotherapy or elastic band ligation (superior effect) of esophageal varices or surgery according to gastroenterologist's decision.
- Plan for long-term management:
    - Prevention of variceal bleeding by periodic band ligation. Porto systemic shunt in selected situations.
    - Start oral propranolol to reduce the portal venous pressure on long-term basis.
    - Treat the underlying liver disease.
- Specific therapy for other causes of upper GI bleed.

LOWER GASTROINTESTINAL BLEEDING

- Lower GI bleeding indicates bleeding from a site below the ligament of Treitz. Evaluation and management of lower gastrointestinal bleeding (LGIB) is more complex and difficult.
- *Hematochezia* is red or maroon blood in stools and signifies lower gut as the bleeding site or massive hemorrhage above the distal ileum.
- *Melena* is blackened stools of tarry consistency and indicates moderate or mild bleeding from sites above the distal ileum.

Note: Massive bleeding from the duodenum or above can cause melena. Hence, in all LGIB, upper GI causes should be excluded by USG and endoscopy.

Common Causes of LGIB beyond Neonatal Period

I. Local
- Infectious enteritis/colitis
- Intussusception
- Amebiasis
- Anal fissure
- Meckels diverticulum
- Solitary rectal ulcer syndrome (SRUS)
- Drug-induced ulcer (NSAIDs)
- Cow's milk protein allergy
- Polyps, diverticula, tumors
- Inflammatory bowel disease
- Hemorrhoids, vascular malformations
- Hirsch sprung disease

II. General
As for UGIB

Clinical Presentation

- Passing frank or altered or tarry blood per rectum. Associated abdominal pain and fever indicate infective or inflammatory disease of the bowel.
- Evidence of UGIB may be perceived clinically or by investigations in 10% cases.
- Features of hypovolemic shock indicate massive bleeding that may not be obvious.
- Associated symptoms and signs of underlying disease can be elicited.

Patient Approach

- As in the case of UGIB, assess from history the possibility of food, medicines or colors inducing black/maroon color to stool. Confirm the presence of blood by guaiac test if needed.
- Proceed as in UGIB for severity assessment, initial stabilization followed by detailed evaluation, and subsequent management.
- History and physical examination are extremely important to detect the causes and severity of bleeding.
- Fever, colicky abdominal pain, and frequent loose stools with blood and mucus point to colitis of infectious or inflammatory etiology.
- Episodes of abdominal pain, vomiting, red currant jelly stools, and sausage-shaped mass in the abdomen are features of intussusception.
- Bleeding is painless in polyps, Meckel's diverticulum, vascular anomaly, and ulcers.
- Cow's milk protein allergy occurs in infants fed with cow's milk and present with loose bloody stools, colic, anemia, and poor weight gain.
- Delayed passage of meconium followed by constipation, abdominal pain, and distension are features of Hirschsprung disease.

- Bloody diarrhea following antibiotic use indicates pseudomembranous colitis.
- Inflammatory bowel disease has to be suspected in presence of recurrent aphthous ulcers, joint pain, and iritis.
- History of painful defecation and hard stools with blood streaking is suggestive of anal fissure.
- History of constipation, straining at stools, and digital evacuation indicates SRUS.
- Children with human immunodeficiency virus infection or immune suppression following chemotherapy can develop cytomegalovirus enterocolitis or polymicrobial inflammation of cecum (typhlitis) causing significant LGIB.
- Palpable purpura of lower limbs in Henoch–Schönlein vasculitis, rectal prolapse on straining, fissure and fleshy anal tags on Crohn's disease, orobuccal pigmentation in Peutz–Jeghers syndrome, and skin lesions of blue rubber bleb nevus syndrome are some of the findings to be searched to detect the etiology.

Physical Examination

Apart from general and GIT examination, a gentle per rectal examination to detect polyps, impacted stool, anal fissure, and anal tags should be done.

Diagnostic Workup

Proceed to all investigations stepwise as in UGIB after stabilization and subsequent evaluation. Additional investigations should be selected as in Box 66.1 based on clinical assessment.

Subsequent Management

Supportive therapy—as in UGIB
Specific therapy—as per etiology.

CONCLUSION

Gastrointestinal bleed can be upper or lower or combined but all lower GI bleeds should be investigated to exclude upper GI involvement.

Chapter 67

Acute Pancreatitis

S Sushamabai

ABSTRACT

Acute pancreatitis is an abdominal emergency increasingly observed in children. Early diagnosis and appropriate treatment can prevent multiorgan failure and death. The diagnostic criteria are any two of the three—acute abdominal pain, three-fold rise in serum amylase/lipase, and radiological evidence of pancreatitis. The main cause is viral infection, the others being drugs and toxins, inborn errors of metabolism and autoimmune disorders. Clinical categorization is as mild and severe acute pancreatitis (SAP). Immediate airway, breathing and circulation (ABC) stabilization and parallel investigations including early imaging to assess the extent of pancreas damage, pain management with intravenous morphine, broad-spectrum antibiotic therapy if febrile, maintenance of fluid and electrolyte balance, and proton pump inhibitor therapy are the important principles in treatment. Detailed investigations, patient approach and the medical and surgical management are discussed. Early enteral feeding is recommended for rapid recovery. All children with acute pancreatitis should have periodic follow-up and prompt treatment of acute exacerbations. Detailed investigations to exclude surgical conditions should be considered as the child starts recovering.

INTRODUCTION

Acute pancreatitis is an abdominal emergency increasingly observed nowadays in pediatrics. The disease is characterized by inflammation and necrosis of pancreas due to diverse etiology. Early diagnosis and appropriate management can prevent death as well as morbidity due to progressive damage of pancreas.

CLASSIFICATION

Mild Acute Pancreatitis

Symptoms lasting less than 48 hours with complete recovery.

Severe Acute Pancreatitis

Life-threatening pancreatitis with systemic inflammatory response syndrome and system dysfunction such as shock, renal failure, acute respiratory distress syndrome (ARDS), disseminated intravascular coagulation (DIC), massive gastrointestinal (GI) bleeding, and systemic or intra-abdominal infection.

ETIOLOGY

- *Blunt abdominal injuries*
- *Infections:*
  - Viral—mumps, coxsackie, cytomegalovirus, hepatitis A, B, non-A–non-B
  - Leptospirosis
  - Septic shock
  - Reye syndrome
  - Mycoplasma
  - Ascariasis
- *Drugs and toxins:*
  - Acetaminophen over dose
  - Isoniazid, metronidazole, furosemide, and steroids
  - Valproic acid and levetiracetam
  - L-asparaginase, 6-mercaptopurine, azathioprine
  - Spider and scorpion envenomation
  - Organophosphate poisoning
- *Obstructive diseases of biliary tract—stones, sludging*
- *Organ transplantation*
- *Autoimmune diseases*
- *Genetic*
- *Metabolic—hypertriglyceridemia.*

PATHOGENESIS

- Premature activation of trypsin within the acinar cell causes autodigestion of the pancreatic tissue.
- A vicious cycle of enzyme activation, release of active proteases, cytokines and inflammatory mediators occur leading to progressive damage of pancreas.

CLINICAL PRESENTATION

- Severe acute upper abdominal pain radiating to the back, persistent vomiting, and fever.

- Child assumes an antalgic position with hips and knees flexed, sitting upright or lying on the side.
- Abdominal distension, epigastric tenderness, and mass
- High fever, jaundice, shock, respiratory distress (due to ARDS, pleural effusion), bleeding (GI, DIC) herald severe disease
- Cullen sign (bluish discoloration around the umbilicus) and/or Grey Turner sign (discoloration of the flanks) are observed in SAP.
- Severe abdominal pain, jaundice, vomiting, and clay-colored stool indicate biliary obstruction.

DIFFERENTIAL DIAGNOSIS

- Acute cholecystitis
- Acute appendicitis
- Acute pyelonephritis
- Sepsis with shock
- Fulminant hepatic failure.

PATIENT APPROACH

- The diagnostic criteria of pancreatitis should be at least two of the following:
  - Acute abdominal pain
  - Three-fold rise of serum amylase and/or lipase activity
  - Radiological evidence of acute pancreatitis.

Serum lipase activity is more specific than amylase; the value rises by 4–8 hours, peaks at 24–48 hours and remains elevated for 2 weeks longer than amylase.
- Severe acute pancreatitis has to be considered as one differential diagnosis in a sick bleeding child with shock, history of trauma, and high fever, infections as described above, drug intake and poisoning/envenomation.
- Admit in pediatric intensive care unit, stabilize ABC; assess capillary blood glucose, correct hypo/hyperglycemia.
- Send blood for complete blood count, serum amylase, serum lipase, coagulation profile, renal function test, liver function test, fasting lipid profile, serum Na, K, Ca, random blood sugar, culture, blood grouping, typing and crossmatching.
- Coagulopathy, leukocytosis, hyperglycemia, hypocalcemia, hyperbilirubinemia and elevated gamma-glutamyl transpeptidase are the supportive laboratory findings.
- Urine examination for glycosuria and culture.

- Imaging studies should be done urgently:
  - Chest skiagram to detect atelectasis, lung infiltrates, pleural and pericardial effusion, and early ARDS.
  - Abdominal skiagram to detect ileus, pancreatic calcification (indicates chronic pancreatitis), pseudocyst, ascites and peripancreatic extraluminal gas bubbles.
  - Ultrasonography abdomen especially to detect biliary stone impaction.
  - Contrast-enhanced computed tomography abdomen (magnetic resonance imaging if contrast dye is contraindicated)—reveals pancreatic enlargement, edema, abscess, mass and fluid collection. More than 30% damage of pancreas predicts bad prognosis.
  - Magnetic resonance cholangiopancreatography, endoscopic retrograde cholangiopancreatography and endoscopic ultrasonography should be considered in recurrent episodes and nonresolving pancreatitis.

SUBSEQUENT MANAGEMENT

Medical

- Pain management—give any of the following:
  - Intravenous tramadol—1 mg/kg/dose q 6 hr diluted in normal saline (NS) in 20 minutes
  - Intravenous morphine—0.05–0.2 mg/kg q 2–4 hours
  - Intravenous fentanyl—1–3 µg/kg/dose q 30–60 minutes till recovery starts.
- Fluid and electrolyte balance:
  - Initial fluid for correction of dehydration—Ringers lactate is superior to NS
  - Maintenance fluid is 5% dextrose + 1/2 NS with KCl 20–40 mEq/L
  - Add NS to the maintenance fluid volume by volume for gastric aspirate
  - Provide necessary correction for associated complications as shock, renal failure, ARDS, and DIC.
- Nasogastric aspiration till vomiting subsides
- Treatment of associated complications (refer respective chapters)
- Intravenous pantoprazole for gastric acid suppression (Chapter 66) followed by oral
- Broad-spectrum antibiotic therapy if there is pancreatic necrosis as revealed from the imaging studies or if the child has systemic inflammatory response syndrome/high fever/leukocytosis
- Treatment of associated complications
- Start early feeding once vomiting stops and pain subsides as it promotes the regeneration of pancreas and intestines
- Initial fluid can be plain water followed by kanji water and then milk.

Surgical

- In children with nontraumatic acute pancreatitis surgical therapy is rarely required
- Indications of surgical interventions are necrosis of pancreas for debridement or drainage of abscess
- Endoscopic therapy for anatomic abnormalities like stricture or stones.

Follow-up: It is mandatory in all children with acute pancreatitis to detect recurrence and chronic pancreatitis.

CONCLUSION

Acute pancreatitis should be considered as a cause of severe abdominal pain in children, investigated and treated.

Chapter 68

Ascites

S Sushamabai

ABSTRACT

Ascites or peritoneal dropsy is the pathologic collection of fluid within the peritoneal cavity. The leading causes are nephrotic syndrome, portal hypertension, spontaneous bacterial peritonitis, pancreatitis, bowel infarction, severe malnutrition and malignancies. Indications for peritoneal tap and laboratory evaluation of ascitic fluid are detailed. Specific therapy for the underlying cause should be started at the earliest. Therapy for ascitic fluid reduction is salt and fluid restriction, diuretic therapy, good protein diet and therapeutic paracentesis, and intravenous albumin or fresh frozen plasma (FFP) administration.

INTRODUCTION

Ascites is the pathologic collection of fluid within the peritoneal cavity. The fluid can be serous, purulent, hemorrhagic, chylous or bilious based on the etiology (Box 68.1).

Box 68.1: Common causes of ascites.

Hepatic
Cirrhosis
Portal hypertension
Fulminant hepatic failure
Budd–Chiari syndrome

Infectious
Abdominal TB
Bacterial peritonitis
Intra abdominal abscess

Neoplastic
Lymphoma
Leukemia

Cardiac
Constrictive pericarditis
Heart failure

Renal
Nephrotic syndrome
Obstructive uropathy
Perforation of urinary tract
Peritoneal dialysis

Gynecologic
Ovarian tumors
Ovarian torsion, rupture

Contd...

Contd...

Gastrointestinal	Miscellaneous
Protein losing enteropathy	Ventriculoperitoneal shunt
Intestinal lymphangiectasia	Chylous ascites
Bowel infarction/rupture	Eosinophilic ascites
Pancreatitis	Systemic lupus erythematosus
	Severe malnutrition

CLINICAL PRESENTATION

Abdominal Distension

- Rapid fluid accumulation presents with abdominal distension and respiratory distress.
- Gradual collection of fluid produces early satiety and poor eating.
- Dullness to percussion, shifting dullness and fluid thrill are the signs of ascites when the quantity of fluid is large.
- Accumulation of small amount of fluid can be detected by the "puddle sign".
- Umbilical and inguinal hernias occur in tense ascites.
- Features of underlying illness can be elicited by history and clinical examination.

Other causes of abdominal distension mimicking ascites are fecal impaction, flatus, fetus, obesity, ovarian cyst and urine retention. They should be excluded by history, physical examination and ultrasonography (USG) abdomen if needed.

INDICATIONS FOR PEDIATRIC INTENSIVE CARE UNIT ADMISSION

- Tense ascites with respiratory distress
- Fever
- Hepatic, cardiac, respiratory and/or renal diseases
- Electrolyte imbalance
- Refractory ascites
- Edema.

PATIENT APPROACH

- Stabilize airway, breathing, and circulation; assess capillary blood glucose (CBG) and correct hypoglycemia
- Bed rest in 45° propped-up position
- Urgent USG abdomen to confirm ascites and to assess the etiology

Table 68.1: Interpretation of serum ascites albumin gradient.

High gradient (≥1.1 g/dL)	Low gradient (<1.1 g/dL)
Portal hypertension	Nephrotic syndrome
Cirrhosis	Tuberculous peritonitis
Fulminant hepatic failure	Pancreatic ascites
Budd–Chiari syndrome	Peritoneal carcinomatosis
Portal vein thrombosis	Serositis

- Laboratory investigations—complete blood count, coagulation profile, liver function test including serum proteins, renal function test, serum electrolytes, random blood sugar, blood grouping, typing, X matching, chest X-ray, electrocardiography, urinalysis and blood and urine cultures if infection is suspected. The common causes of ascites can be diagnosed by these investigations.
- Tuberculin test
- Diagnostic peritoneal tap if bacterial peritonitis, tuberculosis or malignancy is suspected (Chapter 122).

ASCITES FLUID EXAMINATION

- Color: Straw-colored in cirrhosis
- Cell count: More than 250 white blood cell/mm^3 with neutrophilia indicates bacterial peritonitis
- Histopathological examination to detect malignant cells
- Culture: Directly inoculate into blood culture bottle
- Gram stain to detect bacterial pathogens
- Proteins: Less than 3 and more than 3 g/dL indicate transudate and exudate, respectively
- Sugar
- Serum ascites albumin gradient (Table 68.1)
- If indicated, pH, lactate, amylase and adenosine deaminase estimation.

SUBSEQUENT TREATMENT

- Detect the underlying cause and treat
- Reduction of ascites:
    - Bed rest 16–18 hr/day
    - Mobilization of ascites fluid by creating negative sodium balance in the body:
        - Salt restricted diet 1–2 g/day, no added salt in the diet or salty snacks
        - Water restriction up to 3/4 maintenance if hyponatremia (serum sodium <125 mEq/L)

- Diet: 150% calories of recommended dietary allowance (yielded from protein 15%, fat 30–35%, carbohydrate 50–55%)
- Diuretic therapy: PO spironolactone + furosemide morning OD
    - To achieve weight loss up to 1% of body weight/day and gradual reduction in abdominal girth
    - Increase the dose of spironolactone 1 mg/kg/week up to 6 mg/kg/day + furosemide 1 mg/kg/day every 2–3 days up to 4 mg/kg/day; stop if no response
- Supplemental albumin or FFP
- Large volume abdominal paracentesis: Remove 200–400 mL/kg/day of ascites fluid over 6 hours under cover of 20% albumin at the rate of 6 g/L of fluid removed; 1/2 the dose immediately and the rest in 6 hours; two trials of large volume paracentesis can be considered.

CONCLUSION

Ascites is pathologic collection of fluid in the peritoneal cavity, should be thoroughly investigated and aggressively managed.

Section 10

INFECTIOUS DISEASES

Chapter 69

Dengue Shock Syndrome

S Sushamabai

ABSTRACT

Dengue shock syndrome is a medical emergency occasionally encountered in dengue viral infection. Patients without warning signs can be managed at home with oral fluids and paracetamol. Those with warning signs should be hospitalized and intravenous (IV) normal saline (NS) maintenance therapy (5–7 mL/kg/hr) is advised. Patients with severe dengue need pediatric intensive care unit care, vigilant monitoring, IV fluid therapy, dopamine or dobutamine infusion, and supportive therapy for organ failure. Those with decompensated shock should be given colloid/fresh whole blood transfusion (FWBT) depending on high or low hematocrit (Hct), respectively, along with maintenance fluid therapy till recovery. Indications for platelet transfusion or platelet-rich plasma are also highlighted. Close clinical monitoring for vitals and intake output chart and laboratory assessment for serum electrolytes (SE), renal function test (RFT), Hct, and platelet count (PLC) are mandatory till recovery.

INTRODUCTION

Dengue shock syndrome is the most serious complication of dengue illness and occurs in a few percentage only. The afebrile period lasting for 24–48 hours as shown in Figure 69.1 is the critical phase of complications.

SEVERITY CLASSIFICATION

As per World Health Organization (WHO) severity classification, the disease can be dengue without/with warning signs or severe dengue leading to plasma leakage, shock, hemorrhage, or multiorgan failure.
- Plasma leakage is heralded by severe abdominal pain, vomiting, ascites, and respiratory distress due to pleural effusion or acute respiratory distress syndrome (ARDS).
- A lateral decubitus chest skiagram or ultrasonogram of the abdomen and/or chest is helpful for early diagnosis (Fig. 69.2).
- Severe bleeding and organ dysfunction like encephalopathy, myocardial failure, ARDS, hepatic, or renal failure are the result of delayed/inadequate/hypotonic fluid therapy.

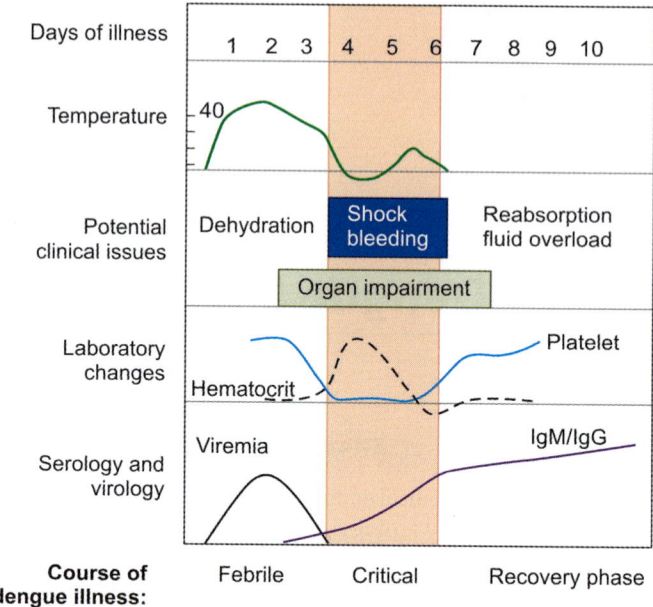

Fig. 69.1: Dengue illness. Critical afebrile phase = bleeding, shock, organ failure. (IgM, immunoglobulin M; IgG, immunoglobulin G. Temperature is given in degrees Celsius (°C))

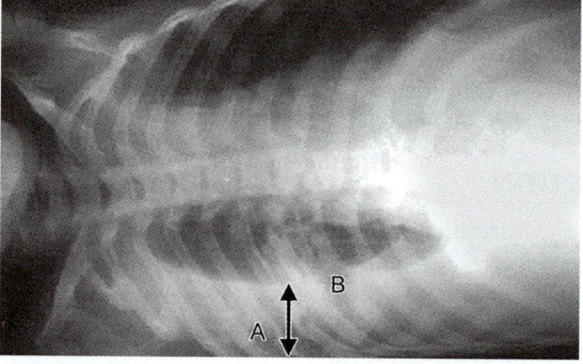

Fig. 69.2: Chest X-ray (R) lateral decubitus view—pleural effusion.

PATIENT APPROACH

- Suspect probable dengue in any child who lives in or travels to an endemic area and presents with fever + two or more of the following features:
  - Myalgia, rash, bleeding tendency, aches and pains, warning signs
  - Positive tourniquet test, leukopenia, or laboratory confirmation
- Categorize as per WHO directions:
  A. No warning signs
  B. With warning signs
  C. Severe dengue

- Warning signs: Abdominal pain/tenderness, persistent vomiting, clinical fluid accumulation, mucosal bleed, lethargy, restlessness, liver enlargement more than 2 cm, increased Hct more than 20%, and/or rapid reduction in platelets
- Assess for bleeding:
  - Clinical—Hess test, anemia, overt bleeding
  - Laboratory—↓Hemoglobin (Hb), ↓Hct, ↓ PLC.

Note: Early bleeding may herald other viral and other hemorrhagic fevers.
- Consider other differential diagnosis of fever and bleeding—meningococcemia, typhoid fever, rickettsial infections, fulminant hepatic failure, malaria, leptospirosis, yellow fever, and influenza
- Confirm dengue virus etiology by nonstructural protein 1 (NS1) antigen Elisa test (in epidemics, laboratory diagnosis is not needed. NS1 antigen remains positive only on days 1–5 of illness)
- Obtain complete blood count on day 1 itself—Hb, total leukocyte, differential leukocyte, PLC, Hct to know the early baseline picture. Pancytopenia is supportive of dengue fever. Persistent leukopenia heralds hectic course
- Consider coexisting infections (dengue + malaria, dengue + influenza A, dengue + leptospirosis) depending on the associated clinical features. Select additional investigations judiciously for diagnostic confirmation
- Proceed to management as per categorization:

Group A—Requires Home Care Only

- Adequate bed rest—avoid schooling till recovery
- Oral fluids 1–2 L/day (oral rehydration solution, Kanji water, milk, fruit juice—avoid excess sugar)
- Give fluids as frequent small feeds
- Treat fever and myalgia—paracetamol 10–15 mg/kg dose q 6 hr
- Avoid nonsteroidal anti-inflammatory drugs—ibuprofen and mefenamic acid—they can predispose to bleeding, liver, and renal failure
- Inform the patient/parent regarding the warning signs, maintaining fluid intake and output chart. If hydration is adequate, child should pass urine four to six times daily. The child should report to the hospital immediately if any warning signs appear (should not wait till next morning)

Note: In Group A, children less than 1 year, those with preexisting chronic diseases like diabetes, asthma, renal, liver, cardiac problems, or having difficulty for medical access need hospitalization.

Flowchart 69.1: Fluid therapy in dengue with warning signs (Group B).

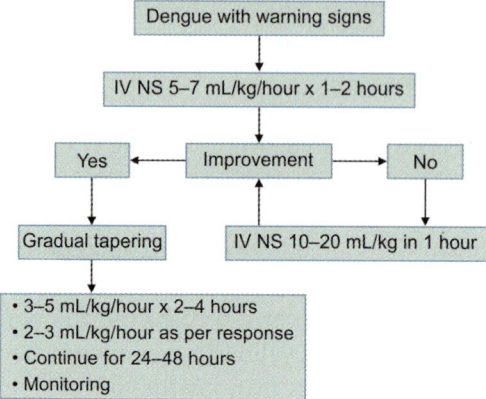

(IV, intravenous; NS, normal saline)

Group B—Need Hospitalization and Intravenous Fluids

- Supportive care is as in Group A
- Intravenous fluids for maintenance requirement as:
  - Normal saline 5–7 mL/kg/hr × 2 hours. Taper as per response in 24–48 hours guided by monitoring (Flowchart 69.1)
  - Other treatment parameters as in Group A.

Group C—Need Hospitalization and Pediatric Intensive Care Unit Care

- Patients with compensated shock:
  - Features—extreme prostration, rapid and thready pulse, cold extremities, delayed capillary refill time (CRFT), normal blood pressure; require high dependency unit care and IV fluid therapy. Fluid recommended is NS 10–20 mL/kg in 1 hour. If improving, gradually taper the IV fluid in 24–48 hours monitoring the clinical signs and urine output which should be maintained at 1–2 mL/kg/hr.
  - If no improvement, assess the Hct; value if less than 40%, give FWBT 10–20 mL/kg in 2–4 hours; if high, give IV colloids (preferred) or NS 10–20 mL/kg in 1–2 hours; on improvement, switch to tapering IV fluid as in Group B (Flowchart 69.2).
- Patients with severe dengue:
  - Present with shock with/without organ or system failure. Assess Hct immediately, start colloid 20 mL/kg in 15 minutes. If improving, repeat colloid 10 mL/kg in 20 minutes followed by gradual tapering with NS in 24–48 hours; those with falling Hct need FWBT transfusion 10–20 mL/kg in 2–4 hours. For patients with continuing low Hct, one or more dose of FWBT may be required (Flowchart 69.3).

Flowchart 69.2: Fluid therapy in severe dengue (Group C) with compensated shock (SBP-N, reduced perfusion)

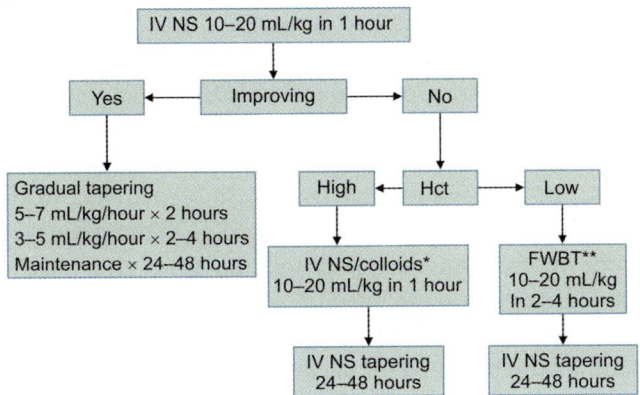

*Colloids—Dextran 40/Gelatin/FFP.
**FWBT—Fresh whole blood transfusion.
(FFP, fresh-frozen plasma; Hct, hematocrit; SBP, systolic blood pressure)

Flowchart 69.3: Fluid therapy in severe dengue (Group C) with hypotensive shock/organ failure.

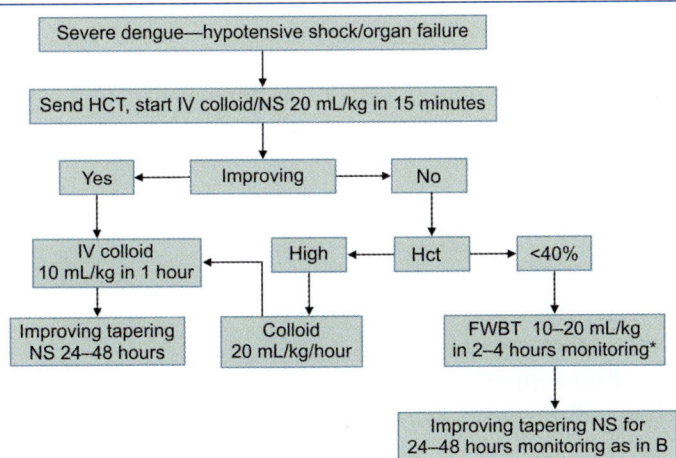

*Rpt bolus colloid/WBT if no improvement.
(FWBT, fresh whole blood transfusion; Hct, hematocrit; IV, intravenous; NS, normal saline; WBT, whole blood transfusion)

Monitoring

- Should be 4-6 hourly or more frequently by an experienced staff nurse. Assess the sensorium, warmth of the extremities, pulse, respiratory rate, CRFT, temperature, blood pressure, and pulse pressure. Pulse pressure

less than 20 mm Hg heralds shock; consider NS bolus and tapering as in Figure 69.1.
- Strict maintenance of intake and output; maintain urine output at 1 mL/kg/hr; rate less than 0.5 mL/kg/hr indicates renal failure; more than 4 mL/kg/hr denotes hypervolemia and polyuria which may cause cardiac failure in the recovery phase.
- Laboratory evaluation—Hct 6 hourly initially, PLC daily, blood glucose, SE, RFT, liver function test, chest X-ray, electrocardiography, ultrasonography, echocardiography according to the situation, if needed.
- Hematocrit more than or equal to 20% from the baseline reveals hemoconcentration and the need for increasing NS infusion rate.
- Hematocrit less than or equal to 20% from the baseline indicates hemodilution and the need for packed red blood cell transfusion.
- Electrocardiography may reveal bradycardia or ventricular extrasystole.
- Echocardiography study is helpful to detect ventricular ejection fraction and the need for dopamine/dobutamine.

Indications for Blood and Blood Products

- Fresh whole blood transfusion:
  - Overt bleeding with shock, shock with low Hct (indicates occult bleeding)
- Platelet transfusion:
  - Platelet count less than 10,000 or less than 50,000/mm^3 with bleeding (in obstetric bleeds and surgery only); ideal preparation is platelet-rich plasma 3–5 U/day.

Dengue with Organ Dysfunction

- Myocardial—fluids, dopamine/dobutamine
- Respiratory—100% O_2, mechanical ventilation
- Renal—fluid therapy, dialysis
- Hepatic—liver supportive therapy
- Encephalopathy—fluids, seizure control, and treatment of brain edema.

Dengue with Fluid Overload

- Manifests during the recovery phase. Features are dyspnea, ascites due to excess or hypotonic fluid therapy.
- Treatment—O_2, lateral decubitus position, reduce/stop IV fluids; administer furosemide 0.1–0.5 mg/kg.
- Hypertonic saline (7.5%) 4 mL/kg administration at the early phase of IV fluid therapy to prevent plasma leakage and hypotension is practiced in some centers.

Discharge Criteria

- Subjective well-being and good appetite
- Afebrile for 48 hours
- Stable hemodynamics
- Adequate urine output on oral fluids
- Platelet count more than 50,000/mm^3, no bleeding.

CONCLUSION

Dengue shock syndrome is a serious complication of dengue viral infection and should be treated with vigilant monitoring, fluid therapy, vasopressors and organ support.

FURTHER READING

1. Kamath SR, Ranjit S. Clinical features, complications and atypical manifestations of children with severe forms of dengue hemorrhagic fever in South India. Indian J Pediatr. 2006;73(10):889-95.
2. Tan GK, Ng JK, Tan KW, et al. Hypertonic saline reduces vascular leakage in a mouse model of severe dengue. issn:2013 April 18 Vol 8(4) Ppe 61621,PMID.
3. World Health Organization. (2012). WHO Guidelines Dengue Fever 2012.

Chapter 70

Fulminant Meningococcemia

S Sushamabai

ABSTRACT

Fulminant meningococcemia is a febrile emergency, especially in infants less than 1 year age. The usual clinical presentation is fever with diarrhea, vomiting, irritability and/or bleeding tendency. The differential diagnoses are viral hemorrhagic fevers, rickettsial infections, drug rashes and vasculitis. Immediate stabilization, investigations, empirical antibiotic therapy with intravenous (IV) ceftriaxone ± vancomycin should be started in the first hour itself. Supportive therapy with fluid and electrolytes, correction of shock by adding hydrocortisone, and treatment of brain edema, hepatic or renal failure are the other complications to be managed. Ideal agent for chemoprophylaxis to close contacts is single dose of ceftriaxone.

INTRODUCTION

Fulminant meningococcemia is the most serious form of invasive meningococcal infection caused by *Neisseria meningitidis* (*Meningococcus*) and is a medical emergency in infants less than 1 year age.

CLINICAL PRESENTATION

- Short febrile illness with vomiting, diarrhea, myalgia, headache, and irritability
- Fever with bleeding, arthritis, and altered sensorium
- Meningitis.

DIFFERENTIAL DIAGNOSIS

- Drug rashes
- Immune thrombocytopenia
- Henoch–Schönlein vasculitis
- Hemorrhagic fevers
- Septic arthritis

- Rickettsial fevers
- Sepsis syndrome.

PATIENT APPROACH

- Admit in pediatric intensive care unit; stabilize airway, breathing, and circulation; assess capillary blood glucose, and correct hypoglycemia.
- Correction of shock by IV normal saline bolus 20 mL/kg in 20–60 minutes × three doses as per the degree of shock. Continue maintenance fluid therapy with 5% dextrose normal saline with KCl. Add inotropes, if fluid-resistant shock.
- Send blood for complete blood count, C-reactive protein (CRP), culture, renal function test, liver function test, arterial blood gas, serum electrolytes, random blood sugar, coagulation profile and for serology as per clinical suspicion.
- Leukocytosis, neutrophilia, raised erythrocyte sedimentation rate/CRP, thrombocytopenia, prolonged coagulation time, hypokalemia and acidosis are observed in fulminant meningococcemia.
- Cerebrospinal fluid, synovial fluid and petechial aspirate studies, including Gram staining and culture are to be done depending on the clinical diagnosis.
- Blood and cerebrospinal fluid for polymerase chain reaction study for meningococcal etiology are reliable for early diagnosis.
- Urinalysis and culture are needed to rule out urinary tract infection and sepsis.

GOLDEN HOUR (1 HOUR) EMPIRICAL ANTIBIOTIC THERAPY

- Third-generation cephalosporins (+vancomycin 60 mg/kg/day div q 6 hourly, if cephalosporin resistance is suspected).
- Alternative drugs in life-threatening beta-lactam allergy are IV chloromycetin, ciprofloxacin or meropenem.
- Administer IV hydrocortisone for children with dopamine-resistant shock.
- Supportive therapy for organ failure includes—mechanical ventilation, fluid and electrolyte therapy, inotropes, dialysis, plasma and blood component therapy for coagulopathy, management of raised intracranial pressure, and liver failure.

SUBSEQUENT MANAGEMENT

- Modify antibiotics as per culture and sensitivity reports; minimum duration of antibiotic therapy is 7 days.

- Persistence of fever after 5 days may be due to endocarditis, septic or autoimmune arthritis.

PREVENTION

- Antibiotic prophylaxis—advised for close contacts of patients at the earliest as detailed below:
    - Rifampicin:
        - Infants less than 1 month age—5 mg/kg/dose q 12 hr four doses
        - Children more than 1 month age—10 mg/kg/dose q 12 hr four doses
        - Adults—600 mg/kg/dose q 12 hr four doses
    - Ceftriaxone less than 15 years—125 mg intramuscular (IM) one dose
        - More than 15 years—250 mg IM one dose
    - Ciprofloxacin more than 18 years—800 mg PO one dose
- Vaccination—As per recommendations.

Note: The ideal antibiotic for therapy and chemoprophylaxis is ceftriaxone, if there is no drug resistance.

CONCLUSION

In infants and children presenting with fever, irritability, diarrhea, vomiting, and bleeding, consider the possibility of meningococcemia and manage.

Chapter **71**

Toxic Shock Syndrome

S Sushamabai

ABSTRACT

Toxic shock syndrome is an acute multisystem disease usually caused by toxic shock syndrome toxin 1 (TSST-1) producing *Staphylococcus aureus* infection and may rapidly progress to shock and death. Clinical criteria are major and minor. The diagnostic triad of major criteria is fever, hypotension, and erythematous desquamating rashes. The empirical antibiotic therapy is first-generation cephalosporins and clindamycin. The details of intravenous (IV) fluid and inotropic therapy as well as corticosteroids and intravenous immunoglobulin (IVIG) administration are discussed.

INTRODUCTION

Toxic shock syndrome (TSS) is an acute multisystem disease rapidly progressing to shock and death, if not diagnosed early and treated promptly.

ETIOLOGY

- Most commonly infection by TSST-1 and some enterotoxin-producing *S. aureus*
- Rarely exotoxin-producing group A streptococcal infection.

CLINICAL PRESENTATION

Menstrual TSS: It occurs in menstruating women of 15–25 years who use tampons.

Nonmenstrual TSS: It is seen in children, nonmenstruating women and men.
- Focus of infection can be sinusitis, infected nasal packing, abscess, osteomyelitis, wound infection, burns and empyema.
- Can be primary bacteremia without any focus of infection.

DIAGNOSTIC CRITERIA

Major criteria (all required):
- Acute fever more than 38.8°C (101.8°C)
- Hypotension
- Erythematous rash with convalescent desquamation.

Minor criteria (any three or more):
- Vomiting and diarrhea
- Myalgia
- Mucous membrane inflammation—vaginal/pharyngeal/conjunctival hyperemia, strawberry tongue
- Liver function abnormalities—bilirubin/transaminase greater than twice the upper limit of normal
- Renal abnormalities—pyuria or elevated renal function test (RFT)
- Central nervous system abnormalities—altered sensorium without focal neurological signs
- Thrombocytopenia 100,000/mm^3 or less.

EXCLUSION CRITERIA

- Absence of another explanation
- Negative blood cultures except occasional growth of *S. aureus*.

Rapid progression to hypotension is the main differentiating feature in TSS as compared to other diseases.

PATIENT APPROACH

- Suspect TSS in any child or in a menstruating adolescent using tampons presenting with high fever, altered sensorium, hypotension, vomiting, diarrhea, skin rashes, mucous membrane congestion, and thrombocytopenia.
- Admit in pediatric intensive care unit; stabilize airway, breathing, and circulation; assess capillary blood glucose; correct hypoglycemia.
- Urgent laboratory investigations—complete blood count; blood, urine and other specimens for culture, RFT, liver function test, coagulation profile and relevant investigations to satisfy the diagnostic criteria.
- Clinical and laboratory evaluation to exclude important differential diagnosis—measles, Kawasaki disease, streptococcal TSS, scarlet fever, leptospirosis, toxic epidermal necrolysis, and sepsis.
- Search for infected focus or foreign body.

FURTHER TREATMENT

- Empirical antibiotic therapy to cover staphylococcal and streptococcal infections—first-generation cephalosporin + clindamycin. Consider vancomycin, if methicillin-resistant *S. aureus* is suspected. Change to appropriate antibiotic as per culture report.
- Aggressive fluid and electrolyte therapy to prevent hypotension, renal failure and cardiovascular collapse.
- Add inotropic support in fluid refractory shock.
- Early IV hydrocortisone therapy 5 mg/kg/dose q 6 hourly.
- Intravenous immunoglobulin therapy in severe infection.
- Remove the infecting tampons, pus or foreign bodies.
- Duration of antibiotic therapy need be minimum of 2 weeks or till the clearance of original focus of infection.

CONCLUSION

Toxic shock syndrome is severe staphylococcal infection leading to shock and death and hence in children presenting with septic shock the possibility should be considered.

Chapter 72

Malaria

S Sushamabai

ABSTRACT

Malaria is a medical emergency requiring urgent diagnosis, clinical categorization and streamlined treatment according to the illness severity and drug resistance. The chapter deals with antimalarial drug therapy as per latest guidelines of World Health Organization and Indian Academy of Pediatrics. Treatment of chloroquine (CQ) responsive and resistant malaria, multidrug resistant *Plasmodium falciparum* infection, treatment failure, artemisinin combination therapy (ACT) and severe complicated malaria are discussed. ACT is superior to other types of drug therapy. Supportive therapy is equally important as chemotherapy and is discussed in detail.

CLINICAL PRESENTATION

- Suspect malaria in any child having fever with malaise, body ache, anemia, jaundice, organomegaly, altered sensorium, convulsions or shock
- Features of severe malaria (caused by *P. falciparum*) are:
  - Varying grades of altered sensorium and recurrent seizures
  - Prostration, shock, and failure to feed
  - Respiratory distress
  - Jaundice, severe anemia [hemoglobin (Hb) <5 g/dL]
  - Bleeding tendency and hemoglobinuria
  - Hypoglycemia and metabolic acidosis
  - Organ failure (liver, kidney)
  - Hyperparasitemia [>2% of infected red blood cells (RBCs) in low-intensity transmission areas or >5% in highly endemic areas]
  - Hyperlactatemia (lactate >5 mmol/L).

DIFFERENTIAL DIAGNOSIS

Typhoid fever, leptospirosis, viral hepatitis, dengue and other hemorrhagic fevers, meningococcemia, septic shock, hemolytic anemia, meningitis, and encephalitis.

PATIENT APPROACH

Malaria is a medical emergency; diagnostic work up and treatment should be started at the earliest even if the features are mild.

Initial Approach

- All severe malaria patients should be admitted in pediatric intensive care unit; stabilize airway, breathing and circulation; assess capillary blood glucose (CBG), correct hypoglycemia and shock urgently.
- Intravenous (IV) fluids and electrolyte therapy as per clinical status. Send blood for confirmation of malaria by thick smear and for species identification by thin smear microscopy (gold standard). Microscopy additionally provides information about the parasite load, prognosis (mature schizonts and pigmented neutrophils indicate poor prognosis) and response to therapy.
- Other tests are quantitative buffy coat (more sensitive than traditional microscopy but costly) and rapid diagnostic tests (costly, lower sensitivity). Polymerase chain reaction is highly sensitive and specific but not available commercially.
- Investigations to assess the disease severity and exclude other differential diagnosis—complete blood count, coagulation profile, serum electrolyte (Na, K, HCO_3, Cl), arterial blood gas/venous blood gas, blood culture, urinalysis and culture, blood grouping crossmatching, coagulation profile, urine routine and culture, blood culture and cerebrospinal fluid (CSF) studies.
- Other relevant investigations to exclude the differential diagnosis and to detect coinfection (dengue, *Leptospira*).

SUBSEQUENT MANAGEMENT

Patient categorization for antimalarial chemotherapy is as follows:
1. Chloroquine sensitive
2. Chloroquine resistant *P. falciparum*
3. Multidrug resistant *P. falciparum*
4. Treatment failure after ACT
5. Severe complicated malaria.

Chloroquine Sensitive Malaria

Refer to Table 72.1 for chemotherapy.

Table 72.1: Therapy in chloroquine sensitive group.

Drug	Plasmodium vivax	Plasmodium falciparum
Chloroquine base	10 mg/kg D1	Same
	10 mg/kg D2	
	5 mg/kg D3	
Primaquin*	0.25 mg/kg OD × 14**	0.75/kg D1

*Contraindicated in infants <1 year, pregnancy, glucose-6-phosphate dehydrogenase (G6PD) deficiency, check G6PD for all; advise preventive therapy in such group with CQ 10 mg/kg weekly.
**5 days as per national malaria-control program.

Chloroquine-resistant *Plasmodium falciparum* Malaria

- Artemisinin-based combination therapy is preferred. It includes artemisinin group of drugs (rapidly acting) and slow-acting drugs (mefloquine, sulfadoxine + pyrimethamine, lumefantrine)
- Artemisinin-based combination therapy is safer, has less side effects compared to quinine, can be given intramuscular (IM) and prevents drug resistance. Three options of ACT in the order of priority are shown below:
    i. Artemether (20 mg)—lumefantrine (120 mg) coformulated tablet × 6 doses
        - First dose at diagnosis, second dose after 8 hours, then one dose bid × 2 days
            5–14 kg   1 tablet/dose
            15–24 kg   2 tablet/dose
            25–34 kg   3 tablet/dose
            >34 kg   4 tablet/dose
        Note—absorption is facilitated by fatty food (milk).
    ii. Artesunate (4 mg/kg/OD × 3 days) + sulfadoxine (25 mg/kg) + pyrimethamine (1.25 mg/kg on D1)
    iii. Artesunate (as above) + mefloquine* 25 mg/kg (15 + 10) as two divided doses on D2 and D3.

Mefloquine safety not established in children; has cross resistance with quinine.

Multidrug-resistant *Plasmodium falciparum*

Indicates CQ + sulfadoxine pyrimethamine resistance
i. Quinine salt 10 mg/kg/dose q 8 hr × 7 days plus
    - Doxycycline (>8 years) 3.5 mg/kg/dose OD × 7 days *or*
    - Clindamycin (<8 years) 20 mg/kg/day in two divided doses × 7 days
ii. If cinchonism:
    - Quinine 3–5 days+
        - Doxycycline or clindamycin × 7 days *or*
        - Single dose of primaquine more than 1 year age *or*
        - Artemether lumefantrine × six doses

Treatment Failure with Artemisinin-based Combination Therapy

- Quinine + doxycycline or clindamycin × 7 days as described in option (3)
  - Treatment failure within 14 days of ACT unusual
  - Assess compliance
  - Confirm diagnosis by blood smear
  - Rule out other causes of fever.

Failure after 14 days of treatment can be retreated with first line ACT.

Severe Complicated Malaria

Artemisinin Combination Therapy

- Artesunate 2.4 mg/kg IV, repeat at 12 and 24 hours followed by once daily oral dose as described for (3); add clindamycin or doxycycline × 7 days
- Artemether—3.2 mg/kg IM followed by 1.6 mg/kg daily × 6 days; if able to swallow, give daily dose as oral; add doxycycline or clindamycin × 7 days as in (3).

Intravenous Quinine Combination Therapy

- Quinine salt 20 mg/kg loading dose in 10 mL/kg normal saline (NS) as infusion in 4 hours. Maintenance dose 10 mg/kg in 10 mL/kg NS, 12 hours after the start of loading dose q 8 hours. Oral if able to swallow for total 7 days.
- Add doxycycline or clindamycin × 7 days as in (3).
- Intramuscular if controlled infusion is not possible—divided as half the dose, dilution 60–100 mg/mL NS, and administer on each anterior thigh.

QUININE—POINTS TO CONSIDER

- Avoid loading dose if quinine, quinidine or mefloquine was received early.
- Infusion rate should not exceed 5 mg/kg/hr.
- If there is no clinical improvement after 48 hours of parenteral therapy, reduce maintenance dose to 5–7 mg/kg.
- Active cardiovascular monitoring is mandatory especially if the patient has cardiac illness or is on antiarrhythmic drugs.
- A single dose of primaquine (0.75 mg/kg) is advised on completion of quinine therapy for gametocyte eradication.

SUPPORTIVE THERAPY IN SEVERE MALARIA

- Oxygenation; mechanical ventilation if needed
- Fluid and electrolyte balance—assess and correct hypo/hypervolemia, hypoglycemia, acidosis and hyponatremia

- Nasogastric tube aspiration and indwelling catheter—strict maintenance of input/output (I/O) chart
- Temperature control—hydrotherapy and paracetamol; avoid aspirin/nonsteroidal anti-inflammatory drugs
- Raised intracranial pressure—propped up position with head in midline, control seizures with lorazepam ± fosphenytoin, hyperventilation; avoid mannitol and steroids
- Respiratory distress—mainly due to metabolic acidosis. IV sodium bicarbonate if blood pH <7
- Disseminated intravascular coagulation—administer vitamin K, fresh frozen plasma, exchange transfusion
- Cardiac failure—fluid volume 2/3 maintenance, treatment of anemia—packed RBC if Hb is less than 5 or less than 7 g/dL with impaired consciousness, hyperparasitemia, respiratory distress, and metabolic acidosis. Exchange transfusion if hyperparasitemia (20% of RBCs parasitized). Judicious use of diuretics and slow transfusion in fluid overload.
- Renal failure—NS challenge followed by IV furosemide 1 mg/kg up to 5 mg/kg. Consider dialysis if no diuresis or other indicators of renal failure present
- Hemolysis—Select artemisinin therapy, packed cell transfusion, consider dialysis if renal failure
- Acute respiratory distress syndrome—O_2, propped up position, restrict fluid intake, add loop diuretics, and mechanical ventilation
- Shock—blood culture, broad-spectrum antibiotics (cefotaxime + amikacin), IV fluids, vasopressors, and respiratory support
- Deepening coma—consider meningitis, encephalitis—CSF study, computed tomography head, lumbar puncture and CSF studies if no contraindication.

MONITORING

- Continuous monitoring of vitals, O_2 saturation till improvement
- 2–4 hourly CBG, I/O chart, Glasgow coma scale, pupils
- 6-hourly Hb, urine Hb
- Daily peripheral smear for parasite load and renal function test.

RESPONSE TO THERAPY

- Clinical—afebrile after 72 hours of specific drug therapy
- Laboratory peripheral blood smear (PBS):
    - Parasite count reduction by 24 hours
    - No parasites after 72 hours of therapy.

Persistent Fever after 72 hours of Chemotherapy

- Thrombophlebitis
- Secondary bacterial infections
- Coinfections—typhoid, leptospirosis
- Immune fever
- Early treatment failure.

Late Treatment Failure

- Reappearance of asexual parasites within 28 days of treatment
- Find out the causes and ensure appropriate therapy.

CONCLUSION

Artemisinin combination therapy (ACT) is superior to other drug therapy in malaria and good supportive therapy is equally important in survival.

FURTHER READING

1. Infectious Diseases Chapter, Indian Academy of Pediatrics, Kundu R, Ganguly N, Ghosh TK. Management of malaria in children: update 2008. Indian Pediatr. 2008;45:731-5.
2. World Health Organization. (2010). Guidelines for the Treatment of Malaria, 2nd edition.

Chapter 73

Leptospirosis

S Sushamabai

ABSTRACT

Leptospirosis, though a zoonotic infection, can cause serious disease in humans and should be considered in the differential diagnosis of flu-like illness, aseptic meningitis, encephalitis, pneumonia, hepatitis, acute kidney injury and fever with bleeding or rashes. The diagnostic investigations are leptospira immunoglobulin M (IgM) or polymerase chain reaction (PCR) test. Microscopic agglutination test is the gold standard but not available for commercial purpose. The choice drug therapy is penicillin G intravenous (IV) 6–8 million IU/m^2/day divided q 4–6 hr for 7 days. Drugs for penicillin allergic patients are cefotaxime, doxycycline, and azithromycin. The fatal complications are cardiorespiratory failure, coagulopathy, renal and hepatic failure. Intensive supportive therapy is needed in such situations.

INTRODUCTION

Leptospirosis is a zoonotic infection occurring as an environmental hazard. 20% of infected humans can have serious illness as anicteric or icteric forms.

PATHOGENESIS

- Organisms enter through cuts and aberrations of skin or intact mucous membranes or by ingestion of contaminated water, proliferate, and circulate in all body organs.
- Endothelial lining of small blood vessels are damaged, followed by secondary ischemia of organs.

CLINICAL PRESENTATION

Anicteric Leptospirosis

Initial septicemic phase: It is common in both groups and lasts for 2–7 days.
- *Symptoms*: High fever, chills, intense headache, orbital pain, and severe myalgia mainly affecting lower limbs and lumbosacral region, nausea, and vomiting.

- *Signs*: Conjunctival suffusion, photophobia, erythematous or urticarial skin rash, lymphadenopathy, hepatosplenomegaly, cholecystitis, orchitis, arthritis, carditis, bradycardia, and hypotension.

Second or immune phase: It can last for several weeks.
- It occurs after a brief asymptomatic period.
- Features are recurrence of fever and manifestations of aseptic meningitis.
- Rare presentations are encephalitis, cranial or peripheral neuropathy or other paralysis.

Icteric Leptospirosis (Weil Syndrome)

- Most severe form—common in adults more than 30 years of age
- Features are jaundice, acute kidney injury, thrombocytopenia and bleeding, and cardiovascular collapse.

DIFFERENTIAL DIAGNOSIS

- Infections—typhoid, malaria, dengue, viral hepatitis, meningitis, encephalitis, cholecystitis, pneumonia, and hantavirus infection.
- Others—hemolytic-uremic syndrome and acute renal failure.

PATIENT APPROACH

- Suspect leptospirosis (especially in endemic areas) in any child presenting with features of flu-like illness, aseptic meningitis, encephalitis, pneumonia, hepatitis, acute kidney injury, and fever with bleeding/rashes.
- Admit in pediatric intensive care unit; stabilize airway, breathing and circulation; assess capillary blood glucose, and correct hypoglycemia.
- Send blood for complete blood count, coagulation profile, renal function test, liver function test, leptospira IgM/polymerase chain reaction test, serological tests for other infections as per differential diagnosis, urinalysis, blood culture, and chest skiagram.
- The gold standard for serologic diagnosis is the microscopic agglutination test, but available at reference centers only.
- Ultrasonography abdomen in icteric type.
- Cerebrospinal fluid (CSF) studies, if neurological symptoms or signs. The CSF findings in leptospirosis are modest elevation of pressure and protein, normal glucose and pleocytosis with mononuclear predominance.

SUBSEQUENT MANAGEMENT

Specific Therapy

- Spontaneous recovery occurs in majority of patients
- Best effect if started before the 7th day of illness
- Drug of choice—penicillin G 6-8 million IU/m^2/day divided q 4 hourly as IV for 7 days
- Other drugs recommended—cefotaxime, doxycycline (>8 years of age 2 mg/kg/day divided q 12 hr maximum 100 mg/day) and azithromycin.

Supportive Therapy

- Maintenance of fluid and electrolyte balance
- Detection and management of respiratory problems, shock, renal/hepatic failure, coagulopathy, meningitis/encephalitis, and polyneuritis.

CONCLUSION

Leptospirosis can present as aseptic meningitis, encephalitis, pneumonia, hepatitis, fever with bleeding or rashes and renal or hepatic failure and should be considered in the differential diagnosis of these clinical situations.

Chapter **74**

Rickettsial Infections

S Sushamabai

ABSTRACT

Rickettsial infections are one of the reemerging hemorrhagic fevers contributing to substantial mortality. The types prevalent in India are scrub typhus, tick typhus (spotted fever) and Q fever. IgM enzyme-linked immunosorbent assay (ELISA) test is the most sensitive and specific investigation for diagnosis. Ideal drug for all age groups is doxycycline for 7–10 days. Azithromycin, clarithromycin, chloromycetin and rifampicin are the other specific drugs. Monitoring and vigilant supportive therapy are mandatory for recovery.

INTRODUCTION

Rickettsial infections are zoonoses transmitted to man by the bite of Arthropod vectors. The types prevalent in India are scrub typhus (*Rickettsia tsutsugamushi*) Indian spotted fever or tick typhus (*Rickettsia conorii*) and Q fever (*Coxiella burnetii*). Mortality is up to 35% if timely treatment is not given.

PATHOGENESIS

The organisms cause microvasculitis especially of brain, myocardium, skeletal muscles, lungs, kidneys, skin and liver and subsequent organ damage and system failure.

CLINICAL PRESENTATION

Disease severity ranges from mild self-limiting illness to life-threatening form.

Suspect rickettsial fever in any child with:
- Short febrile illness and intense unrelenting headache, myalgia, restlessness, calf muscle pain and tenderness

- Fever with abdominal pain, nausea, vomiting and diarrhea
- Fever with rashes—as discrete macules evolving to maculopapular, petechial or hemorrhagic, which appear initially around ankles, legs and wrists, then palms and soles and later spreading to trunk. Can progress to gangrene of ear lobes, nose, fingers, toes and scrotum.
- Acute febrile encephalitis, myocarditis, collapse, and hepatitis
- Fever with eschar and regional lymphadenopathy and hepatosplenomegaly
- Fever with any of the above features progressing to pulmonary edema and renal failure
- Febrile child with tick bite mark or contact with tick infested pet animal
- Fever with painless eschar at the site of parasite bite is pathognomonic but may not be always seen.

PATIENT APPROACH

- Admit in pediatric intensive care unit; stabilize airway, breathing, and circulation if in myocarditis, shock or encephalitis.
- Send blood for complete blood count, coagulation profile, peripheral smear studies, serum electrolytes, renal function test, and liver function test including serum proteins. Leukopenia with relative lymphocytosis, anemia, thrombocytopenia, high erythrocyte sedimentation rate, hyponatremia, elevated transaminases and low serum albumin are the supportive laboratory findings.
- Diagnostic tests:
    - *Less than 7 days*: Polymerase chain reaction test in blood and tissues; this test is species specific and has low sensitivity.
    - *More than 7 days*: IgM ELISA has high sensitivity and specificity and is the preferred one. Immunofluorescence assay test for IgM and IgG against rickettsiae and immunoperoxidase assay are the other tests.
    - Other relevant investigations to rule out the differential diagnosis.

DIFFERENTIAL DIAGNOSIS

- Dengue illness, measles, and infectious mononucleosis
- Leptospirosis, typhoid, and malaria
- Meningococcemia
- Immune vasculitis especially Kawasaki disease.

MANAGEMENT

Subsequent Management

- High index of suspicion is helpful to make early diagnosis and prevent death.

Specific Therapy

- The drug of choice is doxycycline (2.2 mg/kg twice daily <40 kg; 100 mg twice daily >40 kg) for 7 days or at least 3 days after the subsidence of fever. In severe and complicated cases, it is extended up to 10 days.
- Doxycycline is recommended for all children suspected of rickettsial fever.
- Rapid defervescence after choice antibiotic therapy is used as a diagnostic test for rickettsial disease.
- Azithromycin (intravenous/PO 10 mg/kg × 5 days), clarithromycin, chloromycetin and rifampicin are alternate choices.
- Fluoroquinolones, though effective, are contraindicated in pregnancy.

Supportive Therapy

- Strict maintenance of fluid and electrolyte balance. Correction of hyponatremia.
- Blood and blood products—fresh frozen plasma, platelet transfusion, and vitamin K.
- Supportive therapy for hepatic and renal failure.

CONCLUSION

Rickettsial infections should be considered in the differential diagnosis of hemorrhagic fevers and investigated to provide early specific therapy.

FURTHER READING

1. Rath N, Kulkarni A, Yewale V. IAP guidelines on rickettsial diseases in children. Indian Pediatr. 2017;54:223-9.

Chapter 75

Invasive Fungal Infections

S Sushamabai

ABSTRACT

Invasive fungal infections are to be suspected in children with prolonged intensive care unit stay, getting cancer therapy, bone marrow and organ transplant recipients, and in immunocompromised patients. The common infections are candidiasis, cryptococcosis, aspergillosis, and histoplasmosis. They are to be suspected in immunocompromised children, those with cancer, organ transplant and hospital-acquired infections, chronic meningoencephalitis, and persons exposed to avian droppings and decayed woods. Specific diagnostic tests are available for all fungal infections. Specific antifungal therapy includes combination therapy with intravenous (IV) amphotericin B, fluconazole, itraconazole, and flucytosine.

INTRODUCTION

Invasive fungal infections are increasing due to the:
- Survival of immunocompromised children—both primary and secondary
- Advanced treatment like organ transplantation
- Increased international traveling which can transmit such infections from high prevalent areas to uncommon places.

Early diagnosis and prompt treatment are a must to prevent mortality.

The common invasive fungal infections are: (1) Candidiasis, (2) Cryptococcosis, (3) Aspergillosis, and (4) Histoplasmosis.

CANDIDIASIS

Invasive candidiasis should be suspected in:
- Febrile oncology patients on chemotherapy and associated neutropenia.
- Bone marrow and solid organ recipients.
- Catheter-associated (central venous) infections in any patient.

Clinical Presentation

- Prolonged fever not responding to antibiotics.
- Clues for diagnosis are the underlying disease, evidence of superficial candidal infections like mucocutaneous lesions.

Diagnosis

- Have a high index of suspicion in risky patients with prolonged fever.
- Blood culture yields isolation of *Candida* within 72 hours.

Specific Treatment

- Susceptibility testing is mandatory in drug selection.
- Fluconazole 12 mg/kg/day (not effective against *Candida krusei* and *Candida glabrata*) IV/oral once daily × 28 days; and monitor hepatic enzymes.
- Amphotericin B (IV) 0.8–1.2 mg/kg/day × 21 days from the last positive *Candida* culture.

CRYPTOCOCCOSIS

- It is the most common invasive fungal infection worldwide, the strain being *Cryptococcus neoformans* (A, B, C, D).
- Clinical disease is unusual in immune competent individuals and children. Risky groups are pigeon breeders and laboratory personnel.
- Mode of infection—inhalation of soil contaminated with avian droppings (pigeons), through contaminated fruits, vegetables, and eucalyptus tree.

Clinical Presentation

Depends on the route of inoculation and the immune competence of the host:
- Cryptococcal etiology has to be considered in severe progressive pneumonia, cavity lesions of the lung, and pleural effusion in the risky groups.
- Disseminated infection is more common in immune-compromised individuals; can present as meningitis, sepsis syndrome, skin, bone, eye, and lymph node infections.
- Irrespective of the immune status of the patient in chronic meningoencephalitis, consider cryptococcosis as the etiology.

Diagnosis

- Definitive test is culture recovery or histologic demonstration of the fungus from the infected tissue.

- Latex agglutination test for cryptococcal antigen in serum or cerebrospinal fluid (CSF) (titer >1:4) is diagnostic.
- India ink preparation has poor sensitivity.

Specific Treatment

It depends on the site of involvement and the host immune status.

Immunocompetent host:
- Asymptomatic mild disease—observe
- Symptomatic disease—fluconazole PO 6–12 mg/kg/day or itraconazole 5–10 mg/kg/day divided q 12 hours for 3 to 12 months. Duration of therapy as per response.
- Severe illness—induction therapy with amphotericin B plus flucytosine (100–150 mg/kg/day divided q 6 hr) for minimum 2 weeks, continue for 6 to 12 weeks as per situation. Should be followed by consolidation therapy with fluconazole/itraconazole for 6 to 12 months.

Human immunodeficiency virus (HIV)-infected children (any severity illness):
- Induction—amphotericin B (0.7 mg/kg/day) with flucytosine (100 mg/kg/day) for 2 to 10 weeks followed by:
    – Consolidation—with fluconazole (oral) for 6 to 12 months
    – Maintenance—with fluconazole lifelong to prevent relapse. Non-HIV patients with immune suppression are also included in this group.

INVASIVE ASPERGILLOSIS

Aspergillosis occurs due to airborne spore inhalation of *Aspergillus*. The risky groups for invasive aspergillosis are as follows:
- Stem cell and solid organ recipients
- Cancer patients
- Primary immune deficiency patients
- Those receiving immune modulatory therapy.

Clinical Presentation

- Fever despite empirical antibiotic therapy in the risky group.
- Prolonged cough, chest pain, hemoptysis, and persistent pulmonary infiltrates.
- High index of suspicion is needed in patients on steroid therapy with vague symptoms since fever is less likely.

- Invasive sinonasal disease, pancarditis, ophthalmitis, osteomyelitis, and progressive central nervous system (CNS) disease are other clinical situations to suspect aspergillosis.

Diagnosis

Pulmonary Aspergillosis

- Gold standard—culture and isolation of the organism from a normally sterile site or bronchoalveolar lavage (BAL). Enzyme-linked immunosorbent assay test for galactomannan (a component of *Aspergillus* cell wall) is a sensitive test.
- Radiology:
  - Chest skiagram—multiple ill-defined nodules are suggestive but not pathognomonic.
  - Computed tomography chest—*Halo sign*-is hemorrhagic nodule surrounded by ischemia.
  - Magnetic resonance imaging (MRI) chest may reveal target sign: It is nodule with lower central signal compared to rim enhancing periphery.

Central Nervous System Aspergillosis

- MRI brain—characteristic lesions are multiple, located in the basal ganglia, and are of intermediate enhancement with no mass effect.
- Cerebrospinal fluid studies for galactomannan assay are diagnostic.
- Biopsy studies from the affected areas of brain.

Treatment

- Empirical antifungal therapy in high-risk patients, options being:
  - Voriconazole IV (>12 years of age) 6 mg/kg/dose q 12 hr × two doses reduced to 4 mg/kg q 12 hr till improvement
  - Maintenance dose 200 mg (oral)/dose q 12 hr for a total of 12 weeks of therapy
  - Amphotericin B deoxycholate IV 1–1.5 mg/kg/day for 4–12 weeks
  - Amphotericin B lipid complex or voriconazole can be tried in treatment failure or drug intolerance.

HISTOPLASMOSIS

It is caused by the inhalation of spores of histoplasma capsulatum, a dimorphic fungus. Soil rich with bird droppings and decayed wood is heavily contaminated with this saprophyte.

Clinical Presentation

- *Acute pulmonary histoplasmosis (APH):*
  - Occurs in young infants and elderly persons after exposure to large inocula like chicken coops, camping on contaminated soil, chopping decayed wood etc. Features are as follows:
    - Flu-like symptoms, hepatosplenomegaly, progressive and severe respiratory distress requiring intubation and ventilation in severe disease.
    - Sarcoid-like disease with arthritis, keratoconjunctivitis, iridocyclitis, pericarditis, and pleural effusion.
    - Broncholithiasis, stone spitting, wheezing, and hemoptysis.
    - Superior vena cava syndrome and congestive heart failure.
- *Chronic pulmonary histoplasmosis* is an opportunistic infection in adults with centrilobular emphysema but rare in children.
- *Progressive disseminated histoplasmosis (PDH):*
  - Affects infants and immunocompromised patients. It is an acquired immunodeficiency syndrome-defining illness.
  - Present as prolonged fever, hepatosplenomegaly, lymphadenopathy, anemia, thrombocytopenia, mucosal ulcerations, skin nodules, and occasional pneumonia.
  - Extrapulmonary infections are destructive bony lesions, oropharyngeal ulcers, Addison disease, meningitis, chorioretinitis, endocarditis, and cutaneous infection.

Diagnosis

- Culture of sputum, BAL, blood or bone marrow yield variable results depending on the type of infection. It has to be confirmed by DNA probe.
- Histopathological demonstration of yeast forms in tissues.
- Radioimmunoassay for fungal polysaccharide antigen (urine, blood, BAL) is the most accepted diagnostic test for PDH.
- Serum complement fixation test for antibody titer (4–6 weeks after exposure) more than or equal to 1:32 is diagnostic of recent infection in acute pulmonary histoplasmosis.
- Skin testing is applicable for epidemiologic studies only.

Treatment

- Oral itraconazole/fluconazole in APH patients, if no self-recovery by 1 month.
- Serious illness—IV amphotericin till improvement; continue with oral itraconazole in two divided doses for 12 weeks; should be continued for 6–12 months for severe mediastinal disease. Consider surgery, if indicated.

CONCLUSION

Invasive fungal infections are more common in patients with prolonged ICU stay, immune compromised patients, and those exposed to avian droppings and decayed woods.

FURTHER READING

1. Mukerjee SB. Cryptococcal meningo encephalitis—a tale of 50 years. Indian Pediatr. 2015;52:503-4.

Chapter 76

Hospital-acquired Infections

S Letha, S Sushamabai

ABSTRACT

Hospital-acquired or nosocomial infections [modified term–health-care-associated infections (HAI)] are infections acquired in the hospital by the patient admitted for some other reason. The diagnostic criteria are appearance of clinical features 48 hours after admission or within 30 days after discharge. The chapter deals with the host and environmental predisposing factors, causating organisms, types of infection, clinical presentation, patient approach and management. Empirical antibiotic therapy includes piperacillin–tazobactam for gram-negative bacteria, vancomycin for methicillin-resistant *Staphylococcus aureus* (MRSA), coagulase-negative staphylococci (CONS), enterococci and clostridium difficile infection and linezolid for MRSA and enterococci. For invasive fungal infections, IV amphotericin is the drug of choice. Preventive measures are proper handwashing and waste disposal.

INTRODUCTION

Hospital-acquired or nosocomial infections are those acquired in the hospital by a patient admitted for a reason other than the infection. The modified term is HAI the diagnostic criteria being the following:
- Appearance of clinical features within 48 hr, after admission
- And/or within 30 days, after discharge from the hospital.

Hospital-acquired or nosocomial infections are a major cause of death (5–10% mortality) affecting developed and resource-poor countries equally.

PREDISPOSING FACTORS

Host Factors

- Prolonged hospital stay
- Immunocompromise: Newborns, old age, protein–energy malnutrition, malignancy, organ transplantation, broad-spectrum antibiotic and

immunosuppressive therapy, primary and secondary immune deficiency disorders
- Congenital anomalies: Cleft palate.

Environmental Factors
- Other patients spreading airborne infections or through physical contact
- Carrier hospital staff
- Contaminated articles and devices: Nebulizers, resuscitation sets, ventilator tubing, intravascular catheters (arterial, venous), urinary catheters, needles, and suction devices
- Eatables
- Dust
- Vectors.

ORGANISMS

All microorganisms can cause healthcare-associated infection (HAI), common ones being:
- Airborne seasonal viruses—Measles, rubella, influenza, varicella, severe acute respiratory syndrome, and respiratory syncytial virus
- Contact viruses—rotavirus, enterovirus
- Blood-borne viruses—hepatitis B virus, hepatitis C virus, and human immunodeficiency virus
- Bacteria—*Staphylococcus aureus*, CONS, *Salmonella, Pseudomonas, Klebsiella, Clostridium,* and *Acinetobacter*
- Fungi—*Candida, Aspergillus*
- Protozoa—*Entamoeba histolytica*
- Vector transmitted—malaria, dengue.

SOURCE OF INFECTION

- Exogenous—most common
- Endogenous—immunocompromised patients, those on broad-spectrum antibiotics or prolonged acid-suppressive therapy.

TYPES OF INFECTIONS

Device Related
- Ventilator-associated pneumonia
- Catheter related—urinary tract infection
- Cannula related—thrombophlebitis, abscess, and bacteremia
- Implant related—bacteremia and sepsis.

Non-device Related
- Surgical wound infections
- Airborne—hospital-acquired pneumonias and tuberculosis
- Blood transmitted
- Vector transmitted
- Foodborne—*Salmonella*, hepatitis A
- Contact—Rotavirus.

CLINICAL PRESENTATION
- Prolonged fever or recurrence of fever after an initial response
- Unresolved or newly appearing pneumonia
- Diarrhea
- Urinary infections
- Persistent wound infection
- Thrombophlebitis, cellulitis, and abscess
- Sepsis
- Exanthematous fever.

PATIENT APPROACH
- Have an index of suspicion for HAI in children with predisposing factors.
- Admit in pediatric intensive care unit if sick; provide isolation room if there is possibility for airborne or droplet spread.
- Stabilize airway, breathing and circulation; send blood, urine, cerebrospinal fluid, wound swab, stools, pus, bronchial aspirate (in ventilated patients) for culture and sensitivity as per disease picture
- Complete blood count and chest radiograph for all. Other investigations as per clinical picture
- Start empirical antibiotic therapy:
    - Piperacillin—Tazobactam for gram-negative bacteria
    - Vancomycin for MRSA, CONS, *Enterococcus*, and *Clostridium difficile* infections
    - Linezolid for MRSA, *Enterococcus*
    - Antifungal agents (Chapter 75)
    - Switch over to appropriate antibiotic as per culture and sensitivity report
    - Continue antibiotics for 7–14 days or at least 4 days of afebrile period
    - Remove or change the devices in such infections.

PREVENTION

- Healthcare-associated infection rates can be reduced up to 50% by well-directed and systematized infection control program.
- Each hospital should have an infection control committee for surveillance of HAI by implementing strict protocol.
- Handwashing by health staff should be ensured—15 seconds scrub with soap under running water for the first wash, before a procedure, before and after caring a contaminated wound, caring a contagious patient and after visible dirt or soiling with secretion or blood.
- Waterless hand hygiene using 3–5 mL of alcohol containing hand rub between patient contacts; preparations can be isopropyl alcohol, ethanol, and chlorhexidine diacetate.
- Routine wearing of mask and gown should be made compulsory within the intensive care unit (ICU).
- Personal protective equipment, which includes gloves, gown, mask, eye protection goggles and face shield, is recommended when there is chance of contact with infected body fluids.
- Standard precautions of care for all patients and equipment in all healthcare settings should be observed.
- Patients having highly contagious infections should be treated in isolation ICUs.
- Proper waste disposal system should be strictly implemented.
- Preparation and handling of food should be clean.
- Vector control measures should be implemented.

CONCLUSION

Hospital-acquired infections or health care associated infections are acquired from the hospital, should be diagnosed and treated in time and effective preventive measures are to be implemented in all hospitals.

Section **11**

CONNECTIVE TISSUE DISORDERS

Chapter 77

Kawasaki Disease

S Sushamabai

ABSTRACT

Kawasaki disease (KD) is an acute febrile illness mostly affecting children less than 5 years of age, characterized by widespread vasculitis with a predilection for coronary arteries, producing coronary artery aneurysm and rupture. The diagnostic clinical criteria are fever for more than 4 days with four out of five clinical criteria—nonexudative congestion of bulbar conjunctiva, oral mucosal and lip changes, unilateral cervical lymphadenopathy more than 1.5 cm, polymorphous exanthem and extremity changes. Atypical Kawasaki with less than four criteria can occur in infants. There is no diagnostic investigation, many are supportive. Systematic approach in treatment is immediate stabilization if in shock, administration of intravenous immunoglobulin (IVIg) along with aspirin. The indications for IV methylprednisolone, clopidogrel, warfarin and rituximab as well as long-term management are discussed.

INTRODUCTION

Kawasaki disease is an acute febrile illness of infectious origin affecting children (mostly <5 years), characterized by vasculitis with a predilection for the coronary arteries. Delay in treatment can cause coronary artery aneurysm and death or sequelae of coronary artery disease.

CLINICAL PRESENTATION

- Fever at least 4 days *plus*
- Presence of at least four principal features as detailed below:
    - Extremity changes:
        - Acute: Erythema palms, soles, edema hands and feet—first week
        - Subacute: Periungual peeling of fingers and toes—weeks 2 and 3
    - Polymorphous exanthem
    - Bilateral bulbar conjunctival nonexudative injection sparing the limbus

- Changes in the lips and oral cavity—erythema, lip cracking, strawberry tongue, diffuse injection of oral and pharyngeal mucosa
- Cervical lymphadenopathy (>1.5 cm) usually unilateral.

Exclusion of other diseases with similar findings is mandatory.

Atypical Kawasaki Disease

- Fever with less than four criteria
- Subsequent coronary artery disease (mostly seen in infants).

Supportive Clinical Findings

- Cardiovascular system—congestive cardiac failure (CCF), myocarditis, shock, pericarditis, valvular regurgitation, and coronary artery abnormalities
- Vascular:
  - Aneurysms of medium-sized noncoronary arteries
  - Raynaud phenomenon
  - Peripheral gangrene
- Musculoskeletal:
  - Arthritis, arthralgia
- Gastrointestinal tract:
  - Diarrhea, vomiting, and abdominal pain
  - Hepatic dysfunction
  - Hydrops of gallbladder
- Central nervous system:
  - Extreme irritability
  - Aseptic meningitis
  - Sensory neural hearing loss
- Genitourinary system:
  - Urethritis and meatitis
- Others:
  - Erythema and induration at BCG injection site
  - Anterior uveitis (mild)
  - Desquamating rash in the groin.

Laboratory Findings

- Leukocytosis with neutrophilia, immature forms
- Elevated erythrocyte sedimentation rate (ESR), C-reactive protein (CRP), and thrombocytosis (after 1 week)
- Anemia, hypoalbuminemia, and hyponatremia
- Dyslipidemia

- Elevated serum bilirubin, transaminases
- Cerebrospinal fluid (CSF) pleocytosis
- Leukocytosis in synovial fluid
- Sterile pyuria
- Two-dimensional echocardiography (2D Echo)—coronary artery dilatation adjusted for the body surface area:
  - Borderline—2.5–3 mm, abnormal more than 3 mm
  - Aneurysms (internal diameter size in mm)
    - Small: Less than 5
    - Medium: 5–8
    - Giant: More than 8

PATIENT APPROACH

- Have a high index of suspicion of KD in children (especially <5 years) with high fever for more than 4 days and clinical findings as described above.
- Admit in pediatric intensive care unit; stabilize if in shock or CCF.
- Urgent 2D Echo to assess the cardiac status.
- Exclude the differential diagnosis—measles, scarlet fever, drug reaction, staphylococcal scalded skin syndrome, leptospirosis, rickettsial infections, toxic shock syndrome, systemic-onset juvenile idiopathic arthritis, Steven-Johnson syndrome—by history and physical examination.
- Send blood for complete blood count, peripheral blood smear (PBS), ESR, CRP, serum bilirubin, serum glutamic pyruvic transaminase, serum albumin, lipid profile and culture.
- Cerebrospinal fluid studies.
- Ultrasonography abdomen to assess liver and gallbladder.
- Urine routine examination and culture.
- Additional investigations to exclude the differential diagnosis.

TREATMENT

Specific

- *Uncomplicated Kawasaki disease:*
  - Intravenous immunoglobulin 2 g/kg at the earliest after diagnosis; best effect if given within the first 10 days of illness. Response is revealed by rapid defervescence and disappearance of other clinical features.
  - Aspirin 80–100 mg/kg/day divided q 6 hr till the patient is afebrile for 48 hours. Continue with low-dose aspirin (5–8 mg/kg/day as single dose) for 6–8 weeks more, in those with normal echocardiogram.
- *IVIg-resistant KD* is persistence or recrudescence of fever 36 hours after the completion of initial IVIg infusion.

- Administer second dose of IVIg 2 g/kg.
- For subsequent recrudescence, IV methylprednisolone or infliximab are the recommended drugs.
- Aspirin high dose followed by low dose as in uncomplicated KD.
- *Complicated KD* is the disease developing coronary artery aneurysm with or without thrombosis.
  - Small solitary aneurysm—continue small dose of aspirin indefinitely
  - Larger or numerous aneurysms—add clopidogrel 1 mg/kg/day maximum dose 75 mg along with low-molecular weight heparin for initial 5 days
  - Giant aneurysm—add warfarin along with aspirin and clopidogrel to maintain INR 1.5–2.014
- *Atypical Kawasaki disease*—patient with fever for more than 4 days but other clinical criteria are less than 4, finally developing coronary artery aneurysm.
  - Biomarkers like blood: N-terminal pro–B-type natriuretic peptide and interleukin-17 are useful indicators for early diagnosis. Specific therapy is as in typical KD.

FOLLOW-UP AND EVALUATION

- *Uncomplicated KD*—repeat echo is advised after IVIg therapy at intervals of 2 weeks, 2 months, 1 year, and 2 years.
- *Complicated KD*—more frequent echo evaluations are needed in the acute stage depending on the coronary artery complications. After 2 months, echo evaluation is needed every 2 months to detect the status of the coronary artery aneurysm. Periodic echocardiographic evaluation and stress testing are needed thereafter, the duration depending on the extent of structural damage.

CONCLUSION

In young children with fever more than 4 days without focus, consider the possibility of Kawasaki disease and Echo studies to assess the coronary arteries.

FURTHER READING

1. Wi L, Chen Y, Zhong S, et al. Blood N-terminal pro-brain natriuretic peptide and interleukin-17 for distinguishing incomplete Kawasaki disease from infectious disease. Indian Pediatr. 2015;52:477-80.

Chapter **78**

Macrophage Activation Syndrome

S Sushamabai

ABSTRACT

Macrophage activation syndrome (MAS) is a fatal complication of systemic onset juvenile idiopathic arthritis (SOJIA) presenting with high fever, progressive anemia, bleeding tendency, lymphadenopathy, hepatosplenomegaly, and central nervous system (CNS) manifestations as altered sensorium and seizures. The diagnostic criteria are the combination of two clinical and two laboratory parameters. The important differential diagnosis is flare-up of SOJIA which can be excluded by paradoxic improvement in arthritis and low erythrocyte sedimentation rate (ESR) seen in MAS. Immediate stabilization, correction of shock, anemia, bleeding and seizure control, IV methylprednisolone, others being cyclosporine and anakinra are the treatment modalities. Early bone marrow transplantation is needed in resistant cases. Vigilant monitoring, treatment of precipitating factors, and supportive therapy are essential for recovery.

INTRODUCTION

Macrophage activation syndrome is a potentially fatal complication of SOJIA which can be encountered at any stage of the disease. Other terminologies are secondary lymphophagocytic syndrome or hemophagocytic lymphohistiocytosis.

CLINICAL PRESENTATION

- High spiking fever, progressive anemia, mucosal and/or skin bleeds, lymphadenopathy, and hepatosplenomegaly.
- Central nervous system dysfunction—irritability, disorientation, lethargy, headache, seizures, and coma.

PATIENT APPROACH

- Consider the possibility of MAS in a child with SOJIA if three or more clinical criteria as described above are present.

- Admit in pediatric intensive care unit; stabilize airway, breathing, and circulation; urgent correction of shock, severe anemia, bleeding, and seizure control are the priority.
- Send blood for complete blood count, ESR, C-reactive protein, peripheral blood smear (PBS), prothrombin time, activated partial thromboplastin time, serum glutamic pyruvic transaminase (SGPT), serum bilirubin, fibrin degradation products, serum albumin, lactate dehydrogenase, serum lipid profile (SLP), serum sodium, serum ferritin.
- Cultures of blood and other body fluids to rule out sepsis.
- Bone marrow study—hemophagocytosis picture supports the diagnosis.
- Send blood for grouping, typing, crossmatching; keep sample for later cross matching.

DIAGNOSTIC CRITERIA

- Any of the two or more clinical criteria (CNS, hemorrhagic, hepatomegaly ≥3 cm) along with two or more laboratory criteria (thrombocytopenia <26,000/mm^3, elevated SGPT >59 U/L, leukopenia <4,000/mm^3, hypofibrinogenemia) are diagnostic.
- Paradoxic improvement in arthritis and low ESR (due to increased levels of fibrin degradation products) are supportive criteria for MAS and and differentiates from flare-up of SOJIA.
- Bone marrow study for hemophagocytosis is not essential if diagnostic criteria are satisfied.

DIFFERENTIAL DIAGNOSIS

- Flare-up of SOJIA—improvement in arthritis and low ESR, are points suggestive of MAS
- Hematological malignancy
- Histiocytosis
- Hemorrhagic fevers
- Sepsis syndrome by gram-positive and negative bacteria or fungal agents.

SUBSEQUENT MANAGEMENT

- High-dose IV methylprednisolone 10–30 mg/kg/dose to a maximum of 1 g in 30 minutes. Watch for adverse effects as cardiac arrhythmia, hypo/ hypertension and shock during infusion and up to 12 hours after therapy.
- Other effective drugs are cyclosporine and anakinra.
- In severe disease, consider drug therapy as for secondary hemophagocytic lymphohistiocytosis with etoposide and intrathecal methotrexate or allogenic bone marrow transplantation.

- Evaluate for precipitating infections, other rheumatological disorders (systemic lupus erythematosus, Kawasaki disease) or neoplasms and provide specific therapy.
- Supportive therapy for fluid and electrolyte balance, coagulopathies, anemia and thrombocytopenia.

CONCLUSION

Consider the fatal complication of macrophage activation syndrome in SOJIA when the child presents with fever, progressive anemia, bleeding, and organomegaly but with low ESR and improving arthritis.

Section 12

HEMATOLOGY ONCOLOGY

Chapter **79**

Blood and Blood Component Therapy

S Sushamabai

ABSTRACT

Blood and blood component therapy are lifesaving. The products used are whole blood, fresh frozen plasma (FFP), red blood cells (RBCs), platelets, granulocytes, and cryoprecipitate. The use of whole blood and granulocyte transfusion are rare nowadays. Cryoprecipitate can be prepared in blood bank and is a cheap and life-saving alternative for bleeding in hemophilia A, if factor VIII is not available. This chapter deals with the indications, dose, and administration of various blood components presently available.

WHOLE BLOOD TRANSFUSION

The few clinical indications are:
- To maintain stable hemodynamic status with acute blood loss more than 25% of total blood volume; dose 10–20 mL/kg in 2–4 hours
- Exchange transfusion—quantity 160 mL/kg; procedure to be completed in 1 hour.

RED BLOOD CELL TRANSFUSION

Indications

- *Infants ≤ 4-month-old:*
  - Hb < 7 g/dL in symptomatic anemia and postoperative period
  - Hb < 10 g/dL in moderate pulmonary disease, preoperatively and during major surgery.
  - Hb < 12 g/dL with severe cardiac or pulmonary disease and during extracorporeal membrane oxygenation.
- *Children and adolescents:*
  - Hb < 7 g/dL in symptomatic chronic anemia and marrow failure and in the preoperative period.
  - Hb < 12 g/dL with severe cardiac or pulmonary disease or during extracorporeal membrane oxygenation (10–15 mL/kg in 2–4 hours).

Precautions

- Grouping, typing, and crossmatching should be done as per standardized method.
- Before transfusion, record the donor details—name, donor number, age, sex, blood group, date of sample collection, and screening test details.
- Collect pretransfusion sample of the recipient which should be stored for 1 week.
- Record the date and time of transfusion.
- Observe the patient for any untoward reactions; stop transfusion if any adverse reaction; treat the problems (Chapter 80).
- Send back the sample to the blood bank in suspected reaction.

Types of Red Blood Cells

- Fresh RBCs (<7 days pre-storage) ideal for newborns.
- Stored RBCs (7–42 days storage) advised for babies more than 7 days of age. Pre-storage leukocyte-reduced RBCs are suspended in an anticoagulant preservative storage solution at a hematocrit value of 60%; valid for storage up to 42 days.
- Preoperative autologous blood collection from the patient to prepare RBCs though ideal is not commonly practiced because of the difficult procedure.

PLATELET TRANSFUSION

Indications

- *Infants ≤ 4-month age*—if the platelet count is:
  - ≤ 1 L/mm^3 with bleeding or on extracorporeal membrane oxygenation
  - ≤ 50,000/mm^3 requiring invasive procedure, clinically unstable or having bleeding
  - ≤ 20,000/mm^3 and clinically stable
  - Normal platelet count with platelet dysfunction having bleeding or on invasive procedure.
- *Children and adolescents*—if platelet count is:
  - < 50,000/mm^3 with bleeding or major invasive procedure
  - < 25,000/mm^3 with minor invasive procedure
  - < 20,000/mm^3 with marrow failure and hemorrhagic risk factor
  - < 10,000/mm^3 with marrow failure without hemorrhagic risk factors
  - Normal count with platelet dysfunction having bleeding or on invasive procedures.

Type of Platelets

Should be ABO group compatible.

Dose

One unit per 10 kg of body weight as platelet-rich plasma or as platelet concentrate; both can raise the platelet count 5,000–10,000/mm^3.

GRANULOCYTE TRANSFUSION

Indications

- *Infants less than or equal to 4-month age:*
  - Blood neutrophil count less than 3.0×10^9/L with fulminant bacterial infection.
- *Children and adolescents:*
  - Blood neutrophil count less than 0.5×10^9/L and progressive infection (bacterial, yeast, or fungal) unresponsive to treatment.
  - Qualitative neutrophil defect and bacterial or fungal infection unresponsive to antimicrobial therapy.

Dose

- Less than 10-kg weight: $1-2 \times 10^9$ neutrophil/transfusion
- Adolescents: $5-8 \times 10^{10}$ neutrophil/transfusion
- Should be continued till infection is resolved.

PLASMA TRANSFUSION

Each bag of FFP is 100–150 mL volume, each mL containing 1 U of all coagulation factors.

Indications

- Dengue shock syndrome with thrombocytopenia—Platelet-rich FFP is advised
- Snake envenomation with hemorrhage
- Alternative to albumin infusion in children with nephrotic syndrome and severe hypoalbuminemia
- Fulminant/chronic hepatic failure
- Disseminated intravascular coagulation, thrombotic thrombocytopenic purpura, hemolytic-uremic syndrome
- Hemorrhagic disease of the newborn
- Anticoagulant protein (antithrombin III, protein C, protein S) replacement.

Dose and Administration

- 10–15 mL/kg in 1 hr; flow rate should not exceed 10 mL/min; can be refrigerated for 24 hours.
- Coadministration of IV furosemide 1 mg/kg is needed in nephrotic syndrome or other edematous conditions.

CRYOPRECIPITATE

- Blood component which contains mainly factors VIII and XIII.
- Volume of each unit is 10–20 mL.
- The component should be ABO compatible.

Indications

- Hemophilia A—as a cheap replacement therapy, if factor VIII is not available.
- Von Willebrand disease
- Uremia with bleeding
- Factor XIII or fibrinogen deficiency.

CONCLUSION

Instead of whole blood transfusion, blood component therapy is the ideal in most clinical situations.

Chapter 80

Transfusion Reactions

Bibin Sajan, S Sushamabai

ABSTRACT

Blood and component therapy though lifesaving, transfusion-associated risks are not uncommon. The immediate reactions can be hemolytic or nonhemolytic. Hemolytic reactions are characterized by restlessness, chest pain, respiratory distress, shock, jaundice, and renal failure. Nonhemolytic reactions are fever, itchy rashes, or varying grades of anaphylaxis. Fluid overload, acid–base and electrolyte disorders, and transfusion-induced lung injury are the other nonhemolytic reactions. Delayed risks are donor-transmitted infections, graft-versus-host disease, immune modulation, and iron overload in repeated transfusions. The chapter deals with diagnostic parameters, monitoring, and management of the immediate reactions.

INTRODUCTION

Transfusion-related problems can occur after blood or component therapy. Such reactions can be classified as immediate and delayed.

IMMEDIATE RISKS

Hemolytic Reactions

- Occur due to errors in grouping and crossmatching of donor and recipient blood samples.
- Clinical features are restlessness, chest or lumbar pain, respiratory distress, nausea, rapid deterioration in general condition, shock, jaundice, hemoglobinuria, and renal failure.

Management

- Transfer the patient to pediatric intensive care unit.
- Check the identity of blood.
- Start intravenous (IV) normal saline (NS) bolus followed by maintenance fluid therapy.

- Send blood for complete blood count, peripheral smear for spherocytes and crenated red blood cells, direct Coombs test, renal function test (RFT), serum electrolytes (SE), prothrombin time, activated partial thromboplastin time, and fibrin degradation products.
- Urine hemoglobin and microscopy
- Send pretransfusion and posttransfusion blood and urine samples, current blood bag, and infusion set used, with clinical details to the blood bank.
- Blood culture from blood bag, tubing, and recipient's blood for bacteria and fungi
- Intravenous furosemide 1 mg/kg can be given to ensure diuresis
- Oxygen therapy and inotropic support
- Cardiorespiratory support
- Monitor 12 hourly RFT, SE, and coagulation profile; make appropriate corrections.
- Treat disseminated intravascular coagulation and renal failure.
- Further transfusion, if needed, should be after appropriate screening.

Nonhemolytic Reactions

Febrile Reaction

It is induced by pyrogens in the transfusion set.

Management

- Stop the transfusion temporarily
- Paracetamol administration and slow restarting
- Monitor for recurrence of adverse effects and manage accordingly.

Mild Reaction—Itchy Rash

Treatment

- Slow transfusion, IV hydrocortisone 5 mg/kg, intramuscular (IM) chlorpheniramine 0.1 mg/kg
- Continue transfusion, if no more symptoms.

Moderate Reaction

Severe itchy rash, flushing, fever more than 38°C, rigors, restlessness, tachycardia, and wheezing.

Treatment

- Stop transfusion; remove the infusing set
- Keep IV access; continue with IV NS infusion as per hydration status

- Intravenous hydrocortisone and IM chlorpheniramine as above
- Salbutamol nebulization, if wheezing
- Restart transfusion slowly; continue if no more symptoms
- If no improvement, treat as life-threatening reaction.

Severe or Life-threatening Reaction

Characterized by fever more than 38°C, rigor, restlessness, tachycardia, tachypnea, hemoglobinuria, unexplained bleeding, confusion, and collapse.

Treatment

- Stop transfusion; continue IV fluid therapy with NS.
- Clear the airway; give oxygen.
- Inject adrenaline (1:1,000) subcutaneous or IM 0.01 mL/kg.
- Treatment of shock
- Intravenous hydrocortisone + chlorpheniramine as above
- Salbutamol nebulization, if wheezing
- Maintain renal blood flow with IV furosemide 1 mg/kg
- Send blood for culture; start IV antibiotics as for sepsis. IV ceftriaxone + amikacin + cloxacillin empirically
- Inform the blood bank with blood sample as described earlier.

Other Nonhemolytic Reactions

- Fluid overload—seen in cardiac failure, nephrotic syndrome, dengue shock syndrome, and severe anemia; can be prevented by transfusion rate less than 2 mL/min, sitting position, and furosemide administration.
- Electrolyte and acid–base imbalance—make appropriate correction.
- Transfusion-related acute lung injury (TRALI):
  - Syndrome of acute hypoxia within 6 hours of transfusion due to noncardiogenic pulmonary edema, the risk factors being mechanical ventilation, sepsis, severe liver disease, and hematological malignancy.
  - Characterized by sudden onset of dyspnea, hypoxemia, hypotension, and fever within 6 hours of transfusion without evidence of cardiac failure.
  - Chest X-ray reveals diffuse patchy pulmonary densities and no cardiomegaly.
  - Transient leukopenia is supportive laboratory evidence.
  - Treatment—stop transfusion; give O_2, IV fluids, vasopressors, and respiratory support.
  - Avoid steroids, antihistamines, and diuretics.

DELAYED OR LATE RISKS

- Infections: Transmitted through donor blood—viral, bacterial, protozoal, and fungal
- Graft-versus-host disease
- Posttransfusion immune modulation
- Iron overload in repeated transfusion.

CONCLUSION

Blood and its component transfusions are lifesaving but transfusion-associated risks, can occur. They, may be trivial to fatal, should be properly monitored and treated.

Chapter 81

Intravenous Immunoglobulin Therapy

S Sushamabai

ABSTRACT

Intravenous immunoglobulin (IVIg) therapy is increasingly indicated in many childhood diseases of serious nature to prevent death and disability. About 25% of the total use is for replacement therapy in children with congenital and acquired immune deficiency disorders, the usual dose being 400–500 mg/kg every 3–4 weeks. Almost 75% is for immune modulation, the common conditions being immune thrombocytopenic purpura (ITP), Kawasaki disease, Guillain-Barr'e syndrome, neonatal sepsis, juvenile idiopathic arthritis, and dermatological disorders. The dose varies in different clinical situations. Serious untoward reactions include anaphylaxis, renal failure, aseptic meningitis, thromboembolic stroke, pulmonary embolism, and myocardial infarction.

INTRODUCTION

Intravenous immunoglobulin therapy has been established for more than four decades and has reduced the mortality and morbidity in children. IVIg is a therapeutic compound prepared from pools of plasma collected with all safety precautions from several thousand (should be >60,000) healthy blood donors.

COMPOSITION AND MODE OF ACTION

- Contains IgG more than 95%, unmodified with intact function.
- Trace amounts of IgM, IgA, and cytokines will be present.
- It inactivates toxins, microbes, and parasites.
- Available in concentrations of 2%, 5%, 10%, 20% as liquid or lyophilized forms.
- Liquid preparations require refrigeration and should be brought to room temperature prior to administration.
- Lyophilized forms need careful reconstitution to prevent aggregation and should be utilized within 2–3 hours after reconstitution.

INDICATIONS

Replacement Therapy (25% of Therapy)

- *Primary immune deficiency disorders, which include:*
  - X-linked agammaglobulinemia
  - Common variable immunodeficiency
  - X-linked hyper IgM
  - Wiskott–Aldrich syndrome
  - Severe combined immunodeficiency
  - Selective IgG class deficiency
- *Secondary immune deficiency:*
  - Congenital acquired immunodeficiency syndrome with recurrent infections
  - Protein-losing disorders—intestinal lymphangiectasia
  - Myeloma
  - Chronic lymphatic leukemia.

Points to be observed in replacement therapy:
- Dose 400–500 mg/kg every 3–4 weeks
- Trough level for IgG should be maintained more than 500 mg/dL.
- Check IgG trough level every 2 months for initial 6 months and then every 6 months.
- Check blood count and liver function test every 6 months.
- Give extradoses during infections and gastrointestinal or urinary loss.

Immune Modulation (75% of Therapy)

- Immune thrombocytopenic purpura
  - Indications:
    - To increase the platelet count more than 20,000/mm^3
    - To arrest severe and rapid bleeding
    - Chronic ITP
  - Dose:
    - Acute ITP 1 g/kg × 2 days
    - Chronic ITP 1 g/kg every month
- Guillain–Barré syndrome
  - Indications:
    - Rapidly progressing ascending paralysis
    - Chronic relapsing polyradiculopathy
  - Dose:
    - 0.4 g/kg/day × 5 days

- Kawasaki disease:
    - Prevents coronary aneurysm.
    - Most effective in the initial 10 days of fever.
    - Dose:
        - 2 g/kg in 12 hours, repeat dose in non/transient responders
- *Neonatal sepsis*—as an adjunctive therapy to antibiotics
    - Dose:
        - 500–750 mg/kg single dose

Emerging Indications

- Connective tissue disorders (juvenile idiopathic arthritis, systemic lupus erythematosus, vasculitis)
- Dermatologic disorders
- Snake envenomation.

PRECAUTIONS PRIOR TO ADMINISTRATION

- Document the clinical diagnosis and exact indication for IVIg.
- Record the baseline temp, pulse, blood pressure of the patient, and previous history of anaphylaxis to IVIg or blood products.
- Enter the brand and number of the preparation and the dose advised.
- Begin with slow rate of infusion—0.01 mL/kg/min.
- Gradually increase to 0.1 mL/kg/min.
- Monitor vitals and for untoward symptoms or signs.
- Repeat users—do not change the brand.

UNTOWARD REACTIONS

- Trivial—usually dose related; characterized by fever, diaphoresis, vomiting, flank pain, and tachycardia
    - Treatment:
        - Stop the infusion, restart in a slow rate
        - Ibuprofen for pain and fever
        - IV diphenhydramine 5 mg/kg/24 hr div q 6 hr
        - IV hydrocortisone 5 mg/kg q 6 hr
- Anaphylaxis—occurs in IgA-deficient individuals:
    - Treat anaphylaxis immediately
    - Replace with IgA-depleted IVIg
- Renal failure—seen in lupus nephritis:
    - More in sucrose-based preparations
    - Read the instructions and prevent

- Severe reactions rarely encountered are aseptic meningitis, thromboembolic stroke, pulmonary embolism, and myocardial infarction.

CONCLUSION

Intravenous immunoglobulin is a life-saving drug for congenital immune deficiency disorders and is becoming established as the drug of choice for immunomodulation therapy to prevent death and disability.

Chapter 82

Hemolytic Uremic Syndrome

N Krishnan Nampoothiri, S Sushamabai

ABSTRACT

Hemolytic uremic syndrome (HUS) is a common cause of acquired renal failure, mostly seen in preschool children. The diagnostic triad consists of anemia, thrombocytopenia, and renal failure. HUS can be infection induced (*Escherichia coli* diarrhea, *Shigella* dysentery, and pneumococcal pneumonia) and noninfection induced or atypical HUS due to immune-mediated abnormalities of the complement system. Clinical presentation is sudden onset of progressive pallor, jaundice, weakness, reduced urine output and altered sensorium, following diarrhea, pneumonia or a trivial illness. Main treatment is supportive therapy for renal failure by fluid and electrolyte balance, dialysis, and correction of anemia. In atypical HUS, plasma exchange by fresh frozen plasma (FFP) is advised. Antibiotics are advised in pneumococcal pneumonia only. Prognosis is good in diarrhea-related HUS. Eculizumab is indicated in atypical HUS of genetic nature.

INTRODUCTION

Hemolytic uremic syndrome is a common cause of acute kidney injury in young children. The diagnostic triad is hemolytic anemia, thrombocytopenia, and acute renal failure.

ETIOLOGY

Infection Induced

- Shiga toxin-producing *E. coli*
- *Shigella* dysentery Type I
- Pneumococcal
- Human immunodeficiency virus (HIV).

Note: History of diarrhea/dysentery/pneumonia/empyema/features of HIV infection will be present prior to the syndrome in this group.

Noninfection Induced

- Genetic—complement abnormalities
- Drug induced
- Systemic diseases:
  - Systemic lupus erythematosus
  - Malignant hypertension
  - Metabolic—cobalamin C deficiency
  - Transplant associated
  - Malignancy.

Note: A triggering factor is usually present in genetic diseases.

CLINICAL PRESENTATION

- Common in preschool age group
- History of initial disease followed by sudden onset of pallor, jaundice, lethargy, irritability, and reduced urine output
- Altered sensorium and seizures occur in a significant group and indicate poor prognosis.
- Genetic onset HUS is more common in adolescents. In this group, onset is insidious and the triggering event will be mild and may be unnoticed.

PATIENT APPROACH

- Suspect HUS in a child or adolescent with rapid onset of pallor, jaundice, altered sensorium, and progressive reduction in urine output.
- Predisposing factors may not be present in the genetic group.
- Admit in pediatric-intensive care unit; stabilize airway, breathing and circulation; start normal saline 10 mL/kg in 10 minutes for volume expansion, if oliguria or anuria; repeat boluses till stable.
- Intravenous furosemide 1 mg/kg can be tried after volume challenge to induce diuresis.
- Send blood for complete blood count, coagulation profile, peripheral blood smear, direct Coombs test (DCT), renal function test (RFT), liver function test, serum electrolytes, lactate dehydrogenase (LDH), serum C_3, and random blood sugar.
- Anemia, thrombocytopenia, broken and distorted red blood cells (RBCs), increased reticulocyte count, high LDH and elevated RFT are characteristics of HUS. DCT will be positive in pneumococcal infection. Serum C_3 is reduced in atypical HUS.
- Evaluate urine for protein and microscopy. Mild proteinuria and microscopic hematuria are supportive of HUS.

SUBSEQUENT MANAGEMENT

- Antibiotics are advised (IV ceftriaxone), if pneumococcal infection is considered. In diarrhea or dysentery-induced HUS, antibiotics are contraindicated.
- Main treatment is for renal failure and the subsequent complications. Consider peritoneal or hemodialysis as per indications.
- Treat anemia with packed RBCs.
- Repeated plasma exchange with FFP is advised in atypical HUS till recovery.
- Provide good nutrition and maintain proper fluid and electrolyte balance.
- Eculizumab (anti-C_5 antibody) is advised in some forms of atypical familial HUS. Meningococcal vaccine should be administered to such patients.

PROGNOSIS

- Majority of patients with diarrhea-associated HUS recover completely.
- Prognosis is guarded in all other types either ending in mortality or in chronic renal failure. Periodic follow-up and renal supportive therapy should be considered in all children.

CONCLUSION

Hemolytic uremic syndrome is a fatal illness, should be suspected in children with sudden onset of pallor, jaundice and renal failure; early intervention is lifesaving.

Chapter 83

Disseminated Intravascular Coagulation

N Krishnan Nampoothiri, S Sushamabai

ABSTRACT

Disseminated intravascular coagulation (DIC) is an acquired coagulopathy with high mortality. Severe infections (bacteria, viruses, fungi, malaria), venoms and toxins, malignancy, trauma, pancreatitis, hypo/hyperthermia all can precipitate DIC. The clinical criteria of DIC are bleeding manifestations in a critically ill child, progressive pallor and jaundice. The supportive laboratory criteria are anemia, thrombocytopenia, and schistocytes in peripheral blood smear and reduced coagulation factors with fibrin degradation products. The management consists of treatment of the precipitating condition, blood component therapy, supportive therapy with fluid and electrolytes, and for organ failure.

INTRODUCTION

Disseminated intravascular coagulation is an acquired coagulopathy of varying grades of severity with high mortality. The illness is triggered by life-threatening systemic diseases causing hypoxia, acidosis, shock, tissue necrosis, and endothelial damage.

COMMON CAUSES OF DISSEMINATED INTRAVASCULAR COAGULATION

Infections

- Bacterial: Meningococcemia, sepsis by gram-negative/positive bacteria
- Rickettsial: Rocky mountain spotted fever
- Viral: Cytomegalovirus, varicella, ebola, and other hemorrhagic viral fevers
- Protozoal: Malaria
- Fungal: *Candida, Aspergillus*

Tissue Injury
- Polytrauma
- Massive burns
- Hypo- or hyperthermia.

Toxins
Snake or insect bites.

Others
- Fulminant hepatic failure
- Acute pancreatitis
- Collagen vascular diseases
- Malignancy
- Hemolytic transfusion reactions
- Hereditary thrombotic disorders.

PATHOGENESIS
- Systemic diseases release the cytokines which alter the endothelium and activate the extrinsic pathway of coagulation.
- A prothrombotic state occurs with the formation of microvascular thrombosis.
- Subsequent consumption of pro- and anticoagulants occur leading to deficiency of FV, FVIII, FII, FI, and platelets.
- The physiologic anticoagulants protein C, protein S, and antithrombin III are also consumed.
- Fibrin degradation products accumulate in blood.
- All these disrupt the smooth endothelial surface and cause microangiopathic hemolytic anemia.

CLINICAL PRESENTATION
- Appearance of bleeding from venipuncture sites in a critically ill child with toxemia or shock is the initial clinical feature.
- Subsequent progression to spontaneous skin bleeding as petechiae and ecchymosis and from the mucosal areas occurs.
- Progressive anemia and jaundice manifest.
- Areas of necrosis due to thrombosis in skin and body organs may occur.

INVESTIGATIONS

- Complete blood count—reveals anemia and thrombocytopenia.
- Fragmented red blood cells (RBCs), burr cells, and helmet-shaped RBCs or schistocytes in peripheral blood smear are diagnostic of DIC.
- Other diagnostic features are reduced fibrinogen (<50%), prolonged, prothrombin time, activated partial thromboplastin time, and thrombin time.
- Appearance of fibrin degradation products (d dimer) in blood is the most specific test.

TREATMENT

- Treat the triggering event—antibiotics for infection, antisnake venom for snake envenomation, etc.
- Correction of shock, acidosis, and hypoxia—may require mechanical ventilation, central venous cannulation, and inotropic support.
- Blood component therapy (Chapter 79):
    - Platelet transfusion for thrombocytopenia
    - Fresh frozen plasma for replacement of coagulation factors and natural inhibitors
    - Cryoprecipitate for hypofibrinogenemia
    - Packed RBCs for severe anemia
    - Vitamin K therapy
- Supportive therapy for:
    - Fluid and electrolyte balance
    - Renal failure
    - Other organ failure
- Anticoagulant therapy—indicated only in:
    - Large arterial or venous thrombosis.

Note: Replacement therapy is not needed if there are no clinical findings and can be stopped once the platelet count and fibrinogen levels are near normal and FDPs (Fibrin Degradation Products) disappear.

CONCLUSION

Consider DIC in a critically ill child developing bleeding, progressive pallor, and jaundice and the presence of schistocytes in peripheral blood smear are diagnostic.

Chapter 84

Sickle Cell Crisis

N Krishnan Nampoothiri, S Sushamabai

ABSTRACT

Sickle cell crisis indicates acute life-threatening complications encountered in sickle cell disease. They are infections such as pneumonia, osteomyelitis, and aplastic crisis by human parvovirus B infection. Noninfectious complications are splenic and hepatic sequestration and cholelithiasis. Vaso-occlusive complications include acute chest syndrome and hand-foot syndrome, priapism, and ischemic stroke. The child may present with fever with or without cough, chest pain, limb or abdominal pain, vomiting, pallor, and jaundice. Empirical antibiotic therapy in pneumonia is ceftriaxone + macrolide and in dactylitis is ceftriaxone + methicillin. In aplastic crisis, packed red blood cell (RBC) and in vaso-occlusive crisis simple or exchange transfusions are advised. Appropriate fluid and electrolyte therapy, analgesic, and antipyretic administration are also needed.

INTRODUCTION

Sickle cell crisis indicates acute life-threatening painful complications encountered in sickle cell disease. They can be infectious or noninfectious.

INFECTIOUS

Nonspecific Fever

- Often indicates bacterial than viral etiology.
- Specific bacterial infections in sickle cell disease are pneumonia and osteomyelitis which can be made out clinically.
- Indications for hospitalization are sick appearance, fever more than 104°F (>40°C), hypotension, prolonged CRFT more than 3 seconds, severe pain, features of dehydration, tachypnea, hemoglobin (Hb) less than 5 g/dL, total leukocyte count more than 30,000/mm^3, and platelet count less than 1 L/mm^3.

- Bacterial agents often involved are encapsulated organisms—*Haemophilus influenzae* type b, *Streptococcus pneumoniae* and *Neisseria meningitides*, *Salmonella*, and *Staphylococcus*.
- Management is as for sepsis with or without shock:
  - Initial stabilization of airway, breathing, and circulation
  - Appropriate fluid therapy (volume replacement + maintenance)
  - Laboratory tests:
    - Complete blood count, coagulation profile, culture of blood, or other body fluids as per clinical diagnosis
    - Chest X-ray, other imaging studies as per clinical indication
  - Empirical antibiotic therapy—intravenous ceftriaxone in first hour, change later as per culture and sensitivity report.
  - Packed RBC transfusion 5 mL/kg in 2 hours
  - Analgesics and antipyretics
  - Continuation therapy as per investigation reports
  - Consider vaccines after recovery

Aplastic Crisis

- Results from the temporary red cell aplasia following human parvovirus B19 infection.
- Characterized by nonspecific fever, anemia, and reticulocytopenia.
- Associated chest pain, abdominal pain, and stroke can occur.
- Management is by early packed RBC (PRBC) transfusion for severe anemia.
- Usually associated with infection; search for it and give appropriate antibiotics.
- Folic acid therapy should be continued.

Noninfectious

Acute Splenic Sequestration

- Seen more in infants and young children with sickle cell anemia.
- Characterized by rapid onset of anemia, left-sided abdominal pain, and splenomegaly; triggered usually by febrile illness.
- Pathognomonic laboratory features are rapid fall in Hb to less than 3 g/dL from the patient's baseline, reticulocytosis, and thrombocytopenia
- Management is by:
  - Fluid therapy with bolus normal saline followed by PRBCs 5 mL/kg in 2 hours
  - Analgesics as paracetamol ± ibuprofen
  - Treatment of the precipitating event.

Hepatic Sickle Cell Crisis

- Characterized by right upper quadrant abdominal pain, tenderness, fever, leukocytosis, and jaundice.
- Mimics viral hepatitis, cholecystitis, and choledocholithiasis
- Rule out the infections and other hepatobiliary complications
- Management is by:
  - Fluid and electrolyte therapy
  - Antibiotics for infection
  - Red blood cell transfusion
  - Paracetamol for fever.

Cholecystitis and Cholelithiasis

- Clinical features are recurrent right upper quadrant pain with or without fever
- Diagnostic confirmation is by ultrasonography abdomen
- Management is by:
  - Supportive therapy to maintain fluid and electrolyte balance
  - Antibiotics for infection
  - Pain management
  - Cholecystectomy.

Acute Vaso-occlusive Incidents

- It is the cardinal clinical feature of sickle cell anemia.
- Pathogenesis is disruption of blood flow in small blood vessels by sickled cells precipitated by infection, dehydration, hypothermia, and prolonged swimming in cold water.
- Clinical feature is unremitting pain in body parts which includes:
  - Acute dactylitis or hand foot syndrome which has to be differentiated from osteomyelitis.
  - Acute chest syndrome has to be differentiated from pneumonia.
  - Priapism.
  - Acute ischemic stroke.

DIAGNOSIS

It can be established by appropriate imaging studies, blood culture, and blood count.

MANAGEMENT

- Pain management (Chapter 46)
- Fluid resuscitation and simple or exchange transfusion in all conditions

- Empirical antibiotic therapy for pneumonia by ceftriaxone + macrolide to cover pneumococci and mycoplasma
- Urology consultation in prolonged priapism for aspiration of blood from corpora cavernosa followed by irrigation with dilute epinephrine.

CONCLUSION

Children with sickle cell disease are prone to develop life-threatening complications with infections, sequestrations, and vaso-occlusive crisis which should be evaluated and treated when they report with trivial symptoms.

Chapter 85

Hemophilias

S Sushamabai

ABSTRACT

Hemophilias are the most common congenital coagulation disorders. Bleeding manifestations usually appear by 8–9 months of age as easy bruising, ecchymosis, hemarthrosis of ankles or mucosal bleeds, but should be suspected in newborns presenting with intraventricular or subgaleal bleeds. Partial thromboplastin time (PTT) more than two times the upper limit is suggestive of hemophilia; type and degree of deficiency are to be confirmed by the factor assay. Patient approach depends on the severity of bleed. Those having intracranial bleed or severe anemia should be stabilized and factor replacement to attain 100% saturation should be started. Children having anemia require packed red blood cell transfusion additionally. For bleeding due to F XI deficiency, fresh frozen plasma (FFP) transfusion is the therapy of choice. Periodic follow-up in specialized clinics for lifelong is a must for prophylactic factor therapy to reduce death and disability.

INTRODUCTION

Hemophilias are the most common congenital coagulation factor deficiencies.

TYPES OF HEMOPHILIA

- X-linked recessive inheritance
    - Hemophilia A—F VIII deficiency
    - Hemophilia B—F IX deficiency
- Autosomal recessive inheritance
    - Hemophilia C—F XI deficiency.

CLINICAL PRESENTATION

- Bleeding due to hemophilia can occur in fetus, neonate or infant.
- Consider the possibility of hemophilia in newborns with intraventricular or subgaleal hemorrhage.

- Common age of clinical presentation is 8–9 months as the baby becomes ambulant. Bruising, hematoma, hemarthrosis (mainly ankles), and prolonged bleeding from trivial mucosal injuries are the usual features.
- The hallmark of hemophilia is hemarthrosis affecting knee and/or elbow in the older child. Recurrent episodes in a single joint produces the "target" joint due to fibrosis of the joint and subsequent new vascularization and more severe bleeding episodes.
- Life-threatening bleeding in hemophilia can be intracranial, upper airway, gastrointestinal, and iliopsoas regions.
- Severe bleeding is not characteristic of hemophilia C.

PATIENT APPROACH

- All children with life-threatening hemorrhage require pediatric intensive care unit care; stabilize airway, breathing and circulation; proceed to parallel assessment by brief history and quick evaluation to detect the etiology and severity of bleeding.
- Perform laboratory evaluation for complete blood count, peripheral blood smear, coagulation profile, grouping and crossmatching for diagnostic confirmation and to exclude the differential diagnosis if not diagnosed previously.
- Arrange for factor-replacement therapy immediately in a confirmed case of hemophilia since delay in therapy will increase mortality and morbidity.
- Prolonged PTT more than two times the upper limit is the hallmark of hemophilia. Type and severity of the disease is to be assessed by specific factor assay at the earliest.
- Low Hb denotes severe and prolonged bleeding.
- The differential diagnosis to be considered in the first episode of bleeding are idiopathic thrombocytopenic purpura, platelet function disorders, type 3 von Willebrand disease (vWD), vitamin K deficiency, and severe liver disease. History, physical examination, and screening investigations will help to exclude all conditions except type 3 vWD in which both von Willebrand factor (vWF) antigen and vWF assay are needed for diagnosis.
- Imaging studies and other investigations are to be done only after starting the specific factor therapy so as to prevent ongoing severe bleed. The dose and duration of factor therapy depend on the severity of hemophilia and the type of bleeding as shown in below:

Severity of bleeding	Rise in factor (%)
Mild-to-moderate bleed	35–50
Severe/life-threatening bleed	100

- Calculation of the dose of recombinant (r) F VIII or r F IX is as follows:
  - Dose of r F VIII (IU) = Percentage desired (rise in r F VIII) × body wt (kg) × 0.5

Table 85.1: Treatment of hemophilia A and B.

Types of bleeding	Hemophilia A	Hemophilia B
Major surgery, life-threatening hemorrhage	50–75 IU/kg F VIII concentrate, then 25 IU/kg q 8–12 hr to maintain trough level >50 IU/dL for 5–7 days, then 50 IU/kg daily to maintain trough level >25 IU/dL for 7 days	120 IU/kg of F IX concentrate* then 50–60 IU/kg q 12–24 hr to maintain F IX at >40 IU/dL for 5–7 days, then at >30 IU/dL for 7 days
Hemarthrosis[†]	[‡]50–60 IU/kg F VIII concentrate on day 1, then 20–30 IU/kg on day 2, 3, 5 until joint function is normal. Additional treatment on alternate days for 7–10 days. Consider prophylaxis	80–100 IU/kg F IX on day 1, then 40 IU/kg on days 2, 4. Additional treatment on alternate days for 7–10 days. Consider prophylaxis
Iliopsoas hemorrhage	50 IU/kg F VIII concentrate, then 25 IU/kg every 12 hr until asymptomatic, then 20 IU/kg on alternate days for 10–14 days till radiological clearance	120 IU/kg F IX concentrate* then 50–60 IU/kg every 12–24 hr to maintain F IX at >40 IU/dL until asymptomatic, then 40–50 IU/kg on alternate days for 10–14 days
Muscle or significant subcutaneous hematoma	50 IU/kg F VIII concentrate, then 20 IU/kg on alternate day till resolution	80 IU/kg F IX concentrate,* repeat every 2–3 days till complete resolution
Hematuria	Bedrest, 1.5 × maintenance fluids, if no control by 1–2 days, give 20 IU/kg F VIII concentrate; add prednisolone if not controlled. (Avoid in HIV patients)	Supportive therapy as in hemophilia A. If not controlled in 1–2 days, give 40 IU/kg F IX concentrate,* give prednisolone if not controlled
Epistaxis	Apply pressure for 15–20 min, pack with petroleum gauze, give antifibrinolytic therapy,[‡] 20 IU/kg factor VIII concentrate if no response	Initial measures same, give 40 IU/kg factor concentrate* if the initial measures fail
Mouth, deciduous teeth, tooth extraction	20 IU/kg F VIII concentrate,[§] antifibrinolytic therapy, remove loose deciduous tooth	40 IU/kg F IX concentrate, others as in hemophilia A
Prophylaxis	20–40 IU/kg F VIII concentrate on alternate day to achieve a trough level ≥1%	30–50 IU/kg concentrate* to achieve a trough level ≥1%

*Indicates r F IX concentrate; for plasma-derived F IX concentrate, use 70% of the stated dose.
[†]Orthopedic evaluation for aspiration in hip involvement.
[‡]For mild/moderate hemophilia desmopressin 0.3 µg/kg can be tried.
[§]Epsilon aminocaproic acid: 100 mg/kg (PO) loading dose followed by 50 mg/kg q 6 hr.
(F, factor; HIV, human immunodeficiency virus)

- Dose of r F IX (IU) = Percentage desired (rise in r F IX) × body wt (kg) × 1.4

Table 85.1 reveals the treatment of bleeding in hemophilia.

- In hemophilia C, bleeding is not severe. Usual situations are major surgery and oral cavity injuries. FFP infusion (10–15 mL/kg) is the advised therapy.

SUBSEQUENT MANAGEMENT

Register in hemophilia clinic for periodic follow-up. Prophylactic factor therapy, physiotherapy for joint involvement, additional vaccine administration, counseling, and rehabilitation are the problems to be handled.

CONCLUSION

Though bleeding in hemophilia manifests during infancy, the possibility should be suspected in newborns with intraventricular or subgaleal hemorrhage; all hemophiliacs should be placed on long-term prophylactic therapy.

FURTHER READING

1. Allen GA, Glader B. Approach to the bleeding child. Pediatr Clin North Am. 2002;49(6):1239-56.
2. http://de.slideshare.net/Andre kurniawan/haemophilia-a (internet from 2016 Nov 21).
3. Scott JP, Montgomery RR. Hereditary clotting factor deficiencies (bleeding disorders). In: Kliegman R, Nelson WE (Eds). Nelson Textbook of Pediatrics. Philadelphia, PA: Elsevier/Saunders; 2011.

Chapter 86

Oncologic Emergencies

P Jayasree, S Sushamabai

ABSTRACT

Oncologic emergencies are life-threatening adverse effects of treatment in malignant diseases, occurring in the early phase of antimalignant therapy and should be anticipated. It can be metabolic [tumor lysis syndrome (TLS), dyselectrolytemia], bone marrow suppression [anemia, neutropenia, thrombocytopenia, disseminated intravascular coagulation, hyperleukocytosis, graft-versus-host disease (GVHD)] and compression syndromes (of spinal cord, brain, superior vena cava, and trachea). The clinical manifestations are pallor, vomiting, fever, features of dyselectrolytemia, bleeding, headache, focal paralysis, cough and respiratory distress. Relevant investigations and management are discussed.

INTRODUCTION

Oncologic emergencies are life-threatening adverse effects of treatment that occur early in the therapy of malignant diseases.

These can be categorized as:
- Metabolic abnormalities
- Bone marrow suppression
- Compression syndromes.

METABOLIC ABNORMALITIES

Tumor lysis syndrome: It is produced by the release of large quantities of metabolites in the circulation due to tumor cell death. The problems encountered are as follows:
- *Hyperuricemia:*
  - Seen in lymphoma, leukemia, and in malignancies with large tumor burden leading to impaired renal function.
  - Occurs 12–48 hours after starting the therapy.
  - Anticipate the condition; assess serum uric acid (UA) Na, K, Ca, P and creatinine prior to therapy and then frequently till therapy is completed.
  - Provide adequate hydration 2 L/m^2 day for prevention.

- Allopurinol (prevents UA synthesis) 10 mg/kg/day divided q 12 hr till 3 days after completion of initial phase of chemotherapy.
- In established TLS with hyperuricemia or those at high risk for TLS, rasburicase (degrades UA) is advised.
- *Electrolyte imbalances*—include:
  - Hyperkalemia, hyperphosphatemia, and hypercalcemia
  - Management as in Chapter 53.

BONE MARROW SUPPRESSION

Causes

- Chemotherapy-induced suppression
- Bone marrow infiltration by malignant tissues.

Manifestations

- *Anemia*—should be corrected by packed red blood cells transfusion (Chapter 79).
- *Thrombocytopenia*—revealed by bleeding manifestation and low platelet count; should be corrected by platelet transfusion (Chapter 79).

Note: Patients receiving immune suppressive therapy should be given irradiated blood products to prevent GVHD and leukoreduced blood products to prevent transfusion-associated reactions and infections.

- *Neutropenia* is absolute neutrophil count less than 500/mm^3.
- *If asymptomatic:*
  - Avoid infections by providing infection-free environment.
  - Adhere to clean food and fluids.
  - Prophylactic treatment with cotrimoxazole (Chapter 125).
- *Febrile neutropenia:*
  - Always indicates serious infections.
  - Hospitalize the patient; send blood, urine and other relevant samples for culture and sensitivity.
  - Start empirical broad-spectrum intravenous antibiotics piperacillin–tazobactam ± amikacin ± vancomycin depending on the clinical situation; change as per culture and sensitivity reports.
  - Add antifungal agents if there is clinical evidence or if the fever persists for more than 3–5 days.
  - *Pneumocystis jiroveci* pneumonia should be treated with cotrimoxazole high dose along with corticosteroids.
  - Treat viral infections with specific antiviral agents.

- *Disseminated intravascular coagulation* (Chapter 83).
    - Manifests as shock or hemorrhage.
    - Occurs due to sepsis, tumor factors or hypotension.
    - Treat the underlying disorder along with fresh frozen plasma and platelet transfusion.
- *Hyperleukocytosis* is total leukocyte count more than 100,000/mm^3.
    - Manifestations are bleeding, thrombosis, pulmonary infiltrates, respiratory distress, and TLS.
    - Treatment is leukapheresis, chemotherapy, and hydroxyurea.
- *Graft-versus-host disease:*
    - Features are diarrhea, dermatitis, and hepatitis due to immune suppression.
    - Follows after nonirradiated blood administration and bone marrow transplantation.
    - Treatment is by corticosteroids, cyclosporine, tacrolimus, and anti-thymocyte globulin.

COMPRESSION SYNDROMES

- *Spinal cord compression*—characterized by back pain ± radicular pain, lower limb weakness ± sensory loss ± incontinence. Due to metastasis of vertebrae or spinal canal; common in neuroblastoma or medulloblastoma; diagnosed by magnetic resonance imaging (MRI) of the affected area. Treatment is by corticosteroids, radiotherapy, chemotherapy, and laminectomy.
- *Raised intracranial pressure*—features are headache, vomiting, seizures, visual blurring, bradycardia, hypotension, confusion, coma, papilledema, hydrocephalus, third and sixth cranial nerve palsy. Seen in neuroblastoma, astrocytoma and gliomas. Diagnostic confirmation by computed tomography/MRI. Treatment—steroids, phenytoin, radiation, and surgery.
- *Superior vena cava syndrome*—clinical presentation is plethora and edema of head and neck, cyanosis, distended neck veins, proptosis and Horner syndrome; seen in lymphoma causing superior mediastinal mass. Treatment—corticosteroids, radiation, and chemotherapy.
- *Tracheal compression*—presents as cough and respiratory distress due to mediastinal mass compressing trachea. Treatment is corticosteroid and radiation.

CONCLUSION

Oncologic emergencies should be anticipated in all children undergoing antimalignant therapy and timely treatment should be given to prevent mortality.

Chapter 87

Anticoagulant and Thrombolytic Therapy

N Krishnan Nampoothiri, S Sushamabai

ABSTRACT

Anticoagulant and thrombolytic therapies are increasing in pediatrics due to the expansion of critical care services. Low-molecular-weight heparin, vitamin K antagonists, warfarin, and aspirin are the commonly used drugs in children. Heparin flushing is often needed in pediatric intensive care units for maintaining central and peripheral vascular access patency and in total parenteral nutrition (TPN). Aspirin is the drug of choice for anticoagulation in Kawasaki disease, the mechanism of action being prevention of platelet aggregation. Newer oral drugs though available, their safety profile in children is not established. For thrombolytic therapy recombinant tissue plasminogen activator intravenous (IV) infusion is advised.

INTRODUCTION

Anticoagulant and thrombolytic therapy are increasingly required in pediatrics because of the advances in treating critically ill children and the increasing awareness of genetic predisposition to thrombotic disorders.

INDICATIONS

- Thromboembolic diseases which include:
  - Extremity deep vein thrombosis
  - Pulmonary embolism
  - Cerebral sinovenous thrombosis
  - Renal vein thrombosis
  - Arterial thrombosis (AT)
  - Rapidly progressive thrombosis
- Prophylactic anticoagulant therapy as in:
  - Coronary AT (Kawasaki disease)
  - Vasculitis syndromes (systemic lupus erythematous)
  - Central venous catheters
  - Peripheral venous cannulation
  - Postcardiac surgery.

DRUGS USED

- Standard or unfractionated heparin
- Low-molecular-weight heparin
- Vitamin K antagonists
- Acetyl salicylic acid
- Newer drugs.

Unfractionated Heparin

- Acts by enhancing the effects of antithrombin III in neutralizing the activated clotting factors X and thrombin.
- Dose: 75–100 U/kg bolus over 10 minutes followed by 20–28 U/kg/hr (higher dose in newborns) as continuous infusion; increase the dose by 5–10% q 6 hr until adequate level of partial thromboplastin time (PTT) (60–85 s) is achieved; duration of the therapy depends upon the illness.
- Adjust the maintenance dose by keeping PTT between 55 s and 85 s.

Advantages: Short halt-life (30–60 minutes), early reversibility.

Limitations: Frequent laboratory monitoring, heparin-induced thrombocytopenia, and risk of contamination.

Monitoring: Heparin level by anti-Xa assay.

Untoward effects: Anaphylaxis and osteoporosis.

Heparin flushing: As prophylaxis against venous thromboembolism.
- Peripheral IV access—1–2 mL of 10 U/mL up to q 4 hr
- Central IV access—2–3 mL of 100 U/mL up to q 4 hr
- Total parenteral nutrition and arterial access—add heparin to make final concentration in the infusate to 0.5–1 U/mL.

Contraindications: Active major bleeding, use with caution, if platelet count is less than 50,000/mm^3.

Adverse effects: Bleeding (stop the infusion for minor bleeds; for major bleeds, give protamine sulfate 1 mg per 100 U heparin; if not controlled, administer fresh frozen plasma (FFP) 10–15 mL/kg).

Low-molecular-weight Heparin

- Low-molecular-weight heparin is the anticoagulant of choice at present, enoxaparin is the most commonly used one in pediatrics.

- Dose 1.5 mg/kg/dose q 12 hr subcutaneous in babies less than 2 months of age; More than 2 months age babies 1 mg/kg/dose q 12 hr; peak level is attained 4–6 hours following the injection, dose adjusted to achieve anti-Xa factor level 0.5–1.0 IU/mL 4 hr after the second or third dose.
- Can be changed to oral anticoagulant as per indication.

Vitamin K Antagonists

- Most commonly used one is warfarin, an oral anticoagulant. Competitively inhibits vitamin K–dependent factor II, VII, IX and X and protein C and S.
- Start therapy while anti-coagulated on heparin which should be continued for 2 more days after starting warfarin.
- Dose: 0.3 mg/kg in infants, 0.09 mg/kg in older children. International normalized ratio (INR) should be maintained between 2 and 3. For prosthetic cardiac valve and recurrent thrombosis, target INR is 2.5–3.5.
- Contraindications: Severe liver and kidney diseases, bleeding, peptic ulcer disease, and malignant hypertension.
- Side effects: Bleeding, skin necrosis, osteoporosis, drug interaction especially with antibiotics and anticonvulsants like valparin and phenytoin. Adjust the drug dosage as per the situation.
- Treat bleeding with vitamin K 5 mg IV + FFP 10–15 mL/kg.

Acetyl Salicylic Acid or Aspirin

- *Dosage*: 1–5 mg/kg/day
- *Indications*: For the prevention of arterial thromboembolism in children with Kawasaki disease, stroke, ventricular assist devices, single ventricle and cardiac defects
- *Mechanism of action*: Prevents platelet thromboxane A2 production by irreversibly inhibiting cyclooxygenase.

Newer Drugs

- *Direct thrombin inhibitors*—dabigatran
- *Factor Xa inhibitors*—apixaban, rivaroxaban
- *Indications*—mainly in adults with venous thrombosis
- *Advantages*—oral fixed dosing, good safety profile, and less need for laboratory monitoring.

THROMBOLYTIC THERAPY

- *Indications*: When rapid clot resolution is needed as in life or limb threatening thrombosis.
- *Choice drug*: Recombinant tissue plasminogen activator.

- *Mechanism of action*: Conversion of endogenous plasminogen to plasmin which degrades fibrin clot.
- *Dose*: 0.01 mg–0.06 mg/kg/hr up to 0.6 mg/kg/hr as IV infusion.
- *Monitoring*: Maintain fibrinogen more than 100 mg/dL and platelet count more than 75,000/mm^3 during treatment. Lytic stage is assessed by FDPs (Fibrin degradation products) and D-dimer assay.
- Unfractionated heparin as adjuvant initial therapy with 10–20 U/kg/hr is advised in patients with low risk of bleeding.
- *Precautions*: Avoid invasive procedures as urinary catheterization, arterial puncture, and rectal temperature recording.

CONCLUSION

Knowledge regarding anticoagulant and thrombolytic therapy is a must because such therapy is getting increasingly established in pediatrics.

Section 13

ACCIDENTS, POISONING, AND ENVENOMATION

Chapter 88

Drowning and Submersion Injuries

S Letha, S Sushamabai

ABSTRACT

Drowning and submersion injuries are one of the leading causes of childhood death and disability worldwide, irrespective of the socioeconomic and medical facilities available. The pathogenesis involves early hypoxemia and hypothermia. Cerebral hypoxic damage, myocardial ischemia, shock, and multiorgan failure follow. Management is rapid rescue from the area, mouth-to-mouth breathing or O_2 therapy, drying the child, and cardiopulmonary resuscitation (CPR). All children brought to the hospital should be observed in emergency department (ED) at least for 6 hours. Pediatric intensive care unit care is indicated if Glasgow Coma Scale (GCS) is less than 13, apnea, hypoxemia, cardiac arrhythmias, other suspected injuries, and child abuse. Priorities are for ventilation, management of hypothermia, shock, cerebral edema, acute respiratory distress syndrome (ARDS), disseminated intravascular coagulation (DIC), and multiorgan failure. Predictors of poor prognosis are submersion more than 10 minutes, coma, apnea, shock, and failure of response for CPR more than 25 minutes.

INTRODUCTION

Drowning is the process of experiencing respiratory impairment from submersion or immersion in liquid. The outcome can be fatal or nonfatal with complete recovery or with varying degrees of disabilities up to vegetative stage. It is one of the leading preventable causes of childhood death and disability worldwide.

PATHOPHYSIOLOGY

- The main injury following a drowning incident is hypoxia.
- Cold injury or hypothermia is the next major problem which occurs even in lukewarm water submersion and aggravates the hypoxic injury.
- Loss of consciousness occurs first followed by myocardial hypoxia, abrupt circulatory failure, and development of arrhythmias.
- Cerebral edema sets in after cardiopulmonary arrest which aggravates the brain ischemia.

- All organs and systems undergo ischemic injury leading to ARDS, acute kidney injury, DIC, gastrointestinal mucosal injury, liver damage, and hemolysis.
- Metabolic derangements are almost similar in fresh-water and salt-water submersion.
- Added risks of infection, chemical and physical injury, aspiration, and impaction can occur in lungs and airways depending on the situation.
- Cold-water drowning is characterized by early shock.

MANAGEMENT

At the Drowned Area

- Extricate the victim at the earliest from the submersion site.
- Start rescue therapy promptly. Priority is for correction of hypoxia. Clear the mouth and throat for any foreign material or vomitus. Chest compression and back blows can be used to dislodge impacted foreign body of the airway. Abdominal thrust is contraindicated since choking and aspiration into the airway and rupture of viscera may follow.
- Start mouth-to-mouth or mouth-to-nose breathing if apnea or if the breathing is ineffective.
- Remove the wet clothes of the victim, wipe to dry up, and wrap in warm clothes.
- Oxygen if available at the site should be started.
- Transport the victim to the nearest health facility for emergency care while resuscitation is being continued.
- Suspect cervical spine injury in victims on diving practice, vehicle crash, fall from a height, a water spot accident, evidence of other traumatic injuries, and in child abuse.
- Protect the cervical spine by applying cervical collar in neutral position till imaging has excluded the possibility of such injury.

In the Emergency Department

Proceed as follows:
- Children with Glasgow Coma Scale (GCS) more than or equal to 13, spontaneous respiration, and verbalization need observation in ED for 6–8 hours.
- Administer oxygen by face mask to keep SpO_2 92–95%.
- Active external warming with warm bath (40°C), thermal blankets, and keeping the patient under radiant warmer till the core temperature reaches 34°C.
- Monitor vital signs (heart rate, respiratory rate, core temperature, and blood pressure), SpO_2, GCS, and intake output.

- Evaluate the pulmonary system for aspiration pneumonia or development of respiratory distress syndrome.
- Investigations to be done are complete blood count (CBC), chest X-ray (CXR), blood urea (BU), random blood sugar, serum electrolytes (SE), arterial blood gas (ABG), and others as per clinical indication.
- Administer intravenous (IV) normal saline (NS) 10–20 mL/kg as bolus followed by maintenance NS till the child is stable.
- Can be discharged from ED if the patient reveals stable vitals, SpO_2, GCS, and accepts oral fluids and reveals stable hydration status for 6 hours.

In the Pediatric Intensive Care Unit

Indications for Admission

- Coma, apnea, cyanosis, labored respiration, shock, and cardiac irregularity
- Glasgow Coma Scale less than 13, hypoxemia—SpO_2 less than 90% in room air
- Hypothermia
- Submersion in polluted water, chemicals, hot liquids
- Suspected child abuse, vehicle accident
- Other external injuries.

Management

- Clear the airway.
- Supplemental oxygen 100% as positive pressure bag and mask ventilation or by intubation and mechanical ventilation as per situation. Hypoxia should be corrected rapidly.
- Correction of hypothermia—proceed for active internal warming by warm environment, warm humidified oxygen, warm IV fluids, and warm gastric lavage till the core temperature reaches 34°C.
- Cardiovascular support by intubation, mechanical ventilation, central venous access, IV bolus NS 10–20 mL/kg in 1 hour followed by NS maintenance therapy.
- Treat hyperglycemia and dyselectrolytemia. Consider intraosseous (IO) infusion if delay in obtaining IV access.
- Treat brady-asystole with IV epinephrine 0.01 mg/kg of 1:10,000 solution q 3–5 minutes as needed. If delay in getting IV access, administer epinephrine 0.1–0.2 mg 1:1,000 solution intratracheally followed by atropine IV 0.01–0.02 mg/kg.
- Investigations should include CXR to rule out ARDS, pneumothorax and aspiration pneumonia, CBC, ABG, renal function test, frequent capillary blood glucose (BG) SE, computed tomography head, and if

feasible, bedside electroencephalogram, other imaging studies if trauma is suspected.
- Continuous monitoring of vitals, SpO_2, GCS, ECG, and intake output at least 6 hourly.
- Inotropic support and correction of electrolyte imbalance. Consider shock energy for defibrillation—first shock 2 J/kg, subsequent shocks more than or equal to 4 J/kg to the maximum of 10 J/kg or adult dose.
- Manage cerebral edema by head-end elevation, IV mannitol [3% saline (if in shock) anticonvulsants (fosphenytoin, phenobarb)], fluid and electrolyte correction, and control of hyperglycemia.
- Deep coma after 24–72 hours indicates death or survival in vegetative stage. Withdrawal of life support need be considered and counseled. Measures for organ donation should be undertaken if the parents wish for it.
- Other measures include antibiotics for infection, renal support by dialysis, detection and control of DIC, treatment of bloody diarrhea, and management of hyperthermia by paracetamol if core temperature more than 37.5°C.
- Therapeutic hypothermia can be considered with individual discretion in centers as per resources available to prevent brain damage.

PROGNOSTIC INDICATORS

- Poor prognosis if deep coma, apnea, absent pupillary responses, cardiac irregularities, shock, hyperglycemia, submersion duration more than 10 minutes, failure of response to CPR more than 25 minutes.
- Good prognosis with GCS more than or equal to 6 at admission, submersion less than 10 minutes, early resuscitation, and rapid recovery with resuscitation.

PREVENTION

- The most effective way to decrease death and disability in drowning is by prevention.
- Supervision of young infants and children should be vigilant. Responsible caretaker should be with them to supervise every moment.
- For older children, health education as well safety precautions should be taught.

CONCLUSION

The main insult in drowning is widespread hypoxia of all vital organs which, if prolonged, prognosis is grave.

Chapter 89

Burn Injuries

S Letha, S Sushamabai

ABSTRACT

Burn injuries are usually accidental in children and are produced by fire, heat, electricity and chemicals in various ways–special situations being electrocution and lightning injuries. Problems encountered are fluid and electrolyte imbalance, loss of plasma proteins and internal organ damage presenting as cardiac arrhythmias, cardiac arrest, acute respiratory distress syndrome (ARDS), liver, kidney muscle and blood vessel damage especially following electrocution and lightning. Management includes removing the patient from the burn area, airway, breathing, and circulation (ABC) stabilization and assessing the extent of burn as per rule of palm. Patients having more than 10% burn area require inpatient (IP) treatment. Fluid calculation is based on Parkland formula, the initial fluid being 5% dextrose Ringer lactate (DRL).

Plasma or fresh frozen plasma (FFP) administration is indicated in burn >40% and those with coagulopathy. Pain management with morphine, skin care by aseptic precautions and silver sulfadiazine cream application, starting enteral feeds by 48 hr and timely reconstructive surgery are the other modalities of treatment.

INTRODUCTION

Burn injuries are caused by the contact of heat, electricity, fire or chemicals and contribute to substantial number of childhood death and morbidity. The injuries are mostly accidental, rarely suicidal (adolescents) or homicidal (as part of child abuse) and can be sustained from:
- Firewood burning, burning leaves, or other wastes
- Scalding from boiling water
- Chemical ingestion and/or spilling
- Blast injuries.

Scalding from boiling liquids is more common in young infants and toddlers.

SPECIAL SITUATIONS

- Electrocution
- Lightning injuries.

PATHOPHYSIOLOGY

The problems encountered are:
- Fluid and electrolyte loss—mainly Na, K
- Loss of plasma proteins
- Organ damage—cardiac arrhythmias, ARDS, and acute kidney injury
- Paralytic ileus
- Secondary infections.

MANAGEMENT

Care at the Site of Occurrence

- Remove the patient from the burning agent—extinguish the flame by rolling the child on the ground/covering with blanket.
- Assess the patency of the airway.
- Remove the clothing if smoky, having chemicals/hot liquid and all tight jewelry to prevent constriction and vascular compromise.
- Wash the chemicals from the affected body area; for burns by hot tar, use mineral oil for removal.
- Cover the burned area with clean cloth to avoid contamination; apply wet compresses to small injuries to reduce the intensity of burns.
- Administer analgesics—ibuprofen or paracetamol.
- Transport the patient immediately to the medical facility.

Care at the Emergency Department

- Establish ABC.
- Preexisting morbidity such as coronary heart disease, asthma, diabetes, hepatic and renal disease should be enquired and documented.
- Provide humidified oxygen if hypoxic.
- Anticipate early endotracheal intubation in extensive burns and burns over face and neck.
- Assess the extent of burn injury—burns are three-dimensional injuries assessed by length, breadth (together described as surface area), and depth. The surface area from the wrist crease to the finger crease (the palm) in the child is approximately 1% of the child's body surface area (BSA) stated as the *rule of palm*.
- The depth of burn can be first degree (swelling, erythema and pain), second degree (swelling, edema, blisters and severe pain) or third degree (painless and dry area).
- Children with less than 10% burn require only outpatient treatment as cleaning and dressing the wound.

- Indications for inpatient care are burn more than 10% BSA, third-degree burn, electrocution, lightning, chemical burns, inhalational injury, child abuse, burns of face, hands, feet, perineum, genitals or major joints, associated trauma and preexisting chronic diseases. Special burn care unit is ideal.
- Start intravenous (IV) fluids with 5% DRL. Calculate the fluid volume using Parkland formula as:
  First 24 hr = (4 mL/kg × %BSA) + maintenance requirement; give 1/2 the volume in the initial 8 hours starting from the time of burns, and the rest half in subsequent 16 hours. After 24 hours only, maintenance fluid therapy (normal saline or 5% dextrose normal saline) is required.
- Monitor pulse rate, blood pressure, urine output (UOP) and sensorium. Adequate UOP should be more than 1 mL/kg/hr. Adjust the IV fluid infusion accordingly.
- Establish central venous line if burns are more than 30% BSA.
- Add 5% albumin infusion 0.4 mL/kg × %BSA if burns exceeds 40% of BSA.
- Administer FFP in children less than 2 years having burns more than 20% BSA and in those with bleeding or coagulopathy.
- Pain relief: Morphine 0.1–0.3 mg/kg as IV except in respiratory burns. Pentazocine and pethidine are alternatives.
- Nasogastric aspiration and urine catheterization if burns more than 20%.
- Tetanus toxoid 0.5 mL administration for all affected children.
- Wound care: Wash with sterile normal saline, debride nonviable tissues, and apply silver sulphadiazine cream. Systemic antibiotics should be considered if bacterial infection is suspected.
- Nutrition: Start oral feeds after 48 hours—initially liquid diet (kanji, milk, fruit juice) with vitamin supplementation, gradually increasing the calories and proteins. 50% excess calories and proteins predicted for the age are advised till complete healing.

INVESTIGATIONS

Should be selected according to the extent of burn injury, the cause and the added complications.

ELECTROCUTION AND LIGHTNING

- Minor burns reveal features of superficial (first degree) burns in both situations.
- Such patients require observation of vitals at least for 4 hours even if apparently stable and wound care and outpatient follow-up.

- *High-tension electrical wire burn and high-voltage lightning* produce serious internal injuries through the pathway of the current, damaging the internal soft tissues.
- The cutaneous lesions need not indicate the intensity of internal damage produced. Soft tissues are the ones affected. Serious injuries occur to the thoracic structures, nervous system, abdominal viscera, muscles and blood vessels through the pathway of electrical flow. Clinical presentations include confusion, coma (due to cerebral edema), cardiac arrest, ARDS, internal bleeding due to vascular damage, liver damage and acute kidney injury (due to muscle damage and myoglobinuria).

MANAGEMENT

- Cardiopulmonary resuscitation including defibrillation
- Fluid and electrolyte therapy, cardiovascular support including inotrope infusion till recovery
- Mechanical ventilation for cardiopulmonary arrest or ARDS
- Monitoring of renal functions and support
- Liver support and treatment of ileus
- Vascular surgery for blood vessel damage
- Reconstructive surgery as healing starts.

PREVENTION

Burn injuries can be prevented by proper safety precautions and education.

CONCLUSION

All patients with burn injuries should be assessed for internal injuries and the extent and depth of burns and urgent treatment provided for fluid and electrolyte resuscitation and should be maintained in sterile environment till recovery.

Chapter 90

Inadvertent Intra-arterial Injection

Bibin Sajan, S Sushamabai

ABSTRACT

Intravenous (IV) injections may rarely enter intra-arterial (IA) route unexpectedly and produce acute severe ischemia and gangrene of the distal part of the injected extremity. The main reason is "high-rising" vascular anomaly of the radial artery, resulting in a superficial branch in the forearm. The most severe injury follows IA barbiturate injection. Clinical presentation is immediate occurrence of severe pain, erythema, cyanosis, and edema of the injected limb distally followed by gangrene. Can be asymptomatic occasionally. Lack of response to the drug injected is the indication to suspect in that situation. Management is immediate stabilization if in compromise, Doppler Ultrasound sonography (USS) of the affected vessel, get another IV access, and maintain perfusion distal to the site of injury, administration of narcotic analgesic and papaverine, and heparinized saline to the injected artery. Surgical consultation, arteriography, and thrombectomy are the limb-saving procedures.

INTRODUCTION

Intra-arterial injection of drugs is occasionally encountered in clinical practice. This is a medical emergency and can cause:
- Acute, severe extremity ischemia, and gangrene
- Medicolegal problems subsequently.

RISK FACTORS

- Vascular anomalies like "high-rising" radial artery can result in a superficial branch in the forearm.[1] This increases the chance of unexpected IA injection.
- The most severe injury follows barbiturate administration.

CLINICAL PRESENTATION

- Immediate severe pain distal to the site of injection.
- Failure of expected effect of the drug after administration.

Table 90.1: Features of intra-arterial injection.[1,2]

Drugs	Intra-arterial injection effects
Atracurium	Ischemia
Atropine*	None reported
Fentanyl*	None reported
Ketamine	Necrosis
Midazolam*	None reported
Morphine*	None reported
Pancuronium*	None reported
Phenytoin	Ischemia, necrosis, tissue death
Propofol	Hyperemia, distal "blanching"
Rocuronium	Ischemia
Succinylcholine*	None reported
Thiopental	Ischemia, necrosis, tissue death
Amiodarone	Ischemia

*Suspect when desired clinical effects are not perceived.

- Pallor, paresthesia, hyperemia, and cyanosis of the affected limb following the injection
- Profound edema and gangrene of the painful area of the limb.

Table 90.1 shows the reported clinical features that follow IA injection of some drugs used in emergency situations.

PATHOPHYSIOLOGY

- Arterial spasm, either caused by the local release of norepinephrine or directly mediated by the drug.
- Direct tissue destruction by the drug.
- Subsequent chemical arteritis leading to endothelial destruction.
- Release of endogenous substances that mediate deleterious effects themselves, for example, thromboxane.
- Drug precipitation and crystal formation within the distal vessel leading to ischemia and thrombosis.

MANAGEMENT—NO UNIVERSALLY ACCEPTED PROTOCOL

- Doppler USS of the affected area to assess the status of the vessel, if available.[1]
- Get another venous access, stabilize airway, breathing, and circulation if any compromise, do not apply heat/cold to the affected area.

- Administer narcotic analgesics.
- Maintain perfusion distal to the site of injury.
- Elevate the extremity to improve venous and lymphatic drainage.
- Do not remove the cannula; administer injection papaverine 1:20 dilution in heparinized saline (0.5 mL heparin in 500 mL normal saline) immediately through the same cannula.
- Start heparin infusion through a separate access—50 U/kg bolus followed by 15–25 U/kg/hr.
- Monitor coagulation parameters—consider urokinase/streptokinase injection.
- Intra-arterial procaine/Tolazoline HCl injection for vasodilatation.
- Arteriography to determine the extent of injury.
- Surgical opinion for extremity sympatholysis—stellate ganglion blocks and lower extremity sympathetic blocks will produce sustained arterial and venous vasodilatation.
- Surgical consultation for thrombectomy and debridement of gangrenous areas.
- Patient or parent communication, counseling, and proper documentation are very important.

CONCLUSION

The main reason for inadvertent intra-arterial injection is high-rising vascular anomaly of the radial artery resulting in a superficial branch in the forearm which is more prone for unexpected intra-arterial injection.

REFERENCES

1. https://academic.oup.com/bjaed/article/10/4/381097 (internet from 30-Nov-2017).
2. Lake C. Extravasation injuries and accidental intra-arterial injection. BJA Edu. 2010;10(4):109-13.

Chapter **91**

Hanging

Manju George Elenjickal, S Sushamabai

ABSTRACT

Hanging is strangulation that involves suspension by the neck. It is mostly accidental but can be suicidal or autoerotic in adolescents. Sudden cerebral edema, ischemia and widespread hemorrhage cause early loss of consciousness and multiorgan failure. Initial assessment should be for the mental status, cardiovascular and respiratory compromise. Stabilization of the cervical spine is the first priority, followed by respiratory support (intubation and mechanical ventilation) along with cardiovascular support. Fluid and electrolyte therapy should be judicial to prevent cerebral edema and acute respiratory distress syndrome (ARDS). Multidisciplinary care involving ear-nose-throat (ENT), anesthesia, pediatric surgery, orthopedics, neuromedicine and neurosurgery should be provided. After stabilization, detailed evaluation for trauma, chest X-ray, computed tomography (CT) head and neck and other imaging studies should be carried out. Psychiatric evaluation is a must for all suspected suicidal and autoerotic hanging.

INTRODUCTION

Hanging is a form of strangulation that involves suspension by the neck.[1] It can be complete or incomplete.
- *Complete hanging*: When the whole body hangs off the ground and the entire weight of the victim is suspended at the neck
- *Incomplete hanging*: Some part of the body is touching the ground, and the weight of the victim is not fully suspended at the neck.[2]

Hanging is usually accidental in children and suicidal in adolescents but can be homicidal or autoerotic.

Significant cervical spinal cord and bone injuries occur in hanging if the victim falls from a distance greater than the person's height. Such injuries indicate bad prognosis.

PATIENT APPROACH

Stabilize the patient first.

History

- Suicidal, homicidal or accidental while playing
- Infants can be caught by the neck between crib slats, fence slats, hanging window cords or curtains.

PATHOPHYSIOLOGY

- The initial event is acute cerebral edema due to jugular venous compression followed by carotid artery compression. Consciousness is lost immediately so that the victim is unable to escape.
- Widespread ischemia and varying degrees of brain hemorrhage set in soon.
- Cardiac arrhythmias, hypotension, and respiratory compromise follow.
- Multiorgan failure sets in.

Examination—assess quickly:
- Mental status—coma level (alert/verbal/painful/unresponsive/Glasgow Coma Scale)
- Respiratory status—apneic or breathing; record pulse oximetry
- Cardiac status for hypotension, arrhythmias or asystole
- Detailed physical examination after stabilization.

MANAGEMENT

- Stabilize the cervical spine.
- Intubation and ventilation, if airway compromise. Always anticipate intubation and mechanical ventilation in an apparently stable victim with very little warning.
- Fluid resuscitation—Ringer's lactate initial bolus followed by 2/3 maintenance therapy with isotonic fluid—normal saline + KCl. Avoid overhydration to prevent brain edema and ARDS.
- Treat cardiac arrhythmias.
- Evaluate for cerebral edema and implement appropriate therapy.
- ENT, anesthesiology, general surgery, orthopedic, neurosurgery, and neuromedical consultations are a must.
- Proceed to detailed evaluation and legal intimation.

DETAILED EVALUATION

- Head-to-foot examination for abrasions, lacerations, contusions, edema over the neck, depending upon how the patient was strangled.
- Subconjunctival and skin petechiae cephalad to the site of choking (Tardieu spots).
- Severe pain on gentle palpation of the larynx indicating laryngeal damage.
- Cough, strider, and muffled voice all indicate laryngeal trauma.

INVESTIGATIONS

- Arterial blood gas analysis in all patients who require intubation, and for subsequent ventilator management.[1] Pulse oximetry is enough for those who do not require mechanical ventilation.
- Soft-tissue neck radiographs (after securing the airway first) in all victims. A fractured hyoid bone indicates severe, occult soft-tissue damage, and subsequent airway compromise, even if the patient appears stable initially.[1]
- Chest radiographs after endotracheal intubation for appropriate positioning and to assess the baseline status of the lungs since ARDS is a complication of hanging.
- Computed tomography scan of the head and neck to assess the neurological status and to detect subtle fractures and soft tissue damage of the neck.[1] Subtle injuries to the laryngeal cartilage may not be apparent on plain radiographs.[1]
- Doppler vascular imaging, CT angiography or arteriography of the carotids in garroting.[1] The thin wires or cords, used in garroting, often produce deep vascular thrombosis. Magnetic resonance imaging is preferred, if readily available.[1]

OTHER PROCEDURES

- Direct fiberoptic laryngoscopy and microlaryngoscopy by the ENT surgeon to establish the full pattern of injuries in patients without immediate risk.
- Cricothyroidotomy for patients with airway deterioration, if endotracheal intubation is unsuccessful.
- Percutaneous translaryngeal ventilation may be used to temporarily oxygenate a patient, if cricothyroidotomy fails.[3] Definitive airway management should be followed.
- Psychiatry consultation should be obtained in all cases of suicidal or autoerotic strangulation.

CONCLUSION

Hanging produces sudden cerebral edema and early loss of consciousness and multiorgan failure; pediatric intensivist should care the patient along with a multidisciplinary team.

REFERENCES

1. Ernoehazy W. Hanging injuries and strangulation. Available form http://misc.medscape.com/pi/iphone/medscapeapp/html/A826704-business.html [Accessed October 2018].
2. Muthukrishnan L, Raman R, Nagaraju K. An unusual cause of accidental hanging in a toddler. Pediatr Emerg Care. 2012;28(9):924.
3. http://ui.emedicine.com/emerg/topic227.htm (internet from 13-Feb-2006).

Chapter 92

Cold Injuries

Manju George Elenjickal, S Sushamabai

ABSTRACT

Cold injuries do occur in warm localities also. The susceptible groups are newborn babies, children with sepsis, neglected infants, adolescents undertaking sports or skiing and sick or old age people. Hypothermia indicates generalized body involvement with core temperature less than or equal to 35°C. Features are shivering, altered mentation, and cardiac arrhythmias. Localized exposure can lead to chilblain, frostbite, trench foot, etc. Severe hypothermia requires pediatric intensive care unit (PICU) care with active and passive rewarming and cardiopulmonary resuscitation (CPR). For localized lesions, slow rewarming, prazosin administration for vasodilatation, and topical steroids for itching are recommended.

INTRODUCTION

Cold injuries are not uncommon in warm regions with ambient temperature more than 20° C, but poorly perceived.

SUSCEPTIBLE GROUPS

- Extremes of age—preterms, newborns, infants, and old age people
- Those with protein–energy malnutrition, sepsis, underlying cardiac, renal, liver, metabolic diseases
- Sepsis
- Shelterless children—nomads, street children left without cloth covering during night
- Athletes participating in winter sports
- Children subjected to imaging studies [computed tomography, magnetic resonance imaging, radiological procedures, ultrasonography, echocardiography (ECHO)] or procedures in air-cooled rooms
- Adolescents involved in mountain climbing and skiing.

PATHOPHYSIOLOGY

- Ice crystals may form within or between the cold-affected cells, interfering with sodium pump or may lead to rupture of the cell membrane.

- Clumping of red blood cells or platelets leading to microembolism or thrombosis, occurs.
- Shunting of blood away from the cold-affected area follows hypothermia, thus aggravating ischemic damage to the affected cells.
- Spectrum of injury ranges from mild to severe involving skin, blood vessels and nerves.

CLINICAL PRESENTATION

It can be:
- Hypothermia
- Local tissue damage.

Hypothermia

- *Hypothermia*: It is core temperature less than 35°C with systemic features.
    - In *cold stress* (core temperature >35°C), patient reveals shivering only.
    - Mentation and functioning are normal. Treatment is *passive rewarming* as detailed below:
        - Remove the child from the cold area and change the wet clothes.
        - Provide warmth by blankets.
        - Supply calories for shivering by warm drinks.

As such cold stress is not categorized as hypothermia.
- *Mild hypothermia (35–32°C)*: Reveals shivering with lethargy fatigue, in coordination, unable for self-care.
- *Moderate hypothermia (<32–28°C)*: Shivering stops. Reveals mental confusion, irritability, and hallucination.
- *Profound hypothermia (<28°C)*: No shivering. All features of moderate hypothermia with bradycardia or cardiac arrhythmia.

Differential Diagnosis

- Child abuse
- Drug ingestion—beta-blockers
- Substance abuse
- Hypoglycemia, sepsis
- Cardiac disease or sudden cardiac arrest.

Patient Approach

- Quick history, physical examination, and parallel stabilization of airway, breathing, and circulation.
- Assess neurological disability and capillary blood sugar.
- Suspect the possibility of hypothermia from history.

- Record rectal temperature and classify the degree of hypothermia.
- Handle the child gently so as to prevent cardiac arrhythmia.
- Cardiopulmonary resuscitation as per protocol, if in cardiac arrest.
- Remove the wet or cold clothing, place in warm environment and cover with blankets.
- Children having cold stress without any underlying risk factors can be managed in the emergency room; should be observed for 4 hours and sent back.
- Those with cold stress and underlying risk factors and all grades of hypothermia require PICU care.
- While stabilizing the child, assess for trauma, sexual abuse, neurologic impairment, and cardiac decompensation.
- Passive rewarming should be provided for all patients with core temperature more than or equal to 32°C, conscious and able to drink.
- Active rewarming is advised for all with core temperature less than 32°C, those with cardiovascular instability, and other risk factors. Methods include:
  - Active external rewarming—warm bath 45–48°C, apply heat to upper torso, chest, axilla and back
  - Active internal rewarming—intravenous warm normal saline 40–42°C bolus followed by maintenance solution
  - Warm moist air or oxygen
  - Warm nasogastric and/or colonic irrigation
- Target for 0.5°C/hr rise in core temperature.
- Stop active measures once the core temperature is 35°C.
- Detect and treat underlying or aggravating factors.
- Accidental deep hypothermia with circulatory arrest—if facilities are available, try rewarming with cardiopulmonary bypass.
- Extracorporeal membrane oxygenation in resistant cases.

Investigations

- Should be streamlined according to the degree of hypothermia, associated complications, and underlying disease situation.
- All PICU-admitted children require arterial blood gas analysis (corrected for temperature), random blood sugar, serum sodium, K, Ca, P, Mg, complete blood count, renal function test, liver function test, coagulation profile, serum amylase and lipase, chest X-ray, electrocardiography (ECG), and ECHO studies.
- Additional lab tests and toxicology, if needed.

Monitoring

- Vitals, Glasgow Coma Scale, input/output chart, ECG, and core temperature hourly.

Local Tissue Damage

Exposure to Damp Cold

It can manifest as:
- Frostnip—characterized by firm, cold, white area on the face, ears or extremities leading to blisters and peeling. Management is slowly warming the area or immersion in a warm water bath.
- Immersion foot/trench foot—occurs in cold weather, affecting the feet remaining in wet, poorly ventilated boots. Manifest as cold, numb, pale, edematous painful feet, may become macerated and superinfected. Pain and hypersensitivity to temperature changes may persist. Treatment is drying the foot, gentle rewarming and nonsteroidal anti-inflammatory drugs (NSAIDs) administration.

Exposure to Dry Cold

- Frostbite—characterized by feet with cold white anesthetic and numb areas progressing to painful hemorrhagic vesicles on rewarming. Management is slow rewarming by immersing in warm water, NSAID, and prazosin for vasodilatation.
- Chilblain (Pernio) is cold injury following vasoconstriction characterized by itchy painful areas evolving into vesicles or ulcers. Areas affected are ears, tips of fingers and toes. Management is slow rewarming and topical corticosteroids for itching. If recurrence condition has to be prevented by avoiding prolonged chilling, protecting the area with gloves and stocking and prazosin administration.

CONCLUSION

Cold injuries are not uncommon in warm countries, the susceptible group being extremes of age, sick children, shelterless and neglected group and children subjected to imaging studies; appropriate preventive measures and early treatment should be implemented.

Chapter 93A

Poisoning in Children

S Sushamabai

ABSTRACT

Poisoning in children is very common and should be suspected when children are brought with unconsciousness, seizures, abnormal odor, respiratory distress or circulatory failure or if the features cannot be explainable with clinical assessment for any illness. The child should be immediately stabilized, consider gastric decontamination, maintain fluids and electrolyte homeostasis, organ support and antidote therapy, if possible. Parents should be counseled regarding prevention of poisoning in children.

GENERAL GUIDELINES

- Suspect poisoning in children brought with unusual odor, drowsiness, convulsions, respiratory distress or circulatory failure.
- All children less than 6 years with poisoning should be hospitalized for observation for minimum 24 hours.

Clues for Poisons and Drugs/Items

Clues for poisons	Drugs/Items
Ataxia	Phenytoin, phenothiazines, piperazine, Dichlorodiphenyltrichloroeethane (DDT)
Cardiac irregularities	Digoxin, beta blockers, tricyclic antidepressants, phenothiazines, theophylline
Constricted pupils	Opioids, organophosphates, barbiturates
Cyanosis	Dapsone, moth balls
Delirium	Datura, antihistamines
Dilated pupils	Datura, tricyclic antidepressants, oleander, methanol
Dry skin	Datura
Abnormal urine colour:	
Blue or green	Methylene blue poisoning
Orange	Rifampicin, Iron poisoning treated with deferoxamine
Gray/black	Phenols or cresols

PATIENT APPROACH

- *Decontamination*: Remove clothings and wash with soap and water (insecticides/corrosives).
- *Ensure airway, breathing, and circulation*:
  - Airway—clear the secretions
  - Give O_2—intubate and ventilate if needed
  - Secure intravenous (IV) access—start fluid therapy, correction of shock
  - Documentation—vitals, Glasgow Coma Scale, pupil reaction and details necessary for medicolegal procedures while eliciting the history
- *Position the child*—in left lateral decubitus
- *Identify the poison*—careful history, smell, physical examination; assess the type, amount and time of poisoning
- *Emesis*—not presently recommended
- *Gastric lavage*:
  - Useful only if done within 1 hour of poisoning, initial aspirate though retrieves only minimum amount of poison, should be sent for chemical analysis
  - Stomach wash with tap water (four to five times). Contraindicated in patients with convulsions, coma, hematemesis, and in kerosene and corrosive ingestion
- *Cathartics*—sorbitol (10%) 1 g/kg in 5 mL/kg water
- *Prevent gastrointestinal (GI) absorption*:
  - Activated charcoal—1 g/kg/dose (1 g in 8 mL water); better to drink it after adding sweetening agent. Be cautious to prevent aspiration, if given through nasogastric tube. Avoid in acid, alkali, cyanide and iron ingestion, and if there is ileus
  - Egg albumin or milk
  - Whole bowel irrigation—proven efficacy; avoid in ileus, bowel perforation, and GI obstruction.
- *Promote excretion of poison*:
  - Fluid therapy—1.5 times maintenance requirement PO/IV
  - Diuresis—furosemide or mannitol (for barbiturates)
  - Forced alkaline diuresis—useful in salicylate and barbiturate poisoning
  - Ammonium chloride to acidify urine for amphetamines
- *Use specific antidotes*
- Others
  - hemodialysis, extracorporeal membrane oxygenation (ECMO), and intralipid emulsion therapy.

COMMON POISONINGS

Hydrocarbons

Kerosene is the most common poisoning encountered in our area.
- Clues—smell of kerosene, cough, dyspnea, drowsiness, and lethargy
- Signs—ataxia, tremors, seizures, metabolic acidosis, chemical pneumonia (revealed by tachypnea, lung crackles, wheeze), acute renal failure, cardiac arrhythmia, and coma.

Lethal dose of kerosene is 30 mL; aspiration of 1 mL can cause severe chemical pneumonia.

Pathophysiology: Coughing and gagging lead to extensive aspiration into the lungs even with small quantity because of the low viscosity and high volatility of kerosene. Type II pneumatocytes are inactivated resulting in surfactant deficiency and atelectasis. Metabolic and respiratory acidosis, superadded bacterial pneumonia, cardiac arrhythmia, hepatic and renal impairment are the other problems to be anticipated.

Management (Flowchart 93A.1)

Other modalities of treatment—surfactant therapy and ECMO.

Flowchart 93A.1: Management of poisoning due to hydrocarbons.

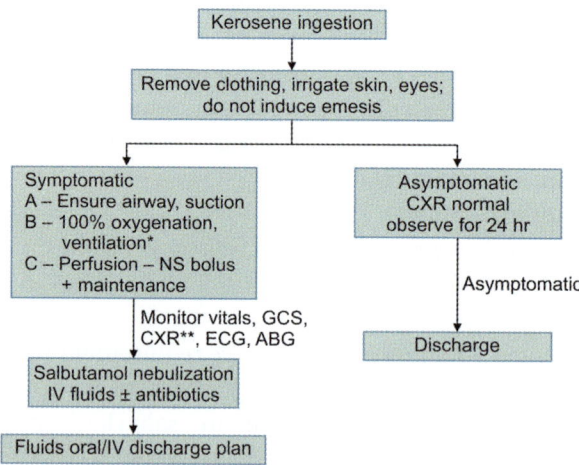

*Mechanical ventilation—If GCS < 8 or falling SpO_2
**CXR can reveal infiltrates in chemical pneumonia by 2 hr after kerosene ingestion.
(ABG, arterial blood gas; CXR, chest X-ray; ECG, electrocardiography; GCS, Glasgow Coma Scale; IV, intravenous; NS, normal saline)

Supportive Management

It is the mainstay of treatment and it includes:
- Throat suction and oxygen therapy
- Intravenous fluids
- Salbutamol nebulization
- Paracetamol
- Antibiotics if lower respiratory tract infection (high fever after 24 hours, signs of pneumonia; start empirical antibiotic therapy- ampicillin+ gentamicin +/- cloxacillin; change as per culture and sensitivity report).
- Corticosteroids if severe stridor.
- Gastric lavage with airway protection using cuffed endotracheal tube may be useful for large recent ingestion.

Cholinesterase—Inhibiting Insecticides

- Inhibit cholinesterase enzymes.
- Commonly used are organophosphates and carbamates.
- Organophosphates permanently inactivate acetyl cholinesterase.
- Carbamates form temporary bond to enzymes for 24 hours only.

Organophosphate Poisoning

Symptoms

- Muscarinic—lacrimation, salivation, bronchorrhea, diarrhea, vomiting, and pinpoint pupils
- Nicotinic—weakness, muscle cramps, fasciculation, hypertension, tachycardia, and respiratory paralysis
- Central—anxiety, restlessness, seizures, cardiac and respiratory depression, coma.

Management

The management of organophosphate poisoning is described in Flowchart 93A.2.

Flowchart 93A.2: Management of organophosphate poisoning.

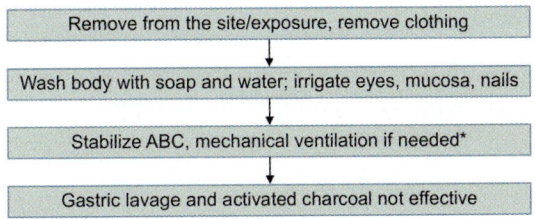

*Avoid succinylcholine, it may cause prolonged paralysis.
(ABC, airway, breathing, and circulation)

Specific Therapy

- *Atropine*:
  - 0.05–0.1 mg/kg IV, repeat q 5–10 minutes until oral and bronchial secretions become dry.
  - Decrease the frequency to q 30–60 minutes and further as per response.

  (Atropine infusion 0.02 mg/kg/hr in severe cases, maintain for 24 hours and then taper off.)
- *Pralidoxime (2-pyridine aldoxime methyl chloride)—not advised in carbamate poisoning*
  - 20–50 mg/kg IV in normal saline over 10 minutes (maximum 200 mg/min).
  - Repeat after 1 hour, if symptoms persist.
  - Repeat q 10–12 hourly for 24–48 hours until all nicotinic symptoms are ablated.

Note:
- Pralidoxime is to be given preferably within 12 hours after ingestion and is contraindicated in carbamate poisoning.
- Pupillary dilatation alone is not an indication of atropinization.
- Tachycardia is not a contraindication for atropine administration.

Supportive Therapy

- Anticonvulsants for seizure control
- Broad-spectrum antibiotics for respiratory infection
- Parenteral fluid therapy till recovery.

Monitoring

- Vitals and pupil size hourly
- Input/output chart 6 hourly
- Renal function test and serum electrolytes 12 hourly
- Chest X-ray when indicated.

CONCLUSION

Poisoning is very common in children, may lead to death, which can be prevented by timely supportive and specific therapy.

Chapter 93B

Other Poisonings: Symptomatology and Management

S Sushamabai

ABSTRACT

The part deals with the clinical manifestations and management of individual poisoning encountered in day-to-day practice; the pattern of poisons can vary in different regions.

INTRODUCTION

The symptoms, signs, and management for different poisons are described below:

Note: Supportive therapy is needed in all.

Other poisonings—Symptomatology and management.

Sr. No.	Poisons	Symptoms and signs	Management
1.	**Acetaminophen**	Stage 1 (12–24 hours): nausea, vomiting sweating, stage 2 (24–48 hours): clinical recovery: Stage 3 (72–96 hours) peak hepatotoxicity, stage 4 (7–8 days): recovery	Avoid activated charcoal, cathartics, monitor liver functions. N-acetyl cysteine 5% solution in fruit juice (O) 140 mg/kg initially then 70 mg/kg q 4 hr. In severe poisoning IV 150 mg/kg in 1 hour, then 50 mg/kg in 4 hours followed by 100 mg/kg in 16 hours in 5%D Methionine -10 mg orally in 4 div doses over 10 hours.
2.	**Acids**	Burns of mouth, esophagus, stomach	Decontaminate skin, eyes; Gastric lavage with milk using soft tube followed by antacids (aluminum hydroxide), endoscopy further procedures depending on the severity of mucosal damage

Contd...

Contd...

Sr. No.	Poisons	Symptoms and signs	Management
3.	**Alkalis** (washing soda, unslaked lime, powerful detergent granules, toilet and drain cleaners, button alkali cells)	Inability to feed, drooling, excessive crying (acute necrosis of esophagus), stridor, hoarseness, respiratory distress (aspiration), chemical burns	Hospitalize, milk or olive oil PO immediately. Gastric lavage contraindicated. Decontaminate skin, eyes, use antibiotics, steroids for 3 weeks to reduce stricture formation. Esophagoscopy by 24 hours, dilatation of strictures, reconstructive surgery.
4.	**Antihistamines** (diphenhydramine, promethazine, chlorpheniramine)	Toxicity mainly due to anticholinergic effects—cardiac arrhythmias, convulsions	As for datura, exchange blood transfusion for severe toxicity
5.	**Barbiturates**	Respiratory depression, hypotension, hypothermia, cerebral edema, coma, acute renal failure. isoelectric EEG tracings can occur	*GD, ventilatory support, volume expansion dopamine, digoxin, forced alkaline diuresis, hemodialysis/hemoperfusion
6.	**Belladona alkaloids** atropine substitutes	As in datura	As for datura
7.	**Benzyl benzoate**	Convulsions, excitement, incoordination	*GD, supportive therapy
8.	**Beta blockers**	Hypotension, bradycardia, hypoglycemia	*GD, glucagon 0.15 mg/kg bolus followed by infusion 0.05–0.15 mg/kg/hr. Fluid therapy
9.	**Calcium channel blockers**	Hypotension, hyperglycemia, hypocalcemia	Insulin 1 U/kg/bolus followed by infusion 0.5–1 U /kg/hr + Ca salts, fluid therapy
10.	**Camphor**	Nausea, vomiting, epigastric pain, muscular irritability, seizures	*GD, resin hemoperfusion, seizure control—phenobarb
11.	**Copper sulfate**	Burning pain in mouth and throat vomiting, watery/bloody diarrhea, hemolysis, anuria, jaundice collapse, convulsions	*GD water/milk /egg white PO, calcium EDTA /d –penicillamine
12.	**Carbamates**	As in organophosphates but milder and no central effects	Supportive, atropine for 6–12 hours

Contd...

Contd...

Sr. No.	Poisons	Symptoms and signs	Management
13.	Dapsone	Cyanosis (due to methemoglobinemia) unresponsive to oxygen. Pulse oximetry unreliable. Other drugs causing methemoglobinemia are nitroprusside, nitrates, chloroquine, local anesthetics.	Gastric lavage, activated charcoal, O_2, ascorbic acid 200–300 mg/day orally, methylene blue 1–2 mg/kg per dose 1% solution IV in 5–10 minutes, may be repeated. Partial exchange transfusion.
14.	Datura	Muscarinic blockade (tachycardia hot dry skin, fever, dilated pupils, urine and bowel retention, initial hypertension then hypotension), ataxia, picking or grasping movements, seizures, psychomotor agitation, hallucinations, coma, cardiovascular collapse	*GD, norepinephrine for hypotension, physostigmine 0.02 mg/kg IV slowly over 5 min, repeat q 10 minutes to maximum 2 mg
15.	Ethylene glycol (EG), and methanol	Nausea, vomiting, CNS depression inebriation, hematuria, acute renal failure. Visual loss in methanol.	Fomepizole 15 mg/kg load,10 mg/kg q 12hr × 4 doses followed by 15 mg/kg q 12 hr till EG level < 20 mg/dL. Sodium bicarbonate for acidosis, folate for methanol, pyridoxine for EG; hemodialysis
16.	Iron salts	Stage 1 (6–12 hours) nausea, vomiting, diarrhea, abdominal pain, hematemesis, melena, shock, coma; Stage 2 (12–36 hours): clinical quiescence; Stage 3 (36–48 hours): hepatic damage/failure; Stage 4: strictures of stomach, intestines; hepatic failure.	Gastric lavage with 5% sodium bicarbonate leaving 50–100 mL in stomach. Fluids and sodium bicarbonate IV. Chelation with deferoxamine 5–15 mg/kg/ hr in 5% dextrose IV, max 6 g. If vin ros color of urine persists give 90 mg/kg in 10–12 hr or till urine clears.
17.	Isoniazid	Convulsions, vomiting	IV pyridoxine 70 mg/kg, max dose 5 g (empirical). If ingested dose known, 1 gm/g INH. *GD, supportive measures, dialysis
18.	Jatropha curcas (Kadallavanakku)	Vomiting, diarrhea, dehydration dyselectrolytemia	*GD, fluid therapy.

Contd...

Contd...

Sr. No.	Poisons	Symptoms and signs	Management
19.	**Lead, Arsenic**	Anorexia, abdominal pain, vomiting constipation, anemia, abnormal behavior, muscle paresis, convulsions, coma, intellectual deterioration	*GD, laxatives, enema. 1. BAL 3–5 mg/kg/dose deep IM q 4 hr first day, further dose depends on toxin. 2. Calcium EDTA 35–50 mg/kg day IV continuous infusion or div q 12 hr. 3. DMSA (O) 10 mg/kg/dose q 8 hr × 5 days, followed by 10 mg/kg q 12 hr ×14 days. Mannitol for cerebral edema.
20.	**Naphthalene**	Nausea, vomiting, hemoglobinuria pallor, jaundice (G-6 PD deficiency), acute renal tubular necrosis	*GD, alkaline diuresis, blood transfusion
21.	**Odollam**	Vomiting, bradycardia, arrhythmia hypotension, hyperkalemia	*GD, IV fluids, atropine, insulin glucose, ECG, cardiac pacing
22.	**Oleander white, yellow**	Dysphagia, burning in throat, vomiting abdominal pain, diarrhea, varying degrees of heart block, muscle twitching, tetany, drowsiness, coma. Lockjaw in white variety.	*GD, and supportive. Two IV drips: one for fluids and lactate/bicarbonate; 2nd for 5% D with atropine 0.4 mg, adrenaline 0.5 mL1:10,000 solution and noradrenaline 0.05 mg/kg to overcome heart block, hypotension
23.	**Opioids** (opium, morphine, pentazocine, diphenoxylate, etc.)	Respiratory depression, coma constricted pupils, paralytic ileus vomiting, cyanosis, convulsions, pulmonary edema	*GD, ventilatory support, IV Naloxone 0. 01–0.1 mg/kg, repeat as needed
24.	**Organochlorines** e.g. DDT, gammexane	Nausea, vomiting, mental confusion, dizziness, muscle twitchings, tremors, convulsions, hypothermia	*GD, activated charcoal, O_2, IV fluids, seizure control. Avoid atropine—can cause arrhythmia.
25.	**Phenol**	Burns, nausea, vomiting, bloody diarrhea, convulsions, pulmonary edema, cardio-respiratory depression	Gastric lavage with vegetable oil, olive oil (O) 30 mL stat and 10 mL/hr to reduce absorption, general supportive measures
26.	**Phenothiazines** Chlorpromazine, trifluoperazine, Metaclopramide	Extrapyramidal movements, especially of tongue, neck retraction, oculogyric crisis, pinpoint pupils (large dose), hypotension, arrhythmias, generalized hypertonia, brisk jerks, coma	*GD, injection diphenhydramine 1 mg/kg/dose followed by orally x 3 days, supportive therapy

Contd...

Contd...

Sr. No.	Poisons	Symptoms and signs	Management
27.	**Plant seeds -castor**	Violent vomiting, abdominal pain bloody diarrhea	*GD, IV fluids, alkaline diuresis hemodialysis or hemoperfusion vitamin K, blood/components
28.	**Phenytoin**	Ataxia, nystagmus, drowsiness	*GD, forced alkaline diuresis, dialysis
29.	**Salicylates**	Tinnitus, fever, sweating, hyperventilation, nausea, vomiting, respiratory alkalosis then metabolic acidosis, restlessness, dehydration, hemorrhage, pulmonary edema, hepatitis	*GD, IV soda bicarb 1–2 mEq/kg bolus followed by continuous infusion to keep urine pH 7.5–8, vitamin K, ranitidine, blood transfusion, dialysis
30.	**Sulphonyl ureas**	Hypoglycemia	Octreotide 1–2 µg/kg/dose q 6-8 hours, IV glucose infusion
31.	**Tincture iodine**	Oral burns, gastric irritation	Gastric lavage with soluble starch solution. Leave 1–5% sodium thiosulfate solution in stomach. Steroids to prevent esophageal stenosis.
32.	**Tricyclic antidepressants**	Features of Datura poisoning, dysrhythmias, hypotension, lethargy, coma, seizures	*GD, ABC stabilization, early airway management, mechanical ventilation, dopamine, seizure control
33.	**Zinc/aluminum phosphide rat poison**	Nausea, vomiting, abdominal pain, hypotension, peripheral circulatory failure, early and high mortality	0.15% copper sulfate solution 200 mL orally followed by gastric lavage. Supportive measures
34.	**Warfarin** (Rat poison)	Abdominal pain, vomiting respiratory distress, hypotension	Monitor coagulation profile, RFT, LFT, saline gastric lavage, vitamin K for bleeding, FFP

(*GD, gastric decontamination)

CONCLUSION

Systematic Approach with general supportive measures and specific antidote therapy are advised for individual poisoning.

Chapter **94A**

Snake Envenomation

S Sushamabai

ABSTRACT

Snake envenomation is the leading environmental hazard observed worldwide and children are at increased risk for mortality due to the relatively higher venom concentration in blood. Clinical presentation can be history of bite, swelling around the bite area, bleeding tendency, altered sensorium, myasthenic paralysis, and multiorgan failure. Grade I (mild) envenomation reveals local changes at the bite area only and normal laboratory values. In grade II (moderate), envenomation, progression of local changes and systemic manifestations occur. Grade III (severe) envenomation is characterized by severe systemic manifestations and multiorgan failure. Antisnake venom (ASV) is the specific drug and should be administered for all patients with grade II and III envenomations at the earliest. For those with grade I categorization, only wound care is needed. Supportive therapy is equally important as specific therapy. Intravenous immunoglobulin (IVIg) is advised in severe envenomation.

INTRODUCTION

Snake envenomation (Sn En) is the greatest environmental hazard in the developing countries but poorly perceived by the public and health authorities. Mortality exceeds death from all the natural calamities worldwide.

VENOMOUS SNAKES OF KERALA

Viper, cobra, krait, and sea snakes.

All medical professionals must know the local types of snakes and their venomous effects.

PATHOPHYSIOLOGY

- Snake venom is a mixture of neurotoxins, cytolysins, anticoagulants, hyaluronidase, cardiotoxins, and histamine. Depending on the type of snakes and their age, the composition and the concentration of toxins differ.
- Viper venom is predominantly hemorrhagic, nephrotoxic, and cardiotoxic. Death is due to early hemorrhage, renal failure, and myocardial damage.
- Cobra venom has neurotoxic, cardiotoxic, and nephrotoxic effects. Death is due to respiratory and myocardial failure.
- Krait venom is mainly neurotoxic; bite is usually painless and presents as gradual onset of creeping myasthenic paralysis and respiratory failure.
- Sea snakes have myotoxins mainly, bites are painless, present as excruciating muscle pain and end up in respiratory impairment and renal failure.

PATIENT APPROACH

Step I

Admit in pediatric intensive care unit; *establish* the diagnosis; *stabilize* airway, breathing and circulation; consider *parallel screening* investigations.

Three groups of patients are encountered following snakebite:
1. Brought with history of alleged snakebite
2. No history of bite, but brought with unusual manifestations
3. History of bite ± snake observed/brought.

Detailed history and examination after stabilization—ask and look for:
- Time of occurrence, local pain, bleeding, edema, necrosis, and treatment given
- Vitals, fluid intake, and output status
- Tender regional lymphadenopathy
- Head-to-foot examination including the pulsations of affected area
- Clinical grading as in Flowchart 94A.1.

Early screening investigations (within 30 min of bite) suggestive of envenomation:
- White blood cell (WBC) more than 20,000/mm^3—all snakes
- Microscopic hematuria -RBCs >20/hpf—viper, cobra
- Decreased cholesterol—cobra and krait.

Flowchart 94A.1: Clinical presentation of snake envenomation.

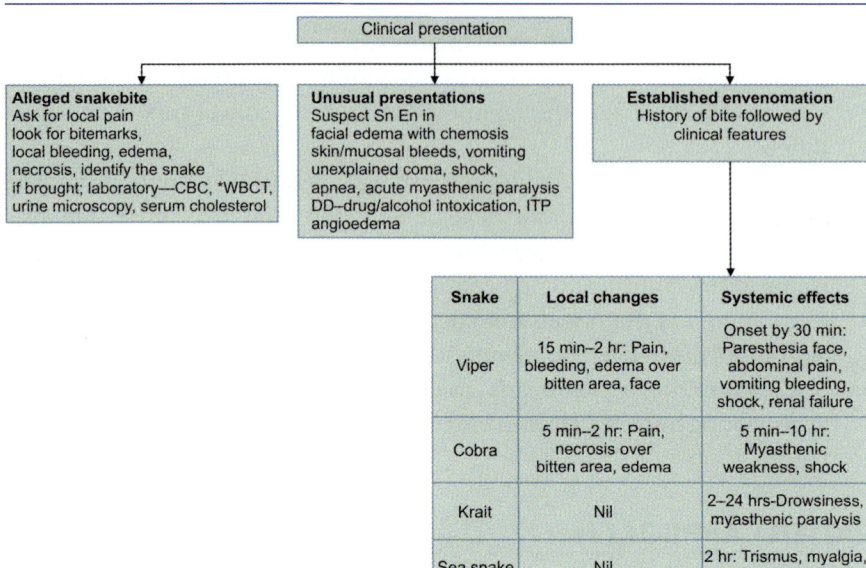

WBCT—Collect 2 mL blood in a clean glass tube. Keep it undisturbed for 20 min and then tilt the tube. If no clot, WBCT is prolonged. The same sample can be used for clot retraction†
†For clot retraction, see footnote ** in Flowchart 94A.2.
(CBC, complete blood count; DD, differential diagnoses; ITP, idiopathic thrombocytopenic purpura; WBCT, whole blood clotting time; Sn En, snake envenomation)

PREHOSPITAL MANAGEMENT

- All bites do not produce envenomation—90% snakes are nonpoisonous, only 50% poisonous snakebites have envenomation. Hence, only 5% of all bites result in envenomation.
- Calm the victim. Allow the limb to rest. Immobilize the limb by crepe bandage—apply it just tight to admit one finger between the limb and the bandage. Keep the limb in level with the heart. Remove the bandage only after starting antisnake venom (ASV) administration.
- Transport the patient to the hospital at the earliest.
- Encourage the patient to drink water so as to facilitate venom excretion.
- Do not manipulate the bitten area.

Step II

Management in the hospital (Flowchart 94A.2).

Step III

Detect and correct complications (Flowchart 94A.3).

Chapter 94A: Snake Envenomation

Flowchart 94A.2: Management of snake envenomation in the hospital.

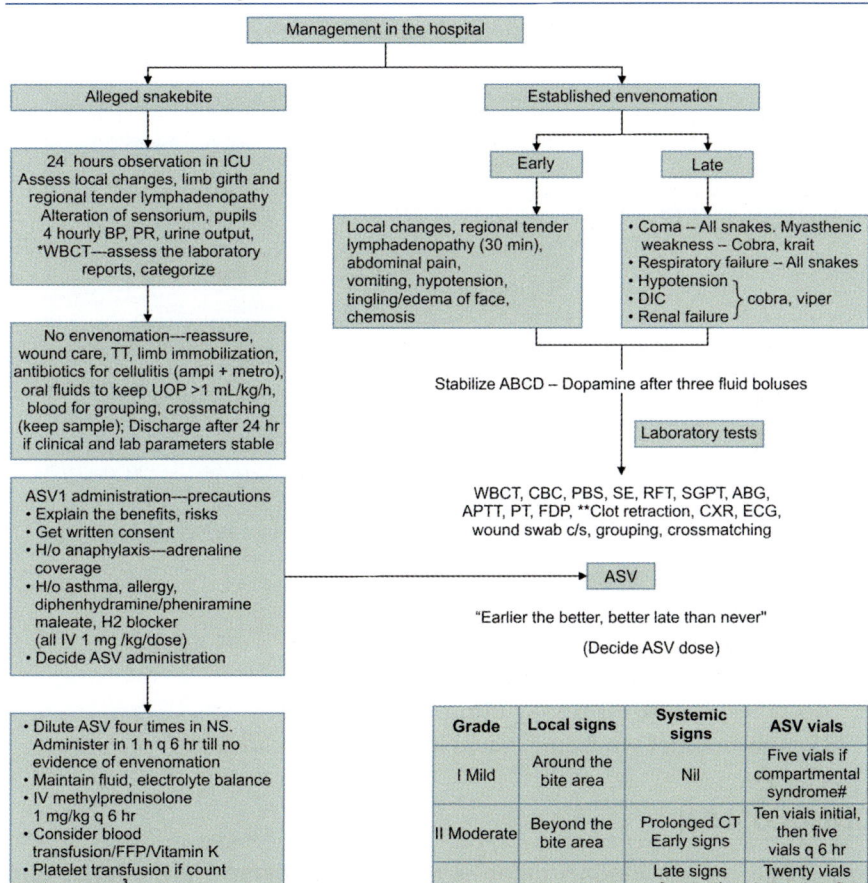

*WBCT - Whole Blood Clotting Time-refer Flowchart 94.A1 for description given as footnote.
**Clot retraction starts 2 hrs after clot formation and completes by 6 hrs. The sample collected for WBCT can be used for this test. See footnote 94.1A.
Consider IVIg 2 gm/kg in 12 hrs in severe cases
Doppler studies to detect vessel wall occlusion.

SUPPORTIVE THERAPY

- Fluid and electrolyte therapy—correction of dehydration and maintenance therapy
- Antibiotics for wound infection—ampicillin + metronidazole
- Paracetamol for pain.

COMPLICATIONS

- Shock and multiorgan failure
- Bleeding and intracranial hemorrhage

Flowchart 94A.3: Management of snake envenomation with complications.

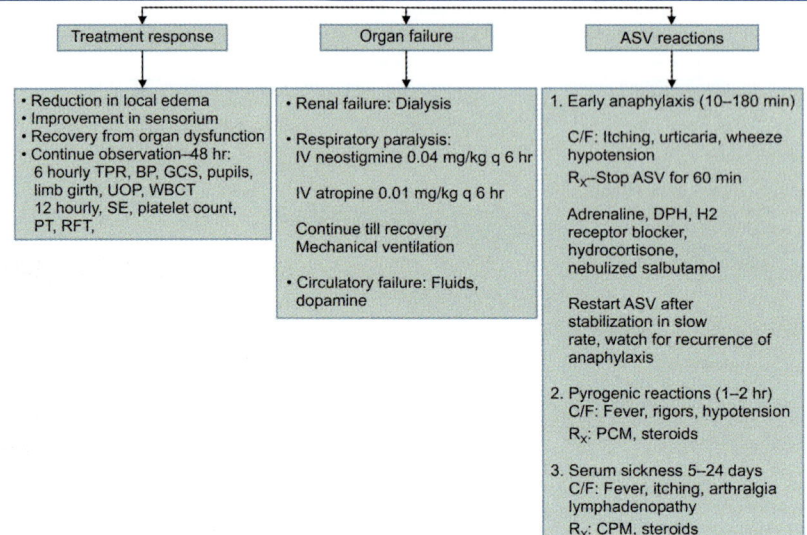

(PCM, paracetamol; CPM, chlorpheniramine maleate).

- Hemolysis
- Disseminated intravascular coagulation
- Acute respiratory distress syndrome
- Compartmental syndrome, necrosis of the bitten area.

CONCLUSION

Anti-snake venom administration is the specific therapy in moderate and severe envenomation, but supportive therapy is equally important.

Chapter **94B**

Scorpion Envenomation

S Letha, S Sushamabai

ABSTRACT

Scorpion envenomation (Sc En) is an acute life-threatening medical emergency. Early diagnosis and appropriate therapy will prevent fatality. The clinical features are early phase of cholinergic storm, late phase of adrenergic stimulation, and in some groups, central nervous system (CNS) manifestations (roving eye movements, cranial nerve palsy, opisthotonos, and emprosthotonos). Pharmacological antidote is prazosin, to be administered within 2 hours followed by nifedipine if hypertension is not controlled. For pain, paracetamol or ibuprofen is advised; morphine is contraindicated. Intensive supportive therapy for fluid and electrolyte maintenance, cardiac and respiratory decompensation, seizures and insulin for hyperglycemia are discussed. Scorpion antivenom if available should be administered in the first hour of therapy.

INTRODUCTION

Scorpion envenomation is an acute life-threatening medical emergency, the fatality rate being 3–22% in India. Stings are often due to accidental contact and usually occur at night. Most stings are not associated with envenomation; severe and fatal envenomation occurs in a few only. Early diagnosis and appropriate management are crucial in lifesaving.

PATHOPHYSIOLOGY

- The poisonous strains in India are the Indian red and the Asian black scorpions.
- Scorpion venom is a complex mixture of mucopolysaccharides, hyaluronidase, phospholipase, acetylcholine esterase, serotonin, histamine, protease inhibitors, histamine releasers, and neurotoxins.
- The net effects of the venom components are:
  - *Neurotoxic* due to direct effect and acetylcholine release
  - *Cardiovascular compromise* due to catecholamine release

– *Autonomic storm, free radical release, and inflammation* leading to myocardial ischemia, pancreatitis, pulmonary edema and insulin suppression, and subsequent hyperglycemia.

CLINICAL PRESENTATION

Note: History of bite may not be obtained.
- Local symptoms vary from screaming due to severe pain, swelling, erythema, edema and necrosis to nil.
- Poisonous stings may become painful after starting treatment due to vasodilatation that relieves ischemia. Painful stings are less poisonous.

SYSTEMIC SYMPTOMS

- *Early phase of cholinergic stimulation*:
  - Starts within 1–2 hours after sting; earlier in infants. Features are vomiting, salivation, sweating, priapism, hypotension, bradycardia, and ventricular premature contractions.
  - Sweating and salivation can last up to 13 hours.
  - Respiratory compromise aggravates due to oral secretions and bronchorrhea.
- *Late phase of adrenergic stimulation*:
  - Starts within 4 hours after sting, can persist for 24–72 hours.
  - Features are tachycardia, hypertension, rhythm disturbances, and left ventricular failure. Prolonged sympathetic stimulation with cold extremities, shock, pulmonary edema, suppression of insulin secretion, and hyperglycemia can be present.
  - Central nervous system manifestations are less common in Indian scorpion stings. They are cranial nerve dysfunctions, roving eye movements, seizures, opisthotonos, emprosthotonos (forward spasm with approximation of face to toes) and encephalopathy.

DIFFERENTIAL DIAGNOSIS

- Organophosphate and methamphetamine poisoning. The differentiating feature is the characteristic roving eye movements in Sc En.
- Acute encephalitic syndrome the differentiating points are sudden stormy onset without constitutional symptoms in scorpion envenomation.

PATIENT APPROACH

- Admit in pediatric intensive care unit; stabilize airway, breathing, and circulation; assess dextrose concentration and make appropriate correction. Consider the following investigations as per clinical situation:

- Complete blood count, random blood sugar (RBS), serum electrolytes, renal function test (RFT), liver function test, creatine phosphokinase, serum glutamic oxaloacetic transaminase, and chest X-ray (to detect pulmonary edema).
- Electrocardiography (changes are peaked T waves in V2–V6), ST elevation in L1, aVL, increased qR duration, and left ventricular hypertrophy by voltage criteria. Low-voltage complexes and left anterior hemiblock indicate poor prognosis.
- Echocardiography—to detect left ventricular systolic dysfunction.

MANAGEMENT

Supportive Therapy

- *Local*—immobilize the limb. Paracetamol/ibuprofen to relieve pain orally or through rectal/nasogastric tube if vomiting
- Oral suction to relieve secretions
- Consider intubation and mechanical ventilation if in respiratory compromise or shock
- *Avoid morphine* since it can aggravate symptoms by histamine release
- *Tetanus toxoid* as per vaccination status
- *Fluid and electrolyte balance* as per cardiopulmonary status. If in shock, provide volume resuscitation with normal saline 10–20 mL/kg in 1 hour followed by maintenance fluid. Consider dopamine or dobutamine infusion (5–15 µg/kg/min) in fluid refractory shock, along with maintenance fluid
- *Pharmacological antidote*:
    - Early administration of prazosin PO/intravenous (IV) (30 µg/kg/dose) competitive postsynaptic alpha 1 adrenoreceptor antagonist is the first-line management for vasoconstriction, hypertension, and tachycardia
    - It increases insulin secretion and also reduces CNS manifestations. Repeat the dose after 3 hours as per clinical response and then every 6 hours, till the extremities are warm and blood pressure is steady. No more than four doses are required.
    - Additional doses of *nifedipine* may be given orally/sublingually *for persistent hypertension.*
    - *Pulmonary edema*:
        - Afterload reduction with dopamine infusion, vasodilatation with sodium nitroprusside (0.4–5 µg/kg/min) or nitroglycerine (1–20 µg/kg/min) as IV infusion.
        - Isosorbide nitrate sublingually 10 mg q 10 minutes can be used as an emergency measure.
        - Intravenous furosemide and aminophylline are the other measures.

- Correction of hyperglycemia with insulin
- Detection and correction of other electrolyte imbalances (refer to respective chapters)
- Intravenous diazepam infusion to counteract pain, irritability and seizures.

Specific Therapy

Scorpion Antivenom

General or species specific should be administered in the initial 1 hour of injury if available. Dose and administration should be as per manufacturer's guidelines.

MONITORING

- Needed for initial 24 hours. To be continued if cardiorespiratory complications or encephalopathy. Most cases recover before 24 hours.
- Should be ideally continuous noninvasive monitoring of vitals, 2–4 hourly intake output, 6 hourly serum electrolyte estimation, and 12 hourly RFT.

POOR PROGNOSTIC INDICATORS

- Delay in initiation of prazosin therapy
- Pulmonary edema, cardiac arrhythmia, myocardial ischemia, and encephalopathy.

CONCLUSION

Scorpion envenomation can present with cholinergic or adrenergic storm or with combined picture; intensive organ supportive therapy is lifesaving.

Chapter 94C

Bee and Wasp Stinging

S Letha, S Sushamabai

ABSTRACT

Wasp and bee stings are commonly encountered. Mostly they produce trivial manifestations but multiple stings (>10) and anaphylaxis can end up fatally. The chapter deals with the pathogenesis, clinical presentation, and management. Treatment for trivial local reactions includes removal of the stingers by scraping, cold compresses over the area, paracetamol for pain, and oral antihistamine. In extensive cutaneous reactions, intramuscular (IM) antihistamine and oral steroids are advised. Anaphylaxis and multi organ dysfunction syndrome (MODS) are to be anticipated and treated accordingly. Late reactions seen are serum sickness, vasculitis, neuritis, encephalopathy, and nephrotic syndrome.

INTRODUCTION

Bees and wasps are insects of the hymenoptera group. Clinical manifestations of their stinging range from mild local reactions to rarely fatal systemic anaphylaxis.

PATHOGENESIS

The components of the venoms are almost common. They include:
- Vasoactive substances—histamine, acetylcholine, and kinins.
- Enzymes—phospholipase, hyaluronidase.
- Apamin and formic acid.
- Melittin—seen in bee venom (50%) is directly cytopathic and nephrotoxic.
- Antigen 5—seen in wasp venom, exact role is not clear.
- Local skin reactions are caused by vasoactive or irritant materials from the insect saliva.
- Systemic reactions are immunoglobulin E-mediated sensitivity to venom antigens and occur if there are more than 10 stinging.

CLINICAL PRESENTATION

History of stinging is usually present.
a. *Local*:
   - Limited swelling and pain, lasts less than 24 hours.
   - Large local—extensive swelling more than 10 cm contiguous with the sting area, develops over hours and days, may last for days.
b. *Generalized cutaneous reactions*:
   - Urticaria, angioedema, and pruritus beyond the site of sting.
c. *Systemic reactions*:
   - As in anaphylaxis: Include urticaria, laryngeal edema, bronchospasm and hypotension. Can occur within 1 hour of stinging.
d. *Toxic reactions*:
   - Fever, malaise, emesis, nausea, acute kidney injury, MODS, rhabdomyolysis, hemolysis; occur in multiple stinging due to direct toxic effect of the venom.
e. *Late reactions*:
   - Serum sickness, nephrotic syndrome, vasculitis, neuritis, and encephalopathy.

DIAGNOSIS

From the history and observing local and systemic manifestations.

INVESTIGATIONS

- Complete blood count, urine routine, renal function test (RFT), liver function test, random blood sugar, and serum electrolytes.
- Others depending on the severity of envenomation.

PATIENT APPROACH AND TREATMENT

Depends on the clinical presentation.
a. *Local*:
- Cold compress, topical agents to reduce itching
- Antihistamines (hydroxyzine), oral analgesics (paracetamol/ibuprofen)
- Stingers should be removed by scraping promptly, should not be squeezed out since the process can release excess venom.
   - *Large local*: Add oral steroids—prednisolone 1 mg/kg/day for 5 days to the above regimen.

Groups (a) and (b) require outpatients care only; (c), (d) and (e) require PICU care.

b. *Generalized cutaneous reaction*:
- Administer epinephrine (1:1,000) 0.01 mg/kg up to 0.5 mg IM to the above regimen (a) and (b).
- Observe for 24 hours for systemic reactions.
- Categorize to group (d) if systemic reactions.

c. *Systemic reactions*—management as in anaphylaxis

d. Management as per organ involvement.

Note: Immunotherapy for hymenoptera venom is available in rare centers.

MONITORING

- Pediatric intensive care unit care for groups (c) to (e) till stable
- Continuous monitoring of vitals and SpO_2 till stable for 24 hours
- Six hourly intake/output chart
- Daily RFT
- Others as per clinical situation.

Follow-up evaluation is needed to exclude nephrotic syndrome.

CONCLUSION

Bee and wasp stings usually produce trivial symptoms but occasionally may end up in anaphylaxis and MODS.

Chapter 95

Rat-bite Fever

S Sushamabai

ABSTRACT

Rat-bite fever is a serious febrile illness caused by *Streptobacillus moniliformis* and *Spirillum minus*. Clinical features are biphasic high fever, headache, vomiting, myalgia, arthritis and polymorphic (including hemorrhagic) rashes. Diagnosis is essentially clinical. Polymerase chain reaction (PCR) test is available for diagnosing *S. moniliformis*. The drug of choice is intravenous (IV) penicillin G × 7 days (plus gentamicin in endocarditis) followed by oral penicillin × 7 days. Alternative ones are doxycycline/gentamicin/streptomycin in penicillin allergic patients.

INTRODUCTION

Rat-bite fever is a febrile emergency with high mortality rate. The illness is poorly perceived since the incidence of rat bite would have been forgotten by the time the clinical manifestations appear.

PATHOPHYSIOLOGY

- The causative organisms are *Streptobacillus moniliformis* and *Spirillum minus*, the latter fever is known as sodoku.
- Infection is caused by the bite/scratch of the rat, handling dead rats or drinking milk contaminated with the bacteria.
- The incubation period is from 3 to 10 days for *S. moniliformis* and 14 to 21 days for *S. minus*.

CLINICAL PRESENTATION

- High fever (105.8°F), chills, intense headache, myalgia and vomiting. May reveal biphasic pattern.
- Polymorphous rash revealing maculopapular to petechial lesions and tender hemorrhagic bullae over hands and feet.
- Migratory polyarthritis.

- Suppurative non-healing ulcer over the bite area is the hallmark of *S. minus* disease.
- Complications encountered are brain and soft-tissue abscesses, myocarditis, endocarditis, persistent arthritis, and pneumonia.

DIFFERENTIAL DIAGNOSIS

- Dengue and other hemorrhagic viral fevers
- Meningitis
- Leptospirosis
- Juvenile idiopathic arthritis
- Pyoderma with sepsis.

PATIENT APPROACH

- Have a strong index suspicion of rat-bite fever as a differential diagnosis, in fever with rashes and migrating poly arthritis.
- History of rat bite has to be elicited in any patient with high fever.
- PCR test in blood or joint fluid is diagnostic for *S. moniliformis*.
- For *S. minus* infection, there are no confirmative diagnostic tests.

TREATMENT

- Drug of choice is penicillin G IV for 5–7 days followed by oral penicillin × 7 days more. High-dose penicillin G × 4 weeks + gentamicin/streptomycin is advised in endocarditis.
- Doxycycline, gentamicin or streptomycin are the alternatives for penicillin allergic patients.
- Fluid and electrolyte therapy.
- Drainage of abscesses.
- Paracetamol for pain and fever.

CONCLUSION

The possibility of rat-bite fever should be considered and investigated in children presenting with hemorrhagic fever; history of rat bite in the recent past is to be enquired.

Section 14

NEONATOLOGY

Chapter 96

Handwashing and Sepsis Prevention

Jacob Abraham, S Sushamabai

ABSTRACT

Handwashing is the cheap and most effective method to prevent sepsis. Both hands should be washed with soap and water for 2 minutes in six steps, each step requiring 20 seconds before and after touching each baby. Use clean and plain water and nonmedicated soap. The order is palms and fingers, dorsal aspect of palms, fingers, thumb, finger tips, wrists, and elbows. Dry the hands with sterile napkin. Rinsing with alcohol is not a substitute for the initial handwashing.

POINTS TO BE OBSERVED IN HANDWASHING

Handwashing is the cheap and effective method of sepsis prevention.
- Use an elbow-operated tap so that the tap is not touched after washing.
  - Washing the hands thoroughly for two minutes in six steps should be insisted as a standard practice in all neonatal units.[1] 20 seconds should be devoted for each step.
  - Both hands should washed before and after touching each baby.
- The staff caring the neonates should maintain their nails clean; long and polished are not allowed.
- Open the tap with hand or elbow.
- Clean and plain water without any added chemicals is advised for handwashing; first wet the hands up to forearm and then apply a nonmedicated soap; wash both hands as detailed below:[2]
  Six steps for effective handwashing (Fig. 96.1):
  1. Palms, fingers, and web spaces
  2. Dorsal aspect of hands
  3. Fingers along with their joints
  4. The first finger or thumb
  5. The tapering end of fingers
  6. From the wrists high up to the elbow.
- Keep elbows always dependent.[3]
- Do not close the tap with hand; close it with the elbow only.[3]

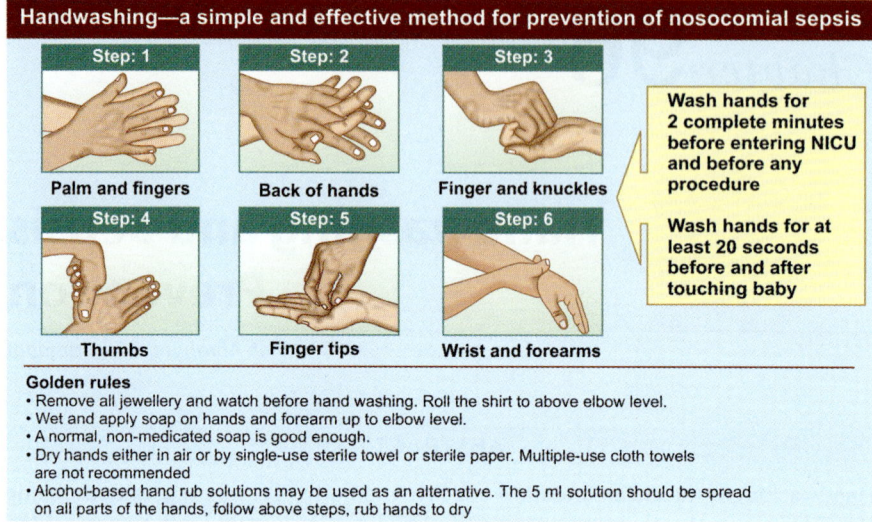

Fig. 96.1: Six steps in handwashing.
Courtesy: Division of Neonatology, Department of Pediatrics, AIIMS, New Delhi.[2]

- The hands should be dried with single-use sterile napkin; sterilized paper is an effective substitute.[3]
- Discard napkin or the paper in the bin kept for the purpose.
- After washing the hands, do not touch pen, door handles, telephones, etc. till the required job is over.
- Rinsing hands with alcohol is not a substitute for the initial handwashing.[2]
- Alcohol (isopropyl alcohol, ethanol, chlorhexidine diacetate) containing cleaning agents can be considered in postnatal wards for the routine ward rounds of apparently normal babies. Use 5 mL solution, apply on both hands and proceed with the same sequence of handwashing.

CONCLUSION

Handwashing with soap and water in six steps is the most effective and cheap method to prevent sepsis. In routine ward rounds of apparently normal babies, alcohol containing cleaning agents can be used in the same sequence of handwashing.

REFERENCES

1. http://www.newbornwhocc.org/pdf/module8_infection_prevention_WD.pdf (Internet 23-Feb-2015).
2. http://www.phishare.org/files/2584_Learners_Guide_Essential_Newborn_Nursing__India.pdf (Internet 21-Dec-2009).
3. http://www.authorsream.com/Presentation/Riccardino-41318-Neonatal-Sepsis3-SEPSIS-Etiology-Education- ppt-powerpoint/(Internet 18-Apr-2016).

Chapter 97

Care of the Normal Newborn

Jacob Abraham, S Sushamabai

ABSTRACT

Normal newborn needs extra care to maintain adequate oxygenation, body temperature, nutrition and to prevent infections. Congenital anomalies are to be picked up at the earliest and solved. Equipment needed for routine care and resuscitation are to be kept ready in the baby care area, easily approachable. Observe sterile precautions in handling the baby, keep warm, care the umbilical cord, practice early and exclusive breastfeeding, administer vitamin K and vaccines as per National schedule.

BASIC PRINCIPLES

- Ensure adequate oxygenation through clear airways
- Prevent hypothermia
- Encourage early breastfeeding
- Prevent neonatal infection
- Identify the newborns with problems at the earliest
- Provide good lighting, cleanliness, and ventilation of the room
- Keep the room adequately warm
- Equipment needed for routine care should be kept ready always in an approachable area
- Equipment for neonatal resuscitation be checked daily, maintained sterile and kept ready in the unit
- Ensure five cleans.

CARE IN THE DELIVERY ROOM

- Observe handwashing.
- Dry the baby completely, keep under warmer, and wrap in a prewarmed sterile sheet.
- Resuscitate (if needed) as per neonatal resuscitation program (NRP) guidelines.
- Cut the cord at 3–4 cm away from skin after applying plastic sterile clamp.

- Assign sex, weigh the baby, give injection vitamin K 1 mg intramuscular (IM).
- Put identification tag and check with mother's tag.

EXAMINE

- From head to toe including palate
- Look for congenital anomalies
- Palpate both femoral pulses
- Umbilical cord vessels—should be two arteries and one vein
- Back of the baby for tuft of hair, swelling, pilonidal sinus
- Orifices—ears, nares (for choanal atresia), and mouth (for esophageal atresia)
- Placenta in high-risk mothers.

INITIATE BREASTFEEDING

Within 30 minutes of normal delivery, within 2 hours in lower segment caesarean section.

POSTNATAL CARE

- Keep mother and baby together (bedding in); keep the baby warm by covering head, body and feet with clean clothes.
- Feed the baby on demand; ensure proper position and latching.
- Provide support and advice to the mother for breastfeeding.

CARE OF THE CORD

- Do not apply anything over the cord; let the cord remain open to dry.
- Watch daily for umbilical discharge, redness, or induration around.

EYE CARE

- No special care needed.
- Use gentamicin/tobramycin eye drops, if any discharge, after sending swab for culture and sensitivity.
- Explain nasolacrimal duct massage.

SKIN CARE

- Do not remove vernix caseosa.
- No baby bath immediately after birth.
- Examine daily for superficial skin infections.
- Look for danger signs daily.

PREVENTION OF INFECTION

- Avoid excess handling and visitors.
- Administer scheduled vaccines—BCG, oral polio, and hepatitis B before discharge.
- Advice the mother regarding exclusive breastfeeding for 6 months and to avoid bottle feeding.

CONCLUSION

Normal newborn requires extra care to establish respiration, maintain body warmth, early and exclusive breastfeeding, and prevention of infection by careful handling and timely vaccines.

Chapter 98

Danger Signs in the Newborn

Jacob Abraham, S Sushamabai

ABSTRACT

Danger signs in newborns indicate serious illness. They are many and should be carefully evaluated.

Danger signs herald the possibility of serious illness; they are:
- Birth weight less than 1,800 g, gestation less than 34 weeks
- Asphyxia—APGAR 0–3 at 1 minute
- Urine not passed for 48 hours
- Delayed passage of meconium more than 24 hours
- Inability to suck and swallow
- Reduced activity/inconsolable cry/convulsion
- Change in color—pale, blue, yellow
- Rapid breathing more than 60/min
- Chest in drawing and apnea
- Persistent or bilious vomiting and diarrhea
- Abdominal distension
- Bleeding from any site
- Foul smelling umbilical discharge
- Premature rupture of membranes more than 24 hours
- Suspected intrauterine infections
- Inability to pass a catheter to stomach or through anal opening
- Hypothermia and hypoglycemia
- Other situations to worry about the baby.

CONCLUSION

Danger signs should be picked up in newborns since they herald serious illness.

Chapter **99**

Neonatal Hypothermia

Jacob Abraham, S Sushamabai

ABSTRACT

Hypothermia, defined as axillary temperature less than 36.5°C, is the leading cause of death in newborns. Clinical grading is mild, moderate, and severe. Features are lethargy, poor feeding, abdominal distension, bleeding, oliguria, hypotension, respiratory distress, and bradycardia. Babies should be investigated to exclude sepsis, hypoglycemia, inborn errors of metabolism, and cyanotic congenital heart disease. Treatment includes removing the baby to warm environment, kangaroo mother care, warm clothing, keeping under radiant warmer, vitamin K injection, and feeding. In severe hypothermia oxygen, IV fluids for maintenance and to prevent hypoglycemia, empirical antibiotics against sepsis are needed. Simple measures to prevent hypothermia should be implemented in all newborns.

INTRODUCTION

Hypothermia is defined as axillary temperature <36.5°C. It is the leading cause of neonatal death.

GRADING

- Mild (cold stress): 36–36.4°C
- Moderate: 32–35.9°C
- Severe: Less than 32°C.

PATHOPHYSIOLOGY

- Hypothermia causes peripheral and pulmonary vasoconstriction, hypoxia, anaerobic metabolism, acidosis, and organ dysfunction. Predisposing factors are prematurity and low birth weight.

CLINICAL PRESENTATION

Restlessness, lethargy, poor feeding, vomiting, abdominal distension, bleeding tendency, and oliguria. Signs are cold extremities, acrocyanosis, delayed capillary refill, bradycardia, hypotension, pulmonary hypertension, and respiratory distress.

Investigations—select as per clinical situation:
- Complete blood count, peripheral blood smear (PBS), sepsis screen, C-reactive protein, and coagulation profile
- Culture—blood, pus, urine, stools, and cerebrospinal fluid
- Serum electrolytes, renal function test, plasma glucose (PG), plasma ammonia, and arterial blood gas
- Ultrasonography abdomen, electrocardiography, and echocardiography studies.

DIFFERENTIAL DIAGNOSIS

- Sepsis
- Hypoglycemia
- Congenital heart disease
- Inborn errors of metabolism.

MANAGEMENT

Warming

- Remove the baby from the source of hypothermia (cold room, cold clothes, wet nappy, cold air, etc.).
- Provide warm room, warm clothes and warm bed.

Mild and Moderate Hypothermia

- Kangaroo mother care and frequent feeding
- Monitor temperature rise (should be 0.5°C/hr) every 2 hourly. Once steady monitor 3 hourly × 12 hr.
- Rule out sepsis if inadequate response.

Severe Hypothermia

- Remove the baby from the source of hypothermia.
- Provide warm clothes and warm bed.
- Keep under preheated radiant warmer/thermostatically controlled heated mattress set at 37–38°C/room heater/200 W bulb (select any one as per situation).

- Measure body temperature every hour (should be 0.5°C/hr rise), then 2 hourly till body temperature is normal and then 3 hourly × 12 hr.
- Once the body temperature is 34°C, slow down the rewarming process.
- Continue routine care as for mild and moderate hypothermia.

SUPPORTIVE MEASURES

- Oxygen
- Fluid therapy—saline bolus followed by maintenance fluids
- Assess blood sugar, give correction if PG is less than 45 mg/dL
- Empirical antibiotics for sepsis pending investigations
- Vitamin K 1 mg intramuscular
- Others as per situation.

PREVENTION

- Warm delivery room and others as in Chapter 97.
- Anticipate hypothermia in low-birth-weight and sick babies.
- Keep baby double clothed with head caps, mittens and socks.
- Keep close to the mother.
- Early and frequent breastfeeding.
- Prevention of sepsis.

CONCLUSION

Hypothermia is a leading cause of neonatal death and should be detected and treated at the earliest. Simple measures are effective to prevent hypothermia and should be implemented in all newborns.

Chapter 100

Neonatal Resuscitation

Ingale Vinod C, Mathew Varghese, Jacob Abraham

ABSTRACT

Resuscitation of the neonate is to be anticipated in all deliveries and be prepared to meet the emergency at any time. Skilled persons (2 in number) should reach the delivery area at least 15 minutes prior to delivery and study the patient details. The resuscitation corner, the equipment, and the drugs needed should be checked. The resuscitation process should be as per guidelines of the country. Term, crying babies with good activity require routine care only. If anyone parameter is absent, dry the baby, keep warm, open the airway and stimulate. If heart rate (HR) is less than 100/min and has respiratory impairment, give positive pressure ventilation (PPV) and chest compression and proceed to intubation. If only labored breathing, administer continuous positive airway pressure (CPAP). Babies with HR less than 60/min, require PPV and chest compression. IV epinephrine, proper fluid therapy, and other supportive measures are needed. Post-resuscitation care should be provided to all such babies.

INTRODUCTION

Five to ten percent of newborns need resuscitation, but this emergency should be anticipated in all deliveries.

PERSONNEL

- One person skilled in initiating neonatal resuscitation for each baby should be present at every delivery.
- An additional skilled person capable of performing a complete resuscitation is desirable.
- Should reach 15 minutes prior to the delivery and assess the clinical details.
- Check the equipment and set the resuscitation area ready.

Chapter 100: Neonatal Resuscitation

EQUIPMENT CHECKLIST

- Warmer or table with a spot light (100 W bulb) 2 ft above, focused on the table.
- Suction equipment *(any one of the following)*:
  - Bulb syringe
  - Mechanical suction catheters 5 or 6 F, 10 or 12 F
  - Meconium aspiration device
  - Feeding tube 6 F and 20 mL syringe
- Bag and mask equipment:
  - Neonatal resuscitation bags (for term and preterm)
  - Face mask for term and preterm
  - Oxygen with flow meter (flow rate up to 10 L/min, tubing and portable oxygen cylinders)

Flowchart 100.1: Neonatal resuscitation algorithm.

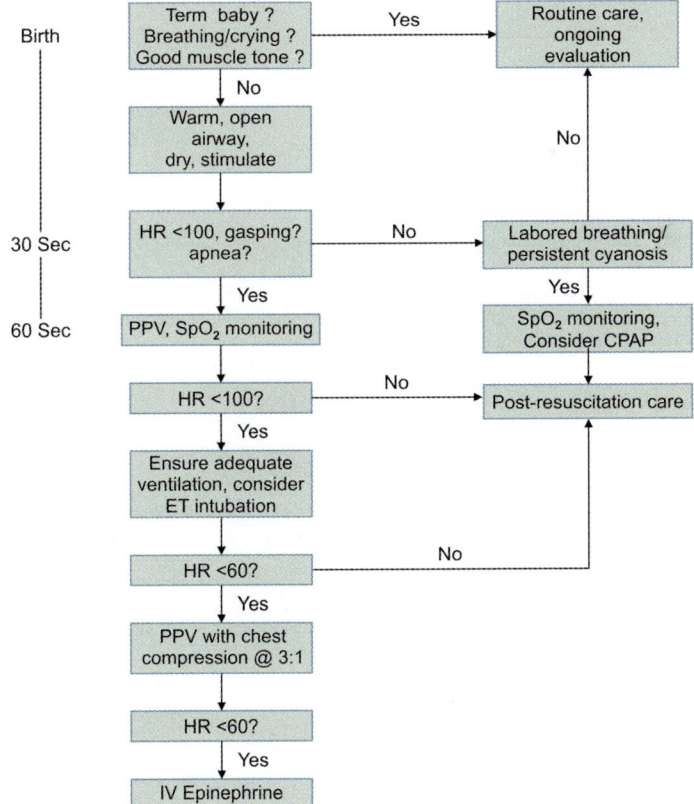

(CPAP, continuous positive airway pressure; ET, endotracheal; HR, heart rate; IV, intravenous; PPV, positive pressure ventilation)

- Intubation equipment:
  - Laryngoscope with straight blades, No. 0 (or preterm) and No. 1 (term)
  - Extra bulbs and batteries for laryngoscope
  - Endotracheal tubes of size 2.5, 3.5 and 4 mm
  - Stylet
  - Scissors
  - Adhesive tape
- Medications:
  - Epinephrine 1:10,000 (1 mg/mL)
  - Normal saline or Ringer lactate
  - 7.5% sodium bicarbonate solution
  - Naloxone hydrochloride
  - Distilled water

Flowchart 100.2: Postresuscitation management.

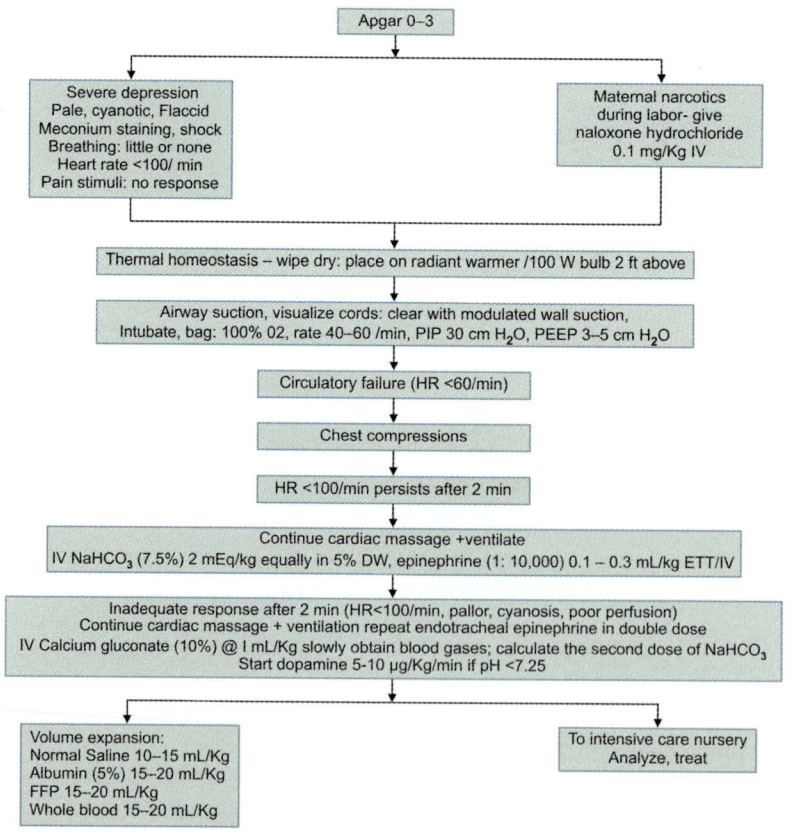

(DW, dextrose water; ETT, endotracheal tube; FFP, fresh frozen plasma; HR, heart rate; IV, intravenous; PEEP, positive end expiratory pressure; PIP, peak inspiratory pressure)

Chapter 100: Neonatal Resuscitation

- Miscellaneous:
  - Prewarmed towels—2
  - Stethoscopes
  - Oropharyngeal airways
  - Syringes 1, 2, 5, 10, 20 and 50 mL
  - Needles 25, 21, 18 G.
  - Shoulder roll
  - Gauze
  - Umbilical clip
- Proceed as per Flowchart 100.1 as the baby is received.

CONCLUSION

Resuscitation of the newborn is to be anticipated in all deliveries. The pediatrician should be updated on the subject; post-resuscitation care is a must in bringing out good results (Flowchart 100.2).

Chapter 101

Neonatal Ventilation

Ingale Vinod C, Mathew Varghese, Jacob Abraham

ABSTRACT

Commonly used ventilator supports in newborns are continuous positive airway pressure (CPAP), pressure-limited time cycled continuous flow and synchronized and patient triggered assist or control support. Indications, contraindications, equipment details, procedure, monitoring and complications to be anticipated are discussed. Ventilator settings and corrections for gas changes are given as tables for CPAP and other modalities of ventilation.

INTRODUCTION

Birth asphyxia is one of the leading causes of mortality in newborns. Pediatricians caring neonates should have sufficient knowledge and hands on experience in neonatal ventilation because at no other time in life one needs the expert help for initiating and maintaining respiration.

Readers are referred to Chapter 16 for more details.

TYPES OF VENTILATORY SUPPORT

- Continuous positive airway pressure
- Pressure limited, time cycled, and continuous flow
- Synchronized and patient triggered (assist/control or pressure support)
- Volume cycled ventilation
- High frequency ventilation.

The initial three modalities are of common use. The points regarding neonate will be briefed in this chapter.

CONTINUOUS POSITIVE AIRWAY PRESSURE

Indications in Newborns

- Respiratory distress syndrome (RDS)
- Apnea of prematurity
- Transient tachypnea of newborn
- Postextubation in preterm very low birth weight babies
- Neuromuscular disorders (occasionally contraindicated)
- To facilitate early extubation at any age.

Less common—pneumonia, meconium aspiration, pulmonary edema/hemorrhage, and laryngo/tracheo/bronchomalacia.

Contraindications to Continuous Positive Airway Pressure

- Progressive respiratory failure
- Congenital malformations of the airway
- Hypotension/hemodynamic instability
- Apnea not improved by CPAP
- Acute RDS.

Types of Ventilators for Continuous Positive Airway Pressure

- Portable stand-alone noninvasive ventilators
- Conventional ventilator by setting the inspiratory and expiratory positive airway pressures.

Mechanism

- Patient controls both the rate and depth of breathing
- Flow through the circuit is increased by the ventilator to maintain a stable preset pressure when the patient's respiratory effort occurs which is sensed by the ventilator.

Initiation of Continuous Positive Airway Pressure (Table 101.1)

- Place a roll under the infant's shoulder to extend the neck slightly.
- Choose the correct size prongs (prongs should fill the nasal opening without stretching the skin or pressing the nasal septum).
- Apply thin strip of transparent adhesive over the nasal septum to avoid trauma
- Place the prongs with the curve downward
- Attach the patient end of the ventilator circuit to the cannula
- Attach pulse oximeter to the infant
- Pass orogastric tube; keep it open for gastric decompression
- Check periodically patency of cannula for mucus plug
- Provide regular gentle nasal suction.

Table 101.1: Protocol for continuous positive airway pressure therapy.

Parameter	Indications		
	RDS	Apnea of prematurity	Postextubation
Initiation of CPAP-starting Pressure FiO$_2$	5–6 cm H$_2$O 0.5, titrate with SpO$_2$	4 cm H$_2$O 0.21–0.4, titrate with SpO$_2$	4–5 cm H$_2$O 0.05 to 0.1 above the preextubation FiO$_2$
What to do if no improvement Pressure	↑in steps of 1 cm Max of 7–8 cm	↑Only up to 5 cm (excess leads to hyperinflation)	↑in steps of 1 cm maximum of 7–8 cm
FiO$_2$	↑in steps of 0.05 maximum of 0.8; keep mean 30%, maximum 40%, then titrate down.	FiO$_2$ increase does not help much	↑in steps of 0.05 maximum of 0.8
Failure of CPAP	Worsening resp PaO$_2$ <50 mm Hg PaCO$_2$ >60 mm Hg Despite CPAP 8 cm, FiO$_2$ 0.8	Recurrent episodes of apnea requiring PPV	Same as in RDS
Weaning from CPAP When	No resp distress SpO$_2$, ABG—normal	No episodes of apnea/desaturation/ bradycardia for 12–24 hours	No resp distress with "decreasing FiO2"
How	Reducing FiO$_2$ in steps of 0.05 to 0.4 Decrease pressure in steps of 1 cm until 4–5 cm, guided by clinical parameters	Same as in RDS	To hood O$_2$ at CPAP and FiO$_2$ to preextubation level

(CPAP, continuous positive airway pressure; RDS, respiratory distress syndrome; PPV, positive pressure ventilation; ABG, arterial blood gas)

Monitoring

- Continuous monitoring—SpO$_2$, respiratory rate (RR), heart rate, and blood pressure
- Six hourly temperature, input/output chart
- Daily weight recording
- Arterial blood gas (ABG) as needed
- Chest—air entry, added sounds
- Abdomen—ileus "CPAP belly".

Complications of Continuous Positive Airway Pressure

- Nasal irritation, damage to septal mucosa
- Pulmonary air leaks
- Decreased cardiac output
- Gastric distension and CPAP belly syndrome
- Impedance of pulmonary blood flow.

MECHANICAL VENTILATION IN NEONATES

Refer to Chapter 16 for detailed explanation.

Indications

- Failure on maximal CPAP
- Recurrent apnea
- Poor respiratory effort
- Extreme prematurity
- Neuromuscular diseases.

Ventilator Controls in Intermittent Mandatory Ventilation

Flow, FiO_2, peak inspiratory pressure (PIP), positive end-expiratory pressure (PEEP), RR, V_T, inspiratory time (T_i), expiratory time (T_e), and inspiratory: expiratory (I:E) ratio.

Normal Ventilation

- Preset depending on clinical condition—PEEP, T_i, RR, flow
- Adjusted according to actual observation—PIP, FiO_2 ensuring V_T
- Initial settings—individualize
- Assess PIP needs by bag ventilation connected to a manometer. Look at chest movement, tidal volume (T_v) and air entry.

Choosing Peak Inspiratory Pressure

- Lowest 10–12, normal compliance—12
- If compliance is less, set PEEP and check chest rise on hand ventilation
- Mildly stiff—14 cm, moderately stiff—16 cm, and severely stiff—18 cm can be assessed by manometer.

Choosing Positive End-Expiratory Pressure

Choosing PEEP—range 3–5 cm water.
- If functional residual capacity is expected to be:
  - Normal—3 cm, moderately reduced—4 cm, severely reduced—5–6 cm
  - If hyperinflation and auto PEEP are expected choose 2–2.5.

Choosing T_i

If inspiratory T_i is expected to be
Normal—0.45 s, mildly short—0.4, moderately short—0.35, severely short 0.3, long—0.5

Rate and I:E ratios—determine minute ventilation
- Initial 40-60 breaths/min (assess work of breathing, asynchrony)
- T_i—0.3-0.5, I:E = 1:2
  Short T_i—decreased ventilation, short T_e air trapping
  Inverse I:E ratio—bad ventilation

Tidal Volume

- Normal 5-8 mL/kg; aim for Tv of 4-6 mL/kg
- Mechanical ventilation—20-48 mL/kg/min

Time Constant

It is the time taken for airway pressure and volume changes to equilibrate throughout the lungs

Time constant (T_c)—Compliance × resistance, for adequate T_i/T_e 3-5 T_c is needed.

Tables 101.2 and 101.3 depict initial ventilator settings and change in ventilator settings as per ABG, respectively.

Monitoring—(*See* Additional Points in Chapter 16)

- Avoid excessive light exposure
- Keep noise level below 45 dB

Table 101.2: Initial ventilator settings.

Disease	PIP (cm H_2O)	PEEP (cm H_2O)	T_i (s)	T_e (s)	V/min (mL)	FiO_2
Mod RDS	18–20	4–5	0.4	0.8	40–50	0.5
Severe RDS	23–25	5–6	0.4	0.8	40–50	0.9–1.0
Apnea of prematurity	12–14	4	0.4–0.5	1.5–2.6	20–30	0.21–0.3
MAS	16–20	2–3	0.4	1.0	30–40	0.9–1.0
Perinatal asphyxia	18–20	3–4	0.4–0.5 Never exceed >0.5	0.8–1.0	30–40	0.5

(MAS, meconium aspiration syndrome; PEEP, positive end-expiratory pressure; PIP, peak inspiratory pressure; RDS, respiratory distress syndrome)

Table 101.3: Changes in ventilator settings as per ABG.

Blood gas abnormality (mm Hg)	Corrective measures				
	FiO$_2$	Rate	PIP	PEEP	T$_i$
Hypercapnia (PaCO$_2$ >50)		↑	↑	↑	
Hypocapnia (PaCO$_2$ <35)		↓	↓		
Hyperoxia (PaO$_2$ >100)	↓		↓	↓	↓
Hypoxia (PaO$_2$ <50)	↑		↑	↑	↑

(ABG, arterial blood gas; PIP, peak inspiratory pressure; PEEP, positive end-expiratory pressure)

Determinants of oxygenation are FiO$_2$ and Mean Airway Pressure (MAP) = $\dfrac{K(PIP \times T_i + PEEP \times T_e)}{T_i \times T_e}$

To increase MAP
↑Flow, ↑PIP, ↑I:E, ↑PEEP

- Assess—core: axillary mismatch, posture: flexed/extended neck, movements: spontaneous vs. induced/paucity
- Tv—lowest possible (5–6 mL/kg)
- Adequate T$_e$
- PaCO$_2$ maintain 40–50 mm Hg.

CONCLUSION

Adequate and updated knowledge in initiating and establishing ventilation in neonates is a must for pediatricians to reduce neonatal mortality as well as birth asphyxia related morbidity in children.

Chapter **102**

Fluid Therapy in Newborns

Jacob Abraham, S Sushamabai

ABSTRACT

Fluid therapy in the newborn period is complex because it has to be initiated as soon as the baby is born and depends on the maturity of the baby at birth and associated problems in this period. Parenteral fluid therapy is needed in preterm babies, those who are unable to feed or have excessive fluid or electrolyte loss or fluid retention or electrolyte imbalance. History of excessive weight loss/gain, presence of edema, clinical features of dehydration and dyselectrolytemia and evidence of cardiac failure are the parameters to be used. The volume of fluid administered is calculated by the weight and maturity of the baby and the associated disease. The composition of the fluid should be 5% dextrose on initial 48 hours of life and then dextrose with electrolytes. Additional fluid should be added for babies under radiant warmer, phototherapy and conditions with fluid loss. The route can be nasogastric in selected situations through feeding tube. Parenteral therapy is by intravenous route using peripheral veins (umbilical vein can be used in first 24 hours as an emergency) or by central veins in critically ill babies.

INTRODUCTION

The normal newborn needs only proper breastfeeding for fluid and electrolyte balance. All high-risk neonates especially preterms, low-birth weight and sick, need careful fluid and electrolyte management because of inherent renal immaturity and deficient concentrating and diluting capacities.

CLINICAL CLUES FOR EXPERT FLUID THERAPY

- Failure to lose weight initially—suspect fluid retention (patent ductus arteriosus and necrotizing enterocolitis in preterm). Normal weight loss is up to 5% in term and 15% in preterm.
- Tachycardia heralds congestive cardiac failure (CCF) or hypovolemia and impending shock.
- Capillary refill time more than 3 s indicates decreased cardiac output.

- Reduced skin turgor, depressed anterior fontanel, and reduced urine output less than 0.5 mL/kg/hr indicate dehydration leading to renal failure.
- Periorbital puffiness, anasarca, and hepatomegaly suggest CCF.

MARKERS OF APPROPRIATE FLUID AND ELECTROLYTE BALANCE

- Normal urine output—1-3 mL/kg/hr
  - Less than 1 mL/kg/hr—inadequate intake or renal impairment
  - More than 4 mL/kg/hr—overhydration or diuresis
- Urine specific gravity—normal 1.008-1.012
  - Less than 1.006 is dilute urine: rule out hyperglycemia—reduce intravenous (IV) fluids
  - More than 1.020 is concentrated urine—increase IV fluids.

MAINTENANCE FLUID

- For first 48 hours, give only dextrose containing fluids
- Concentration of dextrose solution less than 1 kg—5%
  More than 1 kg—10%
- Monitor for hyperglycemia—if present change to 5% dextrose from 10% dextrose
- After 48 hours, electrolyte containing fluid solution should be given: Na, K, Cl at 1-2 mEq/kg/day during first week and thereafter at 2-3 mEq/kg/day
- Do not give potassium-containing fluid till urinary flow is established and normal renal function is ensured
- Baby under radiant warmer or phototherapy—increase fluids by 20 mL/kg/day for birth weight less than 1,500 g and 10 mL/kg/day for those more than 1,500 g
- Replace volume per volume for gastric fluid loss by 1/2 normal saline (NS) (for other body fluid loss replace with NS)
- Table 102.1 reveals fluid requirement for first 7 days of life.

Table 102.1: Fluid requirement for initial 7 days of life.

Body weight (kg)	Days and fluid rate mL/kg/day						
	1*	2*	3	4	5	6	7
<1 kg**	100	120	140	160	180	200	200
1-1.5 kg	80	100	120	140	160	170	170
>1.5 kg	60	80	100	120	140	150	150

*Give only dextrose containing fluid on days 1 and 2.
**Use only 5% dextrose containing fluid.

ROUTE OF ADMINISTRATION

- It can be oral in not sick babies either directly or through nasogastric tube.
- In most emergency situations IV route through peripheral veins or scalp veins can be accomplished.
- Umbilical vein can be used as an emergency for the initial 24 hours of life.
- Central veins should be resorted to critically ill babies.

CONCLUSION

Fluid therapy in newborns is often required in emergency situations, should be calculated according to the maturity, weight, post natal postnatal age, associated disease process and should be strictly monitored clinically and by laboratory parameters. The routes can be nasogastric, peripheral veins, scalp veins or central veins as per situation.

Chapter **103**

Admission to the Neonatal Intensive Care Unit

Jacob Abraham, S Sushamabai

ABSTRACT

There are few newborns requiring special care either in SCNA or neonatal intensive care unit (NICU) depending on the care needed for the sickness and the facilities in these areas. Babies who are preterm, low birth weight, large for gestational age, having congenital anomalies, respiratory distress, cyanosis, significant jaundice, anemia, other danger signs (Chapter 98), asymptomatic hypoglycemia and those with maternal concerns of illness are included in this group. Obstetrical problems warranting special baby care are maternal diabetes requiring insulin, meconium stained amniotic fluid, and maternal seizures. Babies referred from outside hospitals and admitted by consultants also belong to this group.

INTRODUCTION

- Some newborns need monitoring in specialized units which could be special care newborn area (SCNA) or neonatal intensive care unit (NICU) depending on the degree of monitoring or care required.
- Admission criteria will vary from unit to unit based on the patient particulars and the level of care provided at each of these areas.

BROAD INDICATIONS FOR ADMISSION INTO NICU

- Premature babies less than 37 completed weeks of gestation
- Term babies with birth weight less than 2.0 kg and more than 4.0 kg (large for gestational age babies are liable to become hypoglycemic)
- Babies with tachypnea, respiratory distress (respiratory rate ≥60/min or chest retractions) or cyanosis at birth
- Those with or suspected to have life-threatening or major congenital malformations picked up at birth and include:
  - Diaphragmatic hernia, esophageal atresia with or without tracheal fistula
  - Absent or ectopically placed anal opening
  - Bilateral choanal atresia or cleft palate

- Baby subsequently found to have:
  - Respiratory distress
  - Significant jaundice requiring treatment—phototherapy or exchange transition
  - Significant feeding problems—lethargy, refusal to feed, bilious and/or persistent vomiting, marked distension of abdomen postfeeding
  - Hypoglycemia on routine monitoring
  - Fever/seizures in the ward
  - Any concern of the mother which warrants monitoring of the baby.
- The following obstetrical complications in the mother warrant observing the baby in the NICU:
  - Gestational/overt diabetic mother on insulin for her sugar control near the time of delivery
  - Meconium staining of amniotic fluid
  - Maternal seizure just prior to delivery
- Conditions where the mother is unable to care the baby.

The following obstetrical factors do not include NICU observation of the baby:
- Mother, immediate post lower segment cesarian section, shifted to the recovery room (unless she needs observation for anesthetic or other medical problems in the surgical postoperative recovery)
- Twin delivery with good-weight babies if the mother is confident to handle her babies
- Well-controlled psychiatric disorder in the mother.

Other reasons for NICU admission are:
- All admissions by a consultant unless specified otherwise
- Any baby referred from outside
- Admissions after routine working hours unless specified otherwise by a consultant.

CONCLUSION

Some neonates need extra care in the special care unit or neonatal ICU. The parameters for selection though internationally specified, may differ in various hospitals. Such maternal and baby factors should always be noted in newborn care.

Chapter 104

Neonatal Convulsions

Jacob Abraham, S Sushamabai

ABSTRACT

Neonates are more prone for seizures than any other age group. The clinical presentation can be subtle seizures, tonic, clonic or myoclonic. The important causes are hypoxic–ischemic encephalopathy, narcotic withdrawal, metabolic derangements, sepsis, TORCH infections, developmental malformations, inborn errors of metabolism (IEM), perinatal insults and epilepsy. The prioritization of the etiology is related to the age of the baby. Approach should be immediate stabilization of ABC, seizure control, parallel quick history and investigations. In most situations etiology can be made out at this stage. Detailed history, physical examination, and investigations are to be completed after the baby is stabilized. The initial anticonvulsant of choice is IV lorazepam followed by IV phenobarbitone, IV fosphenytoin, IV levetiracetam, and PO topiramate. IV pyridoxine can be given empirically. Fluid and electrolyte therapy, cardiovascular, respiratory and renal support should be given. The etiology should be detected and treated. Tapering or stopping of anticonvulsant depends on the etiology.

DEFINITION

Paroxysmal alteration in neurological function (behavioral and/or autonomic) with or without impairment of consciousness.

CLINICAL PRESENTATION

- Subtle seizures—oral, buccal, ocular, lingual, or limb movements, apnea or autonomic phenomena
- Tonic
- Clonic
- Myoclonic.

CAUSES

- *Age 1–4 days*: Hypoxic ischemic encephalopathy, narcotic withdrawal, accidental injection of local anesthetic, intraventricular hemorrhage,

metabolic [hypocalcemia, hypoglycemia, hypomagnesemia, hypo/hypernatremia, pyridoxine deficiency/dependency, sepsis, inborn errors of metabolism, perinatal insults]
- *Age 4–14 days*: Meningitis, hypocalcemia, hypoglycemia, kernicterus, IEM, developmental malformations, benign neonatal convulsions, and epileptic syndromes
- *Beyond 2 weeks age*: Meningitis; toxoplasmosis, other infections (syphilis, varicella-zoster, parvovirus B19), rubella, cytomegalovirus, and herpes infections; IEM, developmental malformations of brain, and epilepsy.

INVESTIGATIONS

- Plasma glucose, serum electrolytes, complete blood count, coagulation profile, renal function test, and C-reactive protein
- Cerebrospinal fluid studies
- Culture studies as per clinical situation
- Ultrasonography/computed tomography/magnetic resonance imaging brain.

PATIENT APPROACH

- Stabilize airway, breathing, and circulation, parallel quick history and physical examination; in most situations, etiology and severity will be obvious.
- Exclude jitteriness (seen in wake stage only and can be stopped by holding the limb) and benign myoclonus (short-lived jerky movements, normal electroencephalogram).
- Rule out/manage hypoxia, hypoglycemia.
- Start anticonvulsants if the above measures fail—as revealed in Flowchart 104.1.

OTHERS

- Cardiovascular support—fluids, inotropes
- Respiratory support—mechanical ventilation
- Fluid and electrolyte therapy
- Hypomagnesemia—0.2 mL/kg $MgSO_4$ (25%) intramuscular (IM)
- Pyridoxine deficiency/dependency—50 mg pyridoxine IV
- Investigations to establish the cause
- If convulsions recur within 2 days continue phenobarbitone
- If no convulsions for 7 days, stop phenobarbital, observe
- Treatment of etiology.

Flowchart 104.1: Algorithm for anticonvulsant therapy in neonatal seizures.

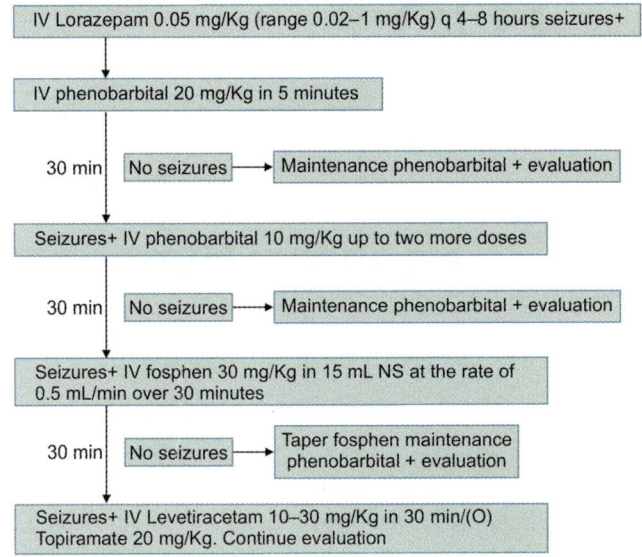

(IV, intravenous; NS, normal saline)

CONCLUSION

Seizures are very common in the neonatal period, can be subtle or classic, are of diverse etiology, should be controlled at the earliest, and the etiology should be detected and treated.

Chapter **105**

Neonatal Hypoglycemia

Jacob Abraham, S Sushamabai

ABSTRACT

Plasma glucose less than 40 mg/dL is considered as hypoglycemia in newborns and is a common complication in preterm, low birth weight, large for gestational age babies, infants of diabetic mothers, sepsis, hypoxia and Rh isoimmunization. Can occur in normal babies also. The features are pallor, sweating, cyanosis, tachypnea, apnea, tachycardia, jitteriness, seizures and altered sensorium. Asymptomatic hypoglycemia can be treated by oral glucose fortified feeds. In symptomatic hypoglycemia IV 10% glucose infusion is given in increasing concentration from 6 mg/kg/min to 12 mg/kg/min, is given till response and then tapered. Hydrocortisone, diazoxide, glucagon, and octreotide are the drugs recommended. Investigations to rule out the underlying etiology should be carried out in resistant cases.

INTRODUCTION

Plasma glucose (PG) less than 40 mg/dL indicates neonatal hypoglycemia.

RISK FACTORS

Low birth weight, preterm, large for gestational age babies, infants of diabetic mothers, sepsis, asphyxia, and rhesus isoimmunization.

CLINICAL PRESENTATION

Pallor, sweating, cyanosis, tachypnea/apnea, tachycardia, jitteriness, seizures, and altered sensorium.

PATIENT APPROACH

- Suspect hypoglycemia in all the risky babies and normal babies with clinical features as described above.
- Assess PG, categorize, and proceed as shown in Flowchart 105.1.

Flowchart 105.1: Management of neonatal hypoglycemia.

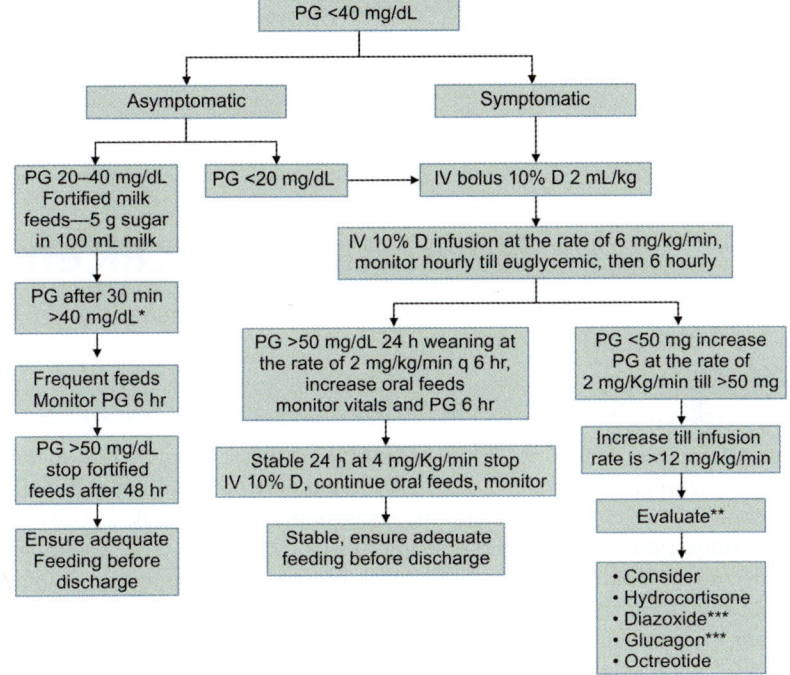

*Switch to symptomatic group, if PG <40 mg/dL.
**Serum insulin, cortisol, growth hormone, plasma ammonia, blood lactate, arterial blood gas, urine ketones and reducing substances, urine aminogram.
***Avoid in small-for-gestational-age babies.
(PG, plasma glucose)

CONCLUSION

Hypoglycemia is a common emergency encountered in normal and high-risk newborns and should be detected in time and treated.

Chapter 106

Neonatal Hypocalcemia

Jacob Abraham, S Sushamabai

ABSTRACT

Serum calcium less than 7 mg/dL is diagnostic of hypocalcemia. This metabolic error is very common in neonates due to several underlying conditions. The clinical manifestations are jitteriness, tremors, exaggerated startle reflex, convulsions apnea, stridor, cyanosis and cardiac failure. Risky groups can have asymptomatic hypocalcemia. Initial stabilization followed by investigation and treatment of hypocalcemia is the approach. 10% IV calcium gluconate 2 mL/kg is the immediate treatment in symptomatic babies. The dose can be increased up to 8 mL/kg/day × 48 hours as infusion and then tapered. Oral calcium 40–50 mg/kg/day has to be continued. Depending on the etiology, vitamin D and phosphorus should be added.

INTRODUCTION

Serum calcium less than 7 mg/dL or ionized calcium less than 4 mg/dL in first 4 weeks of life is diagnostic of hypocalcemia.

CAUSES

- Preterm and low-birth-weight babies
- Severe birth asphyxia
- Infant of diabetic mother
- Vitamin D deficiency
- Hyper- and hypoparathyroidism
- Postexchange transfusion
- Renal failure (acute/chronic)
- Drug induced
- Hypo-/hypermagnesemia
- Hyperphosphatemia.

Flowchart 106.1: Management of neonatal hypocalcemia.

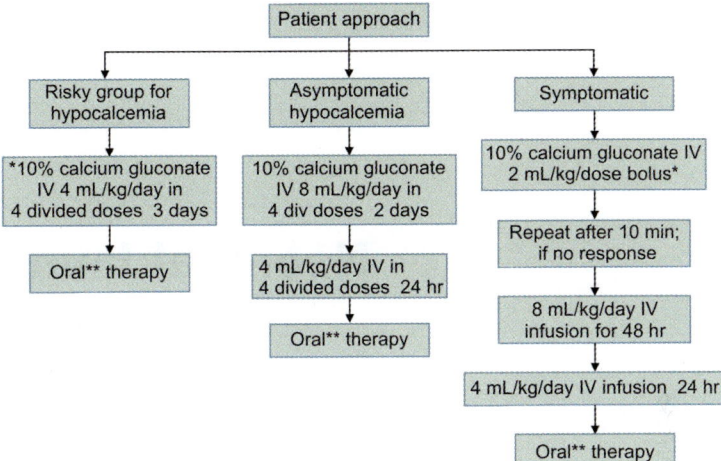

*1 mL/kg of IV 10% Ca gluconate yields 10 mg/kg of elemental Ca. Administer as 1:1 in 5% D; give under cardiac monitoring; safeguard against extravasation.
**Oral replacement—40–50 mg/kg/day elemental calcium. Supplement P, vitamin D as per etiology.
(IV, intravenous)

CLINICAL PRESENTATION

- Jitteriness, myoclonic jerks, exaggerated startle, seizures, apnea, cyanosis, laryngospasm, stridor, and cardiac failure.
- Asymptomatic hypocalcemia can occur in the risky group and should be detected and treated.

INVESTIGATIONS

- Serum calcium, phosphorus, magnesium, and alkaline phosphatase needed in all.
- Consider serum parathyroid hormone and 25(OH)D as per clinical situation to exclude hypoparathyroidism and hypovitaminosis D.
- Others as per clinical situation
- Electrocardiogram for corrected QTc, if more than 0.2 s, is supportive of diagnosis.
- Proceed as given in Flowchart 106.1 for management.

CONCLUSION

Hypocalcemia is a common metabolic error encountered in the neonatal period and should be aggressively treated.

Chapter 107

Neonatal Jaundice

Jacob Abraham, S Sushamabai

ABSTRACT

Clinical jaundice is perceived in newborns when serum bilirubin is more than 7 mg/dL. Patient approach depends on the disease severity. Critically ill babies require initial stabilization along with parallel history, physical examination, and investigations. In most situations, the etiology and type of jaundice can be made out in the first assessment itself. The severity of jaundice in newborns can be made out clinically by Kramer index. Unconjugated hyperbilirubinemia is the most dangerous type of jaundice in the early neonatal period, which should be corrected by phototherapy or exchange transfusion. The chapter deals with the details of therapy, investigations, monitoring, and post-transfusion care.

Newborn appears clinically jaundiced when the serum bilirubin (SBR) is more than 7 mg%.

PATIENT APPROACH

- Stabilize airway breathing and circulation if critically ill; otherwise proceed to detailed history:
  - Onset, activity, feeding problem, fever, lethargy, seizures
  - High-colored urine, clay-colored stools, bleeding tendency
  - Family history of jaundice, blood group incompatibility, phototherapy or exchange transfusion in siblings.

PHYSICAL EXAMINATION

- Assess the degree of jaundice by gentle dermal pressure and observing the yellowish skin color in good daylight.
- Clinical severity of jaundice can be assessed based on Kramer index as – Serum bilirubin: face = 5 mg/dL, mid-abdomen = 15 mg/dL, soles = 20 mg/dL. Jaundice to the mid-abdomen, associated symptoms and/or signs/high-risk factors are indications to investigate.

Flowchart 107.1: Diagnostic approach to neonatal jaundice.

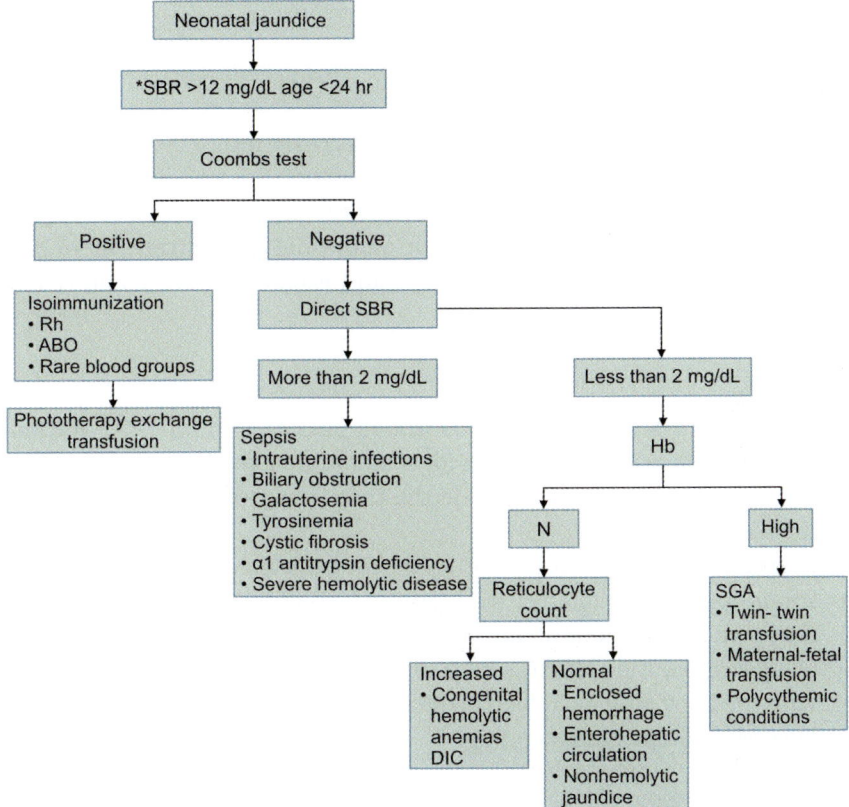

*Serum bilirubin
(DIC, disseminated intravascular coagulation; IU, intrauterine; Rh, rhesus; SBR, serum bilirubin; SGA, small for gestational age; Hb, hemoglobin)

- General examination for activity, pallor, bleeding spots, cephalohematoma, hemangioma, Moro reflex, posture, weight, gestational age
- Abdominal examination for hepatosplenomegaly.

Proceed to screening investigations to categorize the type and severity of jaundice and to decide the intervention needed:
- Blood for complete blood count, SBR (total and direct), reticulocyte count, peripheral blood smear studies for abnormal red blood cells, Coombs test
- Categorize the type of jaundice, probable etiology and severity of jaundice as revealed in Flowchart 107.1.

Proceed to phototherapy or exchange transfusion as detailed.

TREATMENT OF UNCONJUGATED HYPERBILIRUBINEMIA

Phototherapy

- Simple noninvasive treatment to bring down unconjugated hyperbilirubinemia
- Body is exposed to a light of wavelength 427–475 nm.
- Bilirubin breaks down to nontoxic components: Reversible photoisomerization (4Z, 15Z to 4Z, 15E) and irreversible photooxidation (to lumirubin) which are excreted through bile and urine, respectively. Table 107.1 reveals the criteria for phototherapy and exchange transfusion (ET) in neonatal jaundice.

Procedure

- Use blue light with maximum absorption peak of bilirubin (450–460 nm).
- Double surface phototherapy is ideal and more effective.
- Place the baby undressed inside the unit; cover the eyes and genitalia (in males).
- Keep the baby at a distance of 15–20 cm from the light source; provide continuous phototherapy except during feeding.
- Intensive phototherapy includes placing a fiberoptic phototherapy blanket under the neonate's back to increase the exposed area.
- Turn the baby after each feed to obtain exposure in all body areas.
- Ensure adequate breastfeeding.

Supportive Therapy

- Intravenous (IV) fluids for babies with dehydration, poor feeding and with risk factors 20% extra maintenance fluid is required to prevent dehydration as breast feeds or ORS.
- Assess hemoglobin (Hb) and if anemic, provide packed cell transfusion.

Table 107.1: Criteria for phototherapy (PT) and exchange transfusion (ET) in neonates with unconjugated hyperbilirubinemia based on body weight and general condition.

Wt in g	Total serum bilirubin (mg/dL)			
	Healthy baby		Sick baby*	
	PT	ET	PT	ET
<1,000 g	5–7	11–13	4–6	10–12
1,001–1,500 g	7–10	13–15	6–8	11–13
1,501–2,000 g	10–12	15–18	8–10	13–15
2,001–2,500 g	12–15	18–20	10–12	15–18

*Sick baby—asphyxia, hypothermia, sepsis, acidosis, hypoxia, hypercarbia, hemolysis

Chapter 107: Neonatal Jaundice

Quality Assessment of Phototherapy Unit

- Change the lamps at least once in 3 months.
- Verify irradiance of the lamps every 3 months.

Monitoring

- Temperature recording 2 hourly
- Urine output (should be at least every 3-4 hr)
- Daily weight recording
- Serum bilirubin at least daily—more frequently as per situation
- Discontinue phototherapy when SBR is below age-specific phototherapy lower limit.
- Monitor for rebound after 24 hours by repeat SBR estimation.

Untoward Effects

- Rash and diarrhea
- Overheating and dehydration.

Exchange Transfusion

Exchange transfusion is lifesaving as well as reduces disability in neonatal hyperbilirubinemia. The procedure has the risk of a major surgery. Hence, adequate precautions should be undertaken.

Indications

- Clinical
  - Kernicterus, hydrops fetalis, heart failure due to hemolytic disease
- Laboratory
  - Cord bilirubin more than 5 mg/dL and Hb less than 10 g/dL
  - Rise in SBR more than 1 mg/dL/hr despite phototherapy
  - Rise in SBR more than 0.5 mg/dL/hr with Hb 11-13 g/dL
  - Serum bilirubin more than 20 mg/dL.

Requirements

- Transfusion blood—should be as fresh as possible.
- Quantity—double the blood volume of the baby (2 × 85 mL/kg).

Group and Type

- Rhesus (Rh) isoimmunization—Rh negative of baby blood group or O Rh negative, compatible with baby's and mother's blood
- ABO incompatibility—O group, Rh compatible with baby's blood

- Other situations—compatible with baby's blood group and Rh type
- Anticoagulant—heparin (ideal) or citrate phosphate dextrose adenine.

Gradually warm the blood and maintain at a temperature of 35–37°C throughout ET. Keep it well mixed by gentle squeezing or agitation of the bag to avoid sedimentation to prevent anemia.

Procedure

Experienced doctor should do the procedure. A competent assistant should monitor the baby, tally the volume exchanged and perform emergency procedure. Empty the baby's stomach before transfusion to prevent aspiration. Maintain body temperature. Monitor vitals. Immobilize the baby. Cannulate the umbilical vein with a polyvinyl catheter to a distance up to 7 cm to obtain a free flow of blood. Collect the first blood sample to estimate the pretransfusion bilirubin value. Aspirate 20 mL of infant's blood alternating with infusion of 20 mL of donor blood. Smaller aliquots (5–10 mL) may be used in sick and premature babies. The process should be completed in 45–60 min. Parameters to be monitored are body temp, heart rate, respiratory rate, SpO_2, blood pH and blood sugar. Collect the second blood sample for bilirubin estimation at the end of the procedure. Administer 1 mL calcium gluconate IV for each 100 mL blood exchanged. Give IV sodium bicarbonate 1 mEq/kg/100 mL blood if blood pH is less than 7.2.

Post-transfusion Care

- Nil oral for 4 hr; give IV maintenance fluid × 8 hr.
- Start oral feeds after 4 hr.
- Assess the vitals, SBR and blood glucose estimation 4–6 hourly for at least 24 hr after ET.
- Keep the baby warm.

Complications

- Hypothermia, bradycardia, apnea, hypoxia, cyanosis, thrombosis
- Acidosis, hypoglycemia, hypocalcemia, necrotizing enterocolitis, infections.

CONCLUSION

Neonatal jaundice can herald serious illness and hence should be closely observed, investigated, and early specific therapy should be implemented.

Chapter 108

Neonatal Sepsis

Jacob Abraham, S Sushamabai

ABSTRACT

Sepsis is the most important cause of neonatal death and should be considered whenever three risk factors are present—the common pathogens being *E. coli*, *Group B Streptococcus*, *Staphylococcus aureus* and *Klebsiella*. Early-onset sepsis appears before 72 hours postnatal age and late-onset sepsis after that. Clinical features are fever or hypothermia, irritability, poor feeding, sclerema and symptoms pertaining to respiratory system, central nervous system, gastrointestinal tract, renal and/or hematology. Suspect sepsis from clinical assessment. Screening investigations are rapid diagnostic tests. System-wise investigations should be selected. Empirical antibiotics (ampicillin + genta/Cefotaxime + amikacin) should be started at the earliest after sending investigations. Necessary changes should be made after getting the reports. Supportive therapy is as important as specific therapy. IV immunoglobulin is also advised.

INTRODUCTION

Sepsis indicates overwhelming infection without localization and is the most important cause of neonatal death.

RISK FACTORS FOR NEONATAL SEPSIS

Consider sepsis when any of the following risk factors is present:
- Low birth weight/preterm baby
- Febrile illness in the mother during delivery
- Foul-smelling liquor
- Meconium-stained amniotic fluid
- Premature rupture of membranes more than 12 hours
- Frequent vaginal examinations (>3 during labor)
- Prolonged and difficult delivery with instruments
- Birth asphyxia and difficult resuscitation.

ETIOLOGY

Common organisms are *Escherichia coli*, Group B streptococci, *Staphylococcus aureus,* and *Klebsiella.*
- *Early-onset sepsis* (<72 hr): Suspect in babies with perinatal hypoxia, resuscitation difficulties, and respiratory distress due to congenital pneumonia.
- *Late-onset sepsis* (>72 hr).

CLINICAL FEATURES

Clinical features are common in both groups and are:
- Fever or hypothermia, irritability, not doing well, poor feeding, and sclerema.
- Features pertaining to gastrointestinal tract, respiratory and cardiovascular systems, renal, central nervous system or hematology.

DIFFERENTIAL DIAGNOSIS

- Birth asphyxia
- Cold injury
- Hypoglycemia
- Inborn errors of metabolism.

PATIENT APPROACH

- History and physical examination—consider the possibility of sepsis from the symptoms, risk factors, and physical examination findings.
- Screening investigations:
    - Rapid diagnostic tests (RDTs):
        - Absolute neutrophil count (<1,500 or >5,000)
        - C-reactive protein (CRP) more than 8 mg/dL
        - Micro–erythrocyte sedimentation rate (micro-ESR) age in days + 3 (any value >15)

Significant when two out of three RDTs are present.
- Sepsis screen:
    - Leukopenia total leukocyte count(TC) <5,000/mm^3
    - Band cell count: Total neutrophil ratio more than or equal to 0.2.
    - Peripheral blood smear revealing toxic granules in neutrophils
    - RDT (absolute neutrophil count, CRP, micro-ESR) positivity
- Cultures—pus, stool, supra pubic (SP) urine, blood, ± cerebrospinal fluid (CSF)

Flowchart 108.1: Approach to neonatal sepsis.

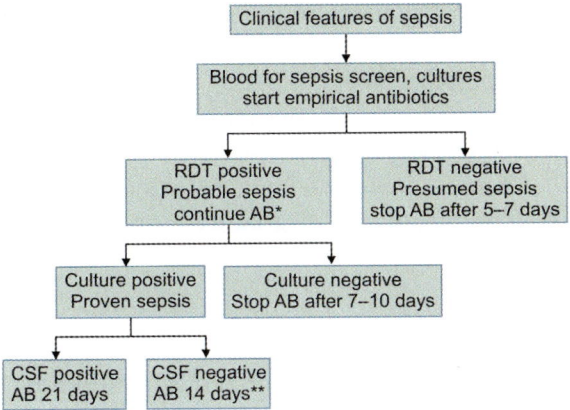

*Antibiotics (AB).
**Pneumonia 14 days, septic arthritis 4–6 weeks.
(RDT, rapid diagnostic tests; CSF, cerebrospinal fluid)

Table 108.1: Empirical antibiotic therapy in neonatal sepsis.

Empirical antibiotic therapy	Drugs	Per dose
First line—ampicillin + gentamicin	Ampicillin	50 mg/kg BD
Second line—cefotaxime + amikacin	Gentamicin	5 mg/kg OD
Third line—ciprofloxacin, cefepime, aztreonam	Cefotaxime	50 mg/kg BD
Meningitis—cefotaxime + amikacin	Amikacin	7.5 mg/kg BD
Staphylococcus infection—cloxacillin/vancomycin	Ciprofloxacin	7.5 mg/kg BD
Necrotizing enterocolitis—cefotaxime + amikacin + metronidazole	Aztreonam	30 mg/kg BD
	Vancomycin	10 mg/kg BD
	Metronidazole	7.5 mg/kg BD

- Chest X-ray, ultrasonography (head, abdomen, bone, joint, soft tissues), Blood glucose (BG), serum bilirubin, serum electrolytes, renal function tests, and liver function test
- Others as per clinical assessment
- Proceed as given in Flowchart 108.1.
- Switch to appropriate antibiotics as per culture reports (Table 108.1).

Supportive Therapy

- Thermoneutral environment
- Oxygenation—hood/continuous positive airway pressure/mechanical ventilation
- Intravenous fluids, stop enteral feeds if very sick or reveals ileus

- Monitor random blood sugar, maintain euglycemia.
- Shock—volume expansion, inotrope
- Vitamin K 1 mg IV
- Treatment of hyperbilirubinemia
- Coagulopathy—fresh frozen plasma/platelets/fresh blood
- Seizures—anticonvulsants
- Increased intracranial pressure—fluid restriction, mannitol
- Intravenous immunoglobulin—1 g/kg/dose—one or two doses in very sick or preterm babies.

CONCLUSION

Sepsis is the leading cause of neonatal mortality; should be anticipated in risky babies and empirical antibiotics and supportive therapy should be started after sending investigations. Intravenous immunoglobulin is recommended in extremely sick babies.

Chapter 109

Apnea in Newborns

Jacob Abraham, S Sushamabai

ABSTRACT

Apnea is cessation of breathing for more than 20 seconds or less than 20 seconds with bradycardia or cyanosis. Extreme prematurity is the leading cause, others being aspiration, sepsis, hypothermia, hypoxic–ischemic encephalopathy, metabolic derangements, inborn errors of metabolism (IEM), airway obstruction, heart failure, and gastroesophageal reflux. Patient approach is initial stabilization, parallel quick history, and physical examination along with investigations. Provide warmth immediately, give tactile stimulation and clear the airway of the baby. Consider bag and mask ventilation. Assess the etiology and severity as revealed in the flowchart. Treat the etiology, provide thermoneutral environment, correct hypoglycemia, maintain fluid and electrolyte balance, and proceed to mechanical ventilation if there are indications. Apnea of prematurity can be treated with theophylline/aminophylline/caffeine citrate/doxapram.

INTRODUCTION

Apnea is cessation of breathing more than 20 or less than 20 seconds with bradycardia or cyanosis.

COMMON CAUSES

- Extreme prematurity
- Sepsis and pneumonia
- Hypothermia
- Intraventricular hemorrhage
- Hypoxic brain injury
- Hypocalcemia
- Hypoglycemia
- Hypomagnesemia
- Inborn errors of metabolism
- Heart failure

- Obstructive airway disease
- Lung collapse
- Gastroesophageal reflux
- Aspiration.

PATIENT APPROACH

Quick history, physical examination, and stabilization.
- Provide warmth and gentle tactile stimulation, clear the airway.
- Bag and mask ventilation if continues to have apnea.
- Assess the gestational age, age at onset of apnea and associated clinical signs.
- Send blood for complete blood count, Blood glucose (BG), serum calcium, Mg, Na, K, arterial blood gas.
- Others as per situation—chest X-ray, ultrasonography head, echocardiogram, blood and body fluids for culture and Gram's stain.
- Proceed as given in Flowchart 109.1.

MANAGEMENT

- Gentle tactile stimulation in mild and intermittent episodes
- Bag and mask ventilation with O_2/intubation if tactile stimulation fails
- Provide thermoneutral environment.
- Maintain euglycemia.
- Treat the etiology.

Flowchart 109.1: Clinical approach to apneic neonate.

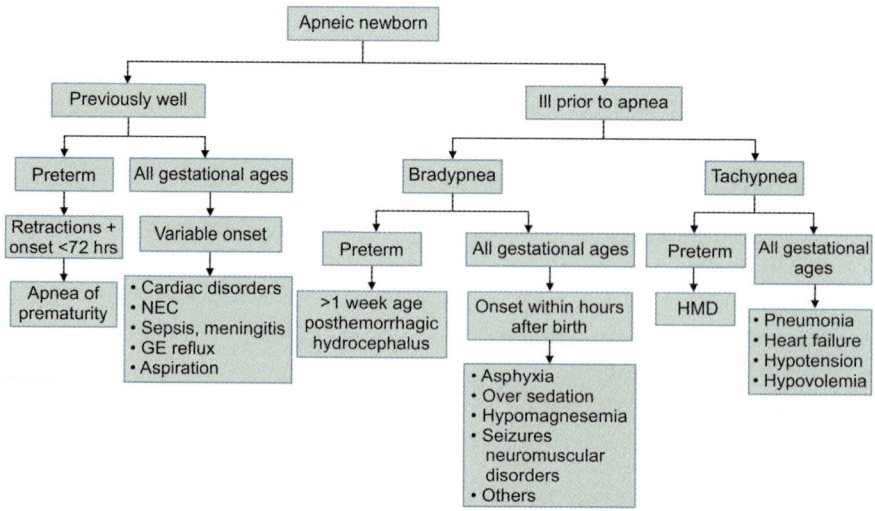

(GE, gastroesophageal; HMD, hyaline membrane disease; NEC, necrotizing enterocolitis)

Flowchart 109.2: Treatment of recurrent apnea of prematurity.

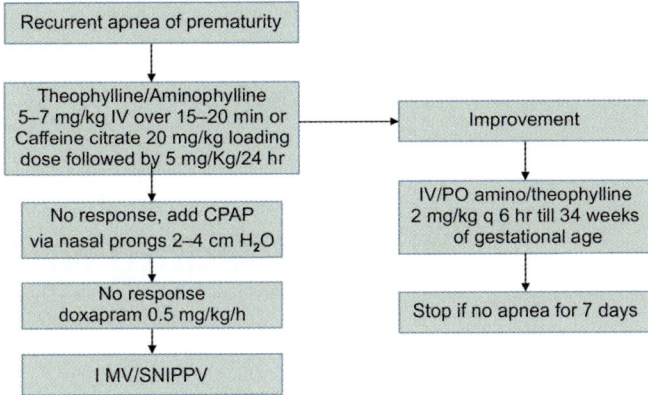

(CPAP, continuous positive airway pressure; IV, intravenous; SNIPPV, synchronized nasal intermittent positive pressure ventilation)

Recurrent apnea of prematurity:
- Onset of apnea in a previously well preterm neonate after the second week of life
- Treatment is by theophylline/caffeine as detailed below (Flowchart 109.2).
- Doxapram or ventilation may be required in resistant causes.

CONCLUSION

Neonates should be closely observed for apnea and corrective supportive as well as specific measures be implemented.

Chapter 110

Bleeding Neonate

Jacob Abraham, S Sushamabai

ABSTRACT

Bleeding neonate is a serious emergency. Proceed to quick assessment, stabilization, collection of blood for investigations, grouping and cross-matching, and arrange for transfusion. Categorize the baby as multiple-site bleeding or bloody stools, sick or not sick in each group. Sick babies with multiple-site bleeding require organ/system-wise investigations to find out the etiology and treat the cause. The most common cause for isolated bloody stool in the neonate is hemorrhagic disease of the newborn (HDN) which can be confirmed by studying the coagulation profile and treated by vitamin K infusion and fresh frozen plasma rarely.

PATIENT APPROACH

Quick assessment, stabilize, categorize, collect blood for complete blood count, peripheral blood smear study, culture, prothrombin time, activated partial thromboplastin time, grouping, cross-matching, and arrange for transfusion (Flowcharts 110.1 and 110.2).

Flowchart 110.1: Approach to newborn with generalized bleeding.

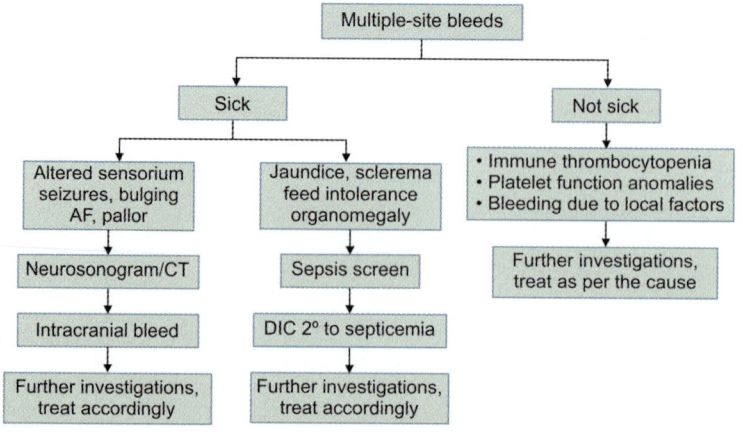

(AF, anterior fontanel; CT, computed tomography; DIC, disseminated intravascular coagulation)

Flowchart 110.2: Approach to newborn with bloody stools.

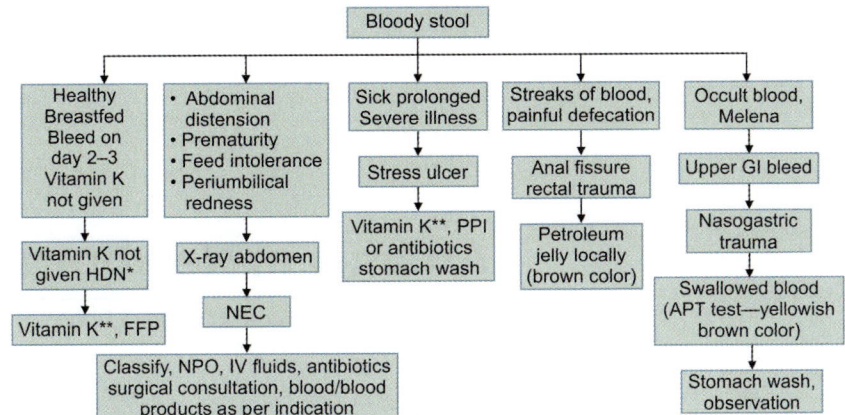

*HDN—Hemorrhagic disease of newborn.
**Vitamin K-1–5 mg as slow IV infusion.
(NEC, necrotizing enterocolitis; PPI, proton pump inhibitor)

CONCLUSION

Bleeding neonate is a medical emergency requiring immediate intervention, can be multiple-site bleeding or isolated bloody stool. The most common cause of bloody stool is hemorrhagic disease of the new born which can be corrected by vitamin K infusion.

Chapter 111

Anemia in Newborns

Jacob Abraham, S Sushamabai

ABSTRACT

Anemia (defined as reduced Hb below 2 SD of mean for the age of the baby) is not uncommon in neonates. In acute severe blood loss, baby presents with pallor and shock; in chronic loss the features are pallor and signs of cardiac failure. In both situations features of underlying cause such as jaundice, hepatosplenomegaly, subgaleal hemorrhage, cephalohematoma, lymphadenopathy, and bleeding manifestations will be present. Baby should be immediately stabilized along with clinical assessment and investigations including blood grouping, Rh typing, and crossmatching. Babies with severe anemia require packed cell transfusion or whole blood transfusion. Less sick babies need to be started on oral iron and folic acid. Recombinant human erythropoietin is advised in chronic anemia. Exclusive breastfeeding and iron-rich complementary feeds should be advised for all babies.

DEFINITION

Anemia is diagnosed if the hemoglobin (Hb) level is more than 2 standard deviations below the mean for the baby's age as shown below:

Age	Hb (g/dL) -2 SD
Birth (cord blood)	13.5
1–3 days (capillary)	14.5
1 week	13.5
2 weeks	12.5
1 month	10

A physiologic decrease in Hb occurs by 8–12 weeks in term babies (Hb = 11 g/dL) and by 6 weeks in preterms (Hb = 7–10 g/dL).

COMMON CAUSES

- Immune hemolytic anemia (rhesus, ABO, rare groups)
- Nonimmune and hereditary hemolytic anemias
- Intrauterine infections—parvovirus

- Blood loss—acute or chronic
  - Intrauterine:
    - Transfusions (twin–twin, fetomaternal)
    - Internal hemorrhage
    - Placental hemorrhage
  - Extrauterine:
    - Hemorrhagic diseases of the newborn
    - Iatrogenic—frequent sampling
    - Concealed hemorrhages, for example, cephalohematoma
    - Umbilical cord bleeding
    - Chronic gastrointestinal bleeding (hemangioma, Meckel's diverticulum).
- Alpha-thalassemias
- Congenital hypoplastic anemias.

CLINICAL PRESENTATION

- Depends on the volume and rapidity of blood loss.
- Acute severe blood loss is characterized by shock and pallor.
- Chronic blood loss presents as pallor and features of cardiac failure (tachycardia, tachypnea, cardiomegaly, flow murmur, hepatomegaly, lung crackles and wheeze).
- Features of underlying cause—jaundice, hepatomegaly ± splenomegaly, bleeding manifestations, lymphadenopathy, cephalohematoma, subgaleal hemorrhage, etc.

PATIENT APPROACH

- Depends on the severity of anemia and the underlying cause.
- Stabilize the baby with oxygen and intravenous fluids while eliciting parallel history and physical examination.
- Send blood for Hb, hematocrit, complete blood count, mean corpuscular volume, reticulocyte count, peripheral blood smear (PBS), Coombs tests, grouping typing, X matching and others as per the clinical situation.
- Proceed to diagnosis as per Flowchart 111.1.

TREATMENT

- Babies with severe anemia require blood/packed cell transfusion (Table 111.1).
- Less sick babies require elemental iron 3–6 mg/kg/day in two divided doses × 3 months, reevaluate and continue with maintenance requirement

Flowchart 111.1: Diagnostic approach to neonatal anemia.

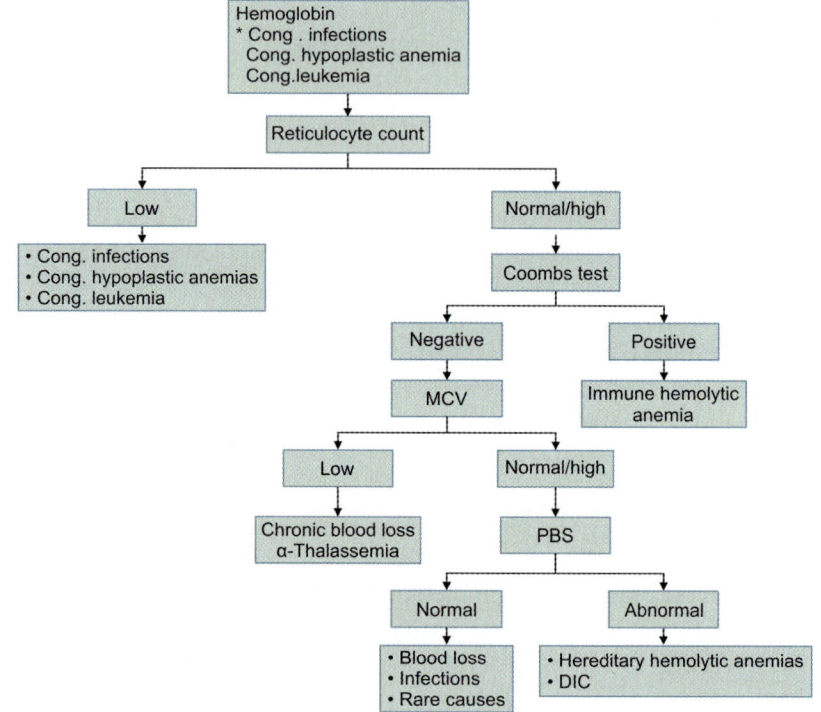

(*Cong, congenital; MCV, mean corpuscular volume; PBS, peripheral blood smear; DIC, disseminated intravascular coagulation)

Table 111.1: Transfusion protocol for newborns with anemia.

Hb (g/dL)	Hct (%)	Newborn details	Transfusion details
≤7	≤20	Asymptomatic	*PRBCs 20 mL/kg in 2–4 hr
≤8	≤25	On supplemental O_2 for cardiac/resp illness Wt gain <10 g/kg/day × 4 days on 100 cal/kg/day Undergoing surgery	*PRBCs 20 mL/kg in 2–4 hr Can be given as two doses
≤11	≤35	On respiratory support	*PRBCs 15 mL/kg in 2–4 hr

*PRBCs (if hemorrhage whole blood transfusion is ideal).
(PRBCs, packed red blood cells)

1 mg/kg/day till Hb is age-appropriate and food intake is adequate for iron requirement.
- Folic acid 0.5–1 mg/day should be supplemented.
- Exclusive breastfeeding for 6 months, and iron-sufficient complementary feeds should be advised.

- Recombinant human erythropoietin may be considered for chronic anemia so as to reduce transfusions.
- The etiology should be detected and treated.

CONCLUSION

Anemia is not uncommon in neonates; if severe, packed cell or whole blood transfusion is lifesaving; in less severe situations, oral iron and folic acid therapy is enough.

Chapter **112**

Neonatal Transport

Jacob Abraham, S Sushamabai

ABSTRACT

Transporting sick neonates to higher centers is required at times depending upon the facility of the hospital in which the baby was cared. In utero transfer is ideal and the reason should be genuine. Select the nearest efficient referral center and shortest route of transport, provide competent care providers and, if possible, allow the mother to accompany. The reason for transport and additional facility available in the referral center are to be explained. Transport the baby in warm condition with appropriate notes. A written consent for transport should be obtained. The faculty of the referral center should be informed prior to transport.

INTRODUCTION

Transporting a sick newborn is infrequently needed; systematized procedure will improve the chance of survival.

POINTS TO CONSIDER

- Transporting sick neonates is not an easy task.
- In utero transport is far more rewarding than the transport of sick neonates after birth.
- Care providers should always be ready, competent and confident to handle this responsibility.
- Select the nearest referral facility for transporting the baby. Use the shortest route, and the fastest possible mode of transport.[1]

PREPARE WELL BEFORE TRANSPORT

Assess[2]

Make sure that there is genuine indication for referral.

Communicate[1]

- Explain the condition, prognosis and reason for referral of the baby.[1]
- Get the written consent for the transport.
- Provide a precise notes of the baby at the time of discharge.
- Explain where to go and whom to contact.[1]
- Inform the referral faculty beforehand, if possible.[1]

Correct Hypothermia

Normalize the temperature of the baby.

Who should Accompany?[1]

- Mother should accompany if possible.[1]
- A doctor and nurse ideally should be present.[1]

Ensure Warm Transport

- Cover the baby with cap, socks, mittens, double-layered cotton dress and blanket.
- Improvised containers or transport incubator may be advised.
- Skin-to-skin care if conditions are feasible.

Additional Care

- Ensure an open airway.
- Check breathing during transport.
- Provide adequate feeds.
- If on intravenous fluids, the accompanying health staff should be able to manage it.

CONCLUSION

Transporting the sick neonates to another center should be undertaken with proper precautions and documentation.

REFERENCES

1. http://www.gmch.nic.in/e-study/e%20lectures/Pediatrics/neonataltransport.pdf (Internet 01-Dec-2017)
2. http://www.sifpsa.org/digitization/cd1_vol2/1.4.pdf (Internet 29-Nov-2009)

Chapter 113

Discharge Protocol

Jacob Abraham, S Sushamabai

ABSTRACT

At the time of discharge of a newborn, the mother should be medically stable, confident to look after and breastfeed the baby. The baby should be stable with SpO_2 more than 95% with no evidence of any systemic disease. The corrected gestational age should be equal to 34 weeks, weight more than or equal to 1.8 kg and feeding technique well demonstrated. Babies at risk for hyperbilirubinemia, serum bilirubin should be collected prior to discharge. Hearing and vision check-up should be done or arranged or completed. Convey clear instructions for follow-up.

POINTS TO CONSIDER

- The mother is medically stable to be discharged, confident to look after and breastfeed the baby without any pain/clinically evident cracked nipples which could prevent breastfeeding.
- No medical problems in the baby—jaundice in the risky range, cyanosis, postductal SpO_2 recorded predischarge is >95%, murmurs and any systemic or local signs of sepsis, including umbilical sepsis and pustules
- Bilirubin levels are to be sent predischarge *in all babies at risk for jaundice, which include:*
  - Rhesus incompatibility
  - ABO incompatibility
  - Babies born to gestational diabetic mothers
  - Born <37 completed weeks of gestation
  - Birth weight <2.5 kg, those with blood collection (cephalohematoma) or extensive bruising
  - Clinically appearing to be significantly jaundiced

- All investigation reports are collected and acted upon/instructions given to follow up on anticipated reports.
- *In a preterm/low-birth-weight baby*, fulfill the following essential criteria:
  - Corrected gestational age = 34 weeks
  - Weight ≥1.8 kg
  - Completed essential tests for neurological status (including ultrasonography head), hearing and vision
  - Feeding technique adequately verified.

CONCLUSION

Discharge protocol of newborns should be properly planned and conveyed when the baby and the mother are stable and clearly documented.

Chapter **114**

Audiology Screening in Neonates

Jacob Abraham, S Sushamabai

ABSTRACT

Hearing evaluation is essential for all newborns even if they are apparently normal. The risky groups for hearing impairment are birth weight less than 1,500 g, family history of deafness, intrauterine infections, those with meningitis, craniofacial anomalies, hyperbilirubinemia, birth asphyxia, mechanical ventilation, features of syndromic malformations and aminoglycoside/furosemide therapy. Presently otoacoustic emission (OAE) prior to discharge is the accepted policy; fail results on two occasions warrant brainstem auditory evoked response (BAER) or automated auditory brainstem response (ABR) for confirmation. Definitive therapy should be started for defective hearing before 6 months of age.

INTRODUCTION

Audiology screening is highly needed in the neonate for early detection of hearing defects and their correction at the earliest.

POINTS TO CONSIDER

- Ideally all neonates should get the benefit of audiology screening.
- The current guideline for audiology screening is *just prior to discharge* using OAE (otoacoustic emission).
- The OAE gives a "Pass"/"Fail" result for each ear.
- A "Fail" on two occasions warrants a BAER (brainstem auditory evoked response).
- A hearing screening to document auditory evoked response in the brainstem is done by a BAER/automated ABR.
- The second test should be done at the earliest, definitely prior to 6 months of age for intervention, if there are definitely impaired evoked responses.
- It is possible to do more definitive tests for hearing, including behavioral audiometry much later.

High-risk Newborns for Hearing Impairment[1]

- Birth weight less than 1,500 g.[1]
- Family history of hereditary childhood sensory neural hearing loss[1]
- Intrauterine infection with cytomegalovirus, rubella, syphilis, and herpes.[1] Toxoplasma can also be a cause.
- Craniofacial anomalies, including morphological abnormalities of the pinna and ear canal.[1]
- Hyperbilirubinemia requiring exchange transfusion.[1]
- Bacterial meningitis[1]
- Apgar scores of 0–4 at 1 minute or 0–6 at 5 minutes[1]
- Mechanical ventilation for more than a week[1]
- Stigmata or other findings associated with a syndrome known to have sensory neural and/or conductive hearing loss[1]
- Aminoglycoside therapy greater than two courses
- Aminoglycoside therapy in combination with loop diuretics (ethacrynic acid, furosemide).[1]

CONCLUSION

All neonates require hearing evaluation at the earliest; corrective steps for impaired hearing should be started before 6 months of age.

REFERENCE

1. http://depts..washington.edu/nicuweb/NICU-WEB/hearscrn.stm (Internet 09-Jan-2010)

Chapter **115**

Visual Screening in Newborns

Jacob Abraham, S Sushamabai

ABSTRACT

All preterm babies and those with suspected intrauterine infections and defective visual fixation require visual screening. Routine check-up at birth for risky babies by an expert ophthalmologist is a must and should be followed by periodic evaluation and correction especially for the preterm and those prone for retinopathy of prematurity (ROP). Treatment for ROP is laser photocoagulation of the avascular retina; propranolol therapy is a newer modality.

INTRODUCTION

Visual screening is an important aspect of newborn care to prevent blindness.

INDICATIONS

- Preterm babies
- Babies with suspected intrauterine infections
- Defective visual fixation on developmental assessment.

PATHOGENESIS

- Retinal angiogenesis begins at 16-week gestation, progresses from optic disk to periphery, reaches outer rim—nasal 36-week, temporal 40-week gestation.
- Any insults during this period, especially less than 32-week gestation, can predispose to retinopathy of prematurity (ROP), characterized by abnormal proliferation of retinal blood vessels into the vitreous, cicatrization and traction on the retina resulting in varying grades of visual impairment.
- Up to 90% of risky babies have self-regression; 10% progress to severe damage.

Table 115.1: Screening age for ROP in preterm babies.

Gestational age at birth (week)	Age at initial examination (week) postmenstrual	
22–27	31	
28	32	
29	33	or 1 month after delivery
30	34	
31	35	
32	36	

CLINICAL MANIFESTATIONS

- Retinopathy of prematurity features can be blindness, squint, cataract, leukocoria to phthisis bulbi.
- Visual defect in newborns should be suspected if there is defective visual fixation and roving eye movements.

DIAGNOSIS

- All babies should have routine eye checkup at birth. Parents should be counseled and informed in the high-risk group regarding follow-up.
- All high-risk babies should be subjected to expert evaluation by an experienced ophthalmologist.
- Retinopathy of prematurity screening should be done in preterm babies at ages specified in Table 115.1.

TREATMENT

- Laser photocoagulation of the avascular retina
- Systemic administration of propranolol is an investigational therapy.
- Periodic follow-up is needed.

CONCLUSION

All preterm babies prone for ROP and the risky ones for visual impairment must have periodic visual screening by experienced ophthalmologist and corrective steps needed to be taken.

Section 15

PROCEDURES

Simple invasive procedures are often required in clinical practice to confirm the diagnosis, exclude the differential diagnosis and to assess the prognosis. Counseling and written consent are a must before doing such procedures. Always take proper sterile precautions before, during, and after the procedure and observe the patient after the procedure, the duration depending on the type of the procedure. Appropriate analgesia/sedation is a must (Chapter 46).

Chapter 116

Lumbar Puncture

S Sushamabai

ABSTRACT

Lumbar puncture (LP) is the procedure done to collect cerebrospinal fluid (CSF) (commonly) and occasionally to administer drugs in spinal canal. Verify the contraindications in the patient and rectify them before the procedure. ABC stabilization is a must before the procedure. The assistant should position the child correctly, observe sterile precautions and introduce the LP needle (size 20–22G) with stylet at L3 or L4 space. Collect four samples of CSF, preserve one for future use. After the procedure press over the area for few seconds and apply sterile dressing. The patient is allowed to rest in prone position after the LP for 2 hours to avoid post-LP headache. The collected CSF should be transported to the laboratory immediately for analysis.

INTRODUCTION

Lumbar puncture (LP) is done to collect cerebrospinal fluid (CSF) or introduce drugs (intrathecal therapy).

INDICATIONS

1. Diagnostic
Meningitis
Encephalitis
Subarachnoid hemorrhage
Guillain-Barré syndrome
Metastatic leukemia
Benign intracranial hypertension

2. Therapeutic
Drug therapy in leukemia
Relieve raised intracranial pressure (ICP)

CONTRAINDICATIONS

- Glasgow Coma Scale less than 8
- Raised intracranial pressure (ICP) with neurologic deficit
- Unstable cardiopulmonary status

- Infection over the puncture site
- Bleeding tendency (LP can be done after correcting the bleeding).

In suspected meningitis, provide empirical antibiotic therapy, if there is contraindication to LP. Procedure can be done when the patient's condition improves.

PROCEDURE

- Correction of dehydration and airway, breathing and circulation stabilization in an unstable patient.
- Position the patient. An experienced assistant should hold the child over a hard surface, the spine brought near the edge of the table. The patient's knees are to be flexed toward his/her chest, the hands placed in between the knees. The assistant should hold the child with one hand at the buttocks so that the back is bent. With the other hand, flex the neck of the child to the chest, making sure that the child is breathing normally (Fig. 116.1).
- Scrub the hands; wear sterile gloves.
- Check the anatomical landmarks; locate the space between L3 and L4 vertebrae (The third lumbar vertebra is at the junction of the line from the highest point of the iliac crests and the vertebral column).
- Prepare the site with povidone iodine and then alcohol from the intended puncture site toward the periphery upto 10 cm, sponging in widening circles. Drape the area with sterile cloth. In older children (>1year), who are alert, 1% lignocaine local anesthetic may be infiltrated into the skin over the area.
- Perform LP. Use an LP needle with stylet (22 G for young infant, 20 G for older child). Insert the needle at the middle of the intervertebral space at 90° and aim the needle toward the umbilicus.

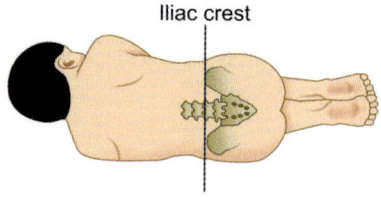

- Apply topical anesthetic 30–45 min prior to procedure
- Spinal cord ends at L1-L2, so sites for puncture are located at L3-L4 or L4-L5
- Restrain patient in lateral decubitus position
  – 'Maximally flex spine' without compromising airway
  – Keep alignment of feet, knees and hips
  – Position head to left if right handed or vice versa

Fig. 116.1: Lumbar puncture—positioning.

- Advance the needle slowly with uniform force. A sudden decrease in resistance will be felt as the dura is punctured.
- Withdraw the stylet and the CSF will drop out of the needle. If no CSF is obtained, the stylet can be reinserted and the needle is advanced slowly once again.
- Collect four samples of 0.5–1 mL CSF in separate sterile containers, one each for culture, biochemistry, preservation for later analysis, and last sample for cell count in the order of collection. The specimens should reach the laboratory within 30 minutes.
- Withdraw the needle quickly after reinserting the stylet. Press over the puncture site for few seconds and cover the area with sterile dressing.
- A traumatic LP revealing bloody CSF occurs when the needle is advanced puncturing the vertebral vein. If so, remove the needle and introduce in the higher space.
- Keep the child in prone position for 2 hours to avoid post-LP headache.

Note—sitting position also is advised for LP.

COMPLICATIONS

- Post-LP headache
- Low-back pain
- Infection
- Brainstem herniation in symptomatic raised ICP.

CONCLUSION

Lumbar puncture is an important investigation to study the CSF to diagnose large number of brain diseases and should be done with proper precautions.

Chapter 117

Central Venous Access

S Sushamabai

ABSTRACT

Central venous access is needed in critically ill patients for multiple drug infusions, fluid therapy, venous pressure monitoring, and total parenteral nutrition. Seldinger technique is the method commonly applied for all central veins. The principle is initial introduction of the needle into the target vessel and then introducing the guidewire through the needle, the needle is then removed, a skin trap is made over the wire, and the flexible catheter is introduced through the wire into the vein with twisting motion. The wire is then removed and the catheter is attached to the infusion set. The common veins selected are internal jugular (right), external jugular, femoral, and subclavian. Catheter care is by daily check-up of the entry area for signs of inflammation, cleaning the area with alcohol solution and applying antiseptic ointment and dressing with sterile gauze. The complications encountered are thrombosis, infection and bleeding.

INDICATIONS

- Patients in shock for central venous pressure monitoring and fluid bolus administration.
- Multiple drug infusions especially for vasopressors.
- Total parenteral nutrition and chemotherapy.

EQUIPMENT

- Skin-cleaning swabs
- 1% lidocaine
- 2 mL syringe, 23 G needle
- Syringe with 0.9% saline
- Seldinger set—cannula size forage
- Suture material
- Infusion set
- Tape
- Towels.

TECHNIQUE

Seldinger technique is used for central venous cannulation.
- The needle is inserted into the target vessel, and flexible end of guidewire is passed freely into the vessel.
- The needle is then removed, leaving guidewire in place.[1] Make skin traps over the wire up to the vein.
- Then, the catheter is advanced with twisting motion into the vessel.
- Remove the wire and occlude the catheter end (to prevent air embolism); attach the catheter end to the infusion set.[2]

VEINS[3]

- Internal jugular
- External jugular
- Subclavian
- Femoral.

PROCEDURE IN GENERAL

- Restrain the child in proper position depending on the vein to be cannulated.
- Identify and mark the point of insertion.
- Scrub hands and put on gloves.
- Prepare the skin with antiseptic solution of povidone iodine.[4] Followed by alcohol and povidone iodine once more. Drape the area; anesthetize the skin with 1% lidocaine, if the child is responsive to pain.[2] Flush with sterile saline after that.
- Secure the catheter by suturing with skin.
- Apply antibiotic ointment and sterile dressing.[4]

Internal Jugular Vein

- Right jugular cannulation is preferred.
- Patient's head is turned to opposite side and placed 30° lower with extension at the neck by keeping a towel beneath the shoulder on the same side.[5]
- There are three approaches for internal jugular cannulation in relation to sternocleidomastoid muscle which are stated next.

Central Approach

- The needle is inserted at the apex of triangle formed by the two lower heads of sternocleidomastoid muscle and the clavicle.[2]

- Direction of the needle is toward ipsilateral nipple 45° posterior until blood appears and the needle is pushed not more than 2 cm.[5]
- Take chest skiagram to verify the needle position and to exclude pneumothorax.

Anterior Approach

Needle is inserted halfway along the anterior border of sternocleidomastoid and is directed toward ipsilateral nipple 45° posteriorly as carotid artery is displaced medially.[5]

Posterior Approach[5]

- Needle is passed behind the posterior border of sternocleidomastoid at one-third of muscle length from its clavicular insertion.
- Direction of the needle is toward suprasternal notch.

External Jugular Vein

- The vein runs from the angle of the mandible to the posterior border of the lower third of sternocleidomastoid muscle
- After restraining the child, turn the head to the opposite side
- Keep the head 30° lower so as to distend the vein
- After cleaning the area, insert the needle followed by cannula at 30° angle with the skin applying negative pressure
- Proceed as in previous vein access.

Subclavian Vein Access

- Ideal position is 30° extension. Keep the towel ball between scapulae and arm adducted by the side.[5]
- Puncture point is just under the clavicle. Locate the junction of middle and medial third of clavicle.[4]
- Syringe with the needle is held perpendicular to the long axis of sternum until blood appears and then pass the guidewire.[5]
- Introduce a dilator with a screwing motion and insert the catheter by Seldinger technique.[5]
- Assess that the tip of catheter is at the junction of superior vena cava and right atrium.[6]

Femoral Vein

- Femoral vein is medial to the femoral artery.[5] It is located by palpating the femoral pulse.[5]
- Restrain the child in supine position and abduct the thigh in frog-leg posture.

- Locate the point 0.5 cm medial to the femoral pulsation which is 0.5 cm below the inguinal ligament.
- Introduce the needle at 45° angle; proceed as in previous descriptions once the vein is entered.
- Catheter position is advanced up to the diaphragm.

CATHETER CARE

- Daily inspection of entry site for signs of inflammation
- Daily clean with alcohol; apply antiseptic ointment and dress with sterile gauze.

COMPLICATIONS

- Thrombosis
- Infection
- Bleeding.

CONCLUSION

Central venous access is often required for caring the critically ill children and should be mastered by all doctors in pediatric intensive care unit.

REFERENCES

1. Butt KMH, Friedman EA. Evolution of vascular access. Artif Organs. 1986;10(4):285-97.
2. Advanced Life Support Group.Practical procedures—circulation. Advanced Pediatric Life Support. 01/01/2005.
3. http://www.mccneb.edu/outlines/healthandpublicservices/NURS/HLTH1210.doc [Internet 27-Mar-2014]
4. Atlas of Emergency Medicine Procedures. Springer Nature. 2016.
5. Praveen K. Procedures in pediatric intensive care unit. Indian J Pediatr. 1993.
6. http://jvir.highwire.org/cgi/cntent/full/11/9/1137 [Internet 18-Feb-2007].

Chapter 118

Peripheral Arterial Cannulation

S Sushamabai

ABSTRACT

Peripheral arterial cannulation is needed in sick children with respiratory problems requiring arterial blood gas (ABG) analysis and for intra-arterial BP monitoring especially in shock. If the patient has coagulopathy, correction has to be done before the procedure. Arteries selected are radial, femoral, dorsalis pedis, and posterior tibial. Radial artery (right) is the common one preferred for collecting blood for ABG. Do Allen test to assess adequacy of collateral circulation prior to puncture. For puncturing the artery, the wrist and hand are kept at 30–45 degree extension by keeping gauze folds under the wrist. Artery is punctured at 30 degree angles at the point of maximum pulsation with a 20 G cannula. Advance the cannula till bright red blood appears in the cannula, remove the needle, and then collect the blood. Seldinger technique can also be applied.

INDICATIONS

- Frequent arterial blood sampling in critically ill children
- Continuous intra-arterial blood pressure (BP) monitoring in the unstable and sick child as noninvasive BP (NIBP) is unreliable in edema, burns, shock and obesity.

CONTRAINDICATIONS

- Negative Allen test
- Coagulation abnormalities—cannulation can be done after correcting the defect.

ARTERIES USED

- Radial
- Femoral
- Dorsalis pedis
- Posterior tibial.

Note: Brachial artery should not be used for puncture or cannulation due to the lack of collaterals. Axillary artery cannulation has the risk of embolization.

PROCEDURE AND EQUIPMENT

General—as for venous cannulation.

Radial Artery

- Right radial artery is ideal since it contains preductal blood.
- Check the adequacy of collateral circulation prior to cannulation by *Allen test* as detailed below:
  Compress and clench the hand to squeeze out the blood. Occlude both the radial and ulnar arteries with manual pressure. The hand will blanch. Release the pressure over the ulnar artery. Disappearance of blanching within 5 seconds indicates adequate collateral circulation from the ulnar artery. Always document the test in patient's record. Continuing observation for digit perfusion is mandatory.
- Stabilize the hand and wrist on a firm board, placing the wrist on 30–45° extension over gauze pads (Fig. 118.1).
- Prepare the area; palpate the artery; locate the pulsation just proximal to the head of radius.
- Select 20 G intravenous cannula (or Seldinger technique); puncture the artery at 30° angle at maximal pulsation.
- Advance the cannula until bright red blood appears; remove the needle and collect blood for ABG observing appropriate precautions.
- Attach a three-way connector with a 10 cm tubing.
- Apply a transparent sterile dressing over the catheter after fixing.

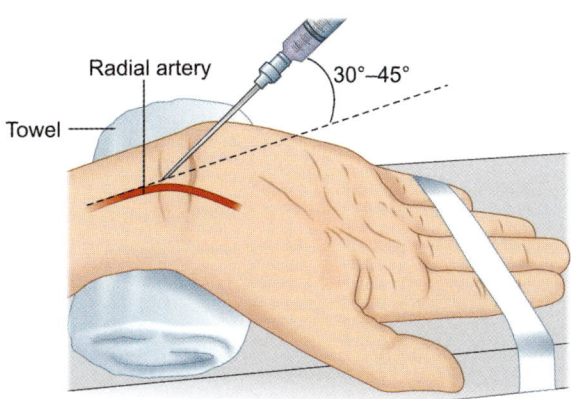

Fig. 118.1: Stabilizing the wrist for radial artery puncture.

- Set up a continuous heparinized saline infusion (1 U heparin/mL saline) at 1 mL/hr.
- Digit perfusion is to be evaluated hourly by capillary refill time, warmth, color and movement.

COMPLICATIONS

- Disconnection of the catheter from the three ways
- Ischemia leading to arteriolar spasm or necrosis
- Emboli formation (blood clot or air)
- Infection of the site leading to sepsis.

CONCLUSION

Peripheral arterial cannulation is often needed in critically ill children to collect blood for ABG analysis and intra-arterial BP monitoring.

Chapter **119**

Intraosseous Access

S Sushamabai

ABSTRACT

Intraosseous (IO) route is selected as an emergency alternative in very sick children to administer drugs and fluids when IV route cannot be obtained. 18G Jamshidi needle or 18G intraosseous needle may be used. Proximal or distal tibia or lower end of femur are the sites advised. After observing sterile precautions the needle is introduced 15 degree angles at vertical direction away from the joint space. As needle enters the marrow the resistance is lost and it stands without support. Remove the stylet and aspirate the marrow. Push heparinized saline to remove clots and connect the IV infusion; the maximum period allowed for IO access is 6 hours.

INTRODUCTION

Intraosseous is approached in critically ill children less than 6 years of age requiring parenteral fluids/drugs, if intravenous (IV) access cannot be obtained.
- Severe hypotension
- Cardiopulmonary arrest
- Failed peripheral vein access in emergency drug therapy as in status epilepticus

REQUIREMENTS (*SEE* CHAPTERS 117 AND 118)

- 18G-bone marrow (Jamshidi) aspiration needle
- 18G-needle with trocar (IO infusion needle).

INFUSION SITES

- Proximal tibia—anteromedial flat surface 1 cm medial and below the tubercle preferred in infants and young children.
- Distal tibia—just proximal to the medial malleolus—preferred in older children.
- Femoral—anterolateral surface 3 cm above the lateral condyle.

Avoid fractured and infected limbs.

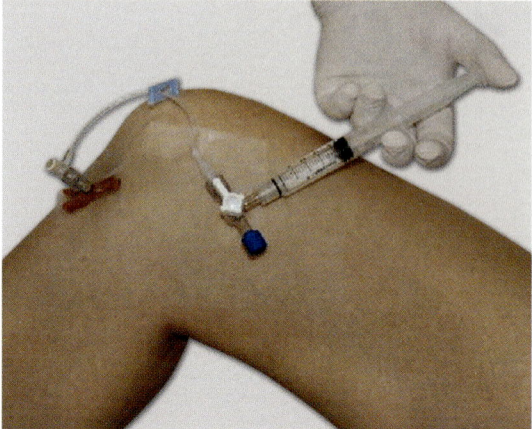

Fig. 119.1: Intraosseous access—upper end of tibia.

PROCEDURE

- Observe aseptic techniques, local anesthesia, if needed.
- Introduce the needle 15° angle to the vertical direction away from the joint space. Penetrate the marrow with a twisting motion until resistance is suddenly lost. The needle should stand without support (Fig. 119.1).
- Remove the stylet and aspirate some marrow to conform marrow space entry.
- Push heparinized saline to ensure location and remove any clot; pressure required is as for IV access.
- Connect the needle to the IV tube and assess free flow.
- Observe the puncture site area for swelling (indicates superficial needle placement/posterior piercing of the bone).
- Secure peripheral or central access. IO access should not be used more than 6 hours.

COMPLICATIONS

- Extravasation of fluid into subcutaneous tissue
- Fat embolism
- Epiphyseal trauma
- Osteomyelitis and subcutaneous abscess.

CONCLUSION

Intraosseous route has to be resorted in sick children when IV access fails; but should not be maintained for more than 6 hours.

Chapter **120**

Needle Thoracocentesis

S Sushamabai

ABSTRACT

Needle thoracocentesis is done to collect pleural fluid for diagnostic study or to remove air or fluid from the pleural space to reduce respiratory distress. For removal of air in tension pneumothorax a large bore cannula is introduced into the second intercostal space in the midclavicular line. A three-way stopcock is attached to aspirate air. For needle aspiration of pleural fluid locate the fluid, quantity and loculations with ultrasonography (USG) or CT. Patient should be properly positioned as recommended for the age and general condition. Mark the puncture point from the inferior angle of the scapula which corresponds to 8th rib or inter space. The needle with a syringe attached is introduced just above the superior margin of the rib. As the needle enters the pleural space, attach a 3-way stopcock to collect adequate fluid in three bottles and transport the specimen for laboratory studies. Remove the needle, place sterile dressing over puncture area, and repeat the chest skiagram. Monitor the patient for 4 hours.

INDICATIONS

- *Diagnostic*—to collect pleural fluid for detailed study
- *Therapeutic*—to remove the fluid or air collection in pleural cavity compromising ventilatory function.

CONTRAINDICATIONS

- Non-cooperative child
- Uncorrected coagulopathy
- Loculated fluid with failed attempts.

Needle Decompression for Tension Pneumothorax

- Observing aseptic precautions, introduce a large bore cannula (16 to 22G as per patient's age) in the second intercostal space in the mid-clavicular line
- Attach a three-way stopcock and syringe and aspirate air
- Consider elective insertion of chest tube.

Needle Aspiration of Pleural Fluid

- Confirm the clinical diagnosis by chest skiagram and ultrasonography/computed tomography scan. Assess the quantity of pus and the presence of loculations.
- Position the patient—sitting and leaning on a wooden support in older children; keep young/sick/sedated children in supine position with the arms placed over the head.
- Observe aseptic precautions.
- Identify and mark the puncture point—angle of scapula corresponds approximately to the eighth rib/interspace.
- Anesthetize the skin, subcutaneous tissue, rib, periosteum, chest wall and pleura with 1% lidocaine.
- Introduce the puncture needle attached to a syringe just above the superior margin of the rib to avoid trauma to the neurovascular bundle; apply slight negative pressure while the needle is advanced.
- Entry into the pleural space is indicated by loss of resistance.
- Attach a three-way stopcock to remove the fluid for diagnostic studies in separate bottles for each laboratory. The maximum fluid aspirated for therapeutic purpose can be up to 20 mL/kg.
- Remove the needle; place a sterile dressing over the puncture site, obtain chest skiagram.
- Transport the fluid immediately for cell count, Gram stain, biochemistry and culture (refer to Chapter 22 for pleural fluid analysis).
- Observe the patient for 4 hours with vitals and SpO_2 monitoring.

COMPLICATIONS

- Trauma to the neurovascular bundle resulting in severe pain and bleeding
- Surgical emphysema.

CONCLUSION

Needle thoracocentesis is an important procedure used in pediatric intensive care units to decompress air in the pleural cavity or collect pus from pleural cavity.

Chapter **121**

Pericardiocentesis

S Sushamabai

ABSTRACT

Pericardiocentesis is the removal of fluid from the pericardial cavity for therapeutic and/or diagnostic purpose. Chest X-ray (CXR), electrocardiography (ECG) and ultrasonography (USG) chest and heart must be evaluated prior to the procedure and if possible 2D echocardiogram (ECHO) of the heart. Patient is placed 30° head elevation, insert 18 to 20G needle with attached syringe 45 degree angles below and left to the xiphoid process; advance it toward the direction of the patient's shoulder applying gentle pressure till pericardial fluid is obtained. Disconnect the needle, attach a three way and aspirate the fluid which should immediately be sent for laboratory studies. Vitals, SpO_2, and ECG should be monitored to detect fatal arrhythmias. Repeat CXR is a must after the procedure.

INTRODUCTION

Pericardiocentesis is the removal of fluid from the pericardial cavity.

INDICATIONS

- *Therapeutic*—impending cardiac tamponade (Chapter 29)
- *Diagnostic*—to detect the etiology of pericardial effusion.

EQUIPMENT/PREAMBLES NEEDED

- 18/20G needle as per the patient's age
- 1% lignocaine, 2 mL, 5 mL, 10 mL syringes, 23 or 24G needles, three-way guard
- Materials and chemicals for sterile procedure (Chapter 116)
- Chest skiagram, electrocardiography (ECG), ultrasonogram of heart
- Two-dimensional echo of heart if feasible.

PROCEDURE

- Obtain consent; give sedation and analgesia as per situation.
- Monitoring—heart rate, blood pressure, respiratory rate, and SpO_2 continuously.
- Keep the patient 30° head end elevation.
- Prepare the area, anesthetize with 1% lignocaine.
- Insert 18 or 20G needle 1 cm below and left to the xiphoid process at 45°.
- Applying gentle suction, advance the needle toward the direction of the patient's left shoulder till pericardial fluid is obtained.
- Disconnect the syringe, attach a three-way guard, and aspirate the fluid.
- Monitor ECG for ST–T wave changes, QRS widening or premature ventricular beats. If such problems are observed, withdraw the needle till ECG reverts to normal and then redirect the needle if further tapping is required.
- Obtain repeat chest radiograph.
- Send the fluid for appropriate laboratory investigations (Gram stain, biochemistry, acid fast staining, culture and sensitivity, adenosine deaminase, etc.).

COMPLICATIONS

- Cardiac arrhythmias
- Pneumo/hemo/pericardium
- Pneumothorax.

CONCLUSION

Pericardiocentesis is an important procedure done in pediatric intensive care unit for diagnostic and therapeutic purposes in pericardial effusion.

Chapter 122

Ascitic Fluid Tap

S Sushamabai

ABSTRACT

Ascitic fluid tap is done for diagnostic evaluation and therapeutic relief of abdominal distension. With peritoneal tap needle and syringe attached, the midpoint between anterior superior iliac spine and umbilicus is punctured using Z tracking technique. Introduce the needle perpendicularly applying negative pressure till peritoneal fluid is obtained. Collect 10–15 mL fluid for laboratory studies. For decompression introduce a catheter through Seldinger technique. After the procedure, allow the patient to rest on lateral position with puncture site upward for 2 hours.

INTRODUCTION

Ascitic fluid tap or abdominal paracentesis is the removal of peritoneal fluid.

INDICATIONS

Therapeutic

To relieve distress in tense ascites.

Diagnostic

To assess the etiology of ascites.

REQUIREMENTS

- Ascitic fluid tap needle or over the needle catheter.
- 1% lignocaine, 23/24 G needles, 2/5 mL syringes, materials and chemicals for sterile procedure (Chapter 116).

PROCEDURE

- Keep the patient 45° head end elevation or supine position.
- Select the site for paracentesis so that the underlying viscera or blood vessels are not damaged.

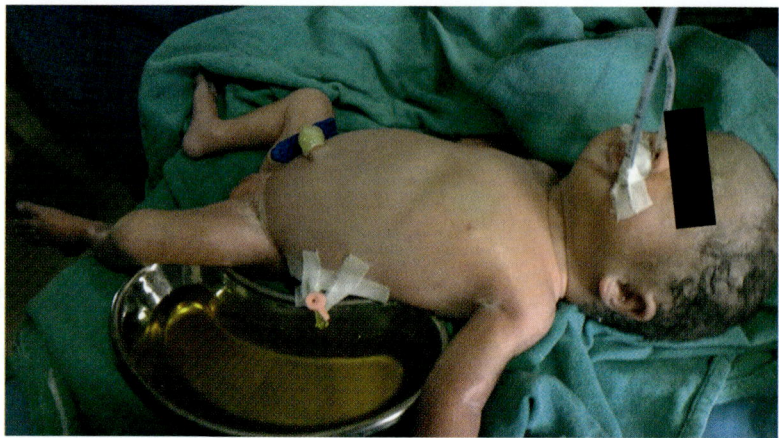

Fig. 122.1: Ascitic fluid tap.

- Ideal site is the midpoint of the line joining the anterior superior iliac spine and umbilicus on right or left iliac fossa (Fig. 122.1).
- In critically ill children, avoid the right lower quadrant since they may have cecal distension.
- Observe sterile precautions (Chapter 116). Administer local anesthesia by "Z" tracking (push the skin anteriorly to infiltrate in the subcutaneous tissue and the muscle).
- The peritoneal tap needle is then advanced in Z tracking technique perpendicular to the abdominal wall applying negative pressure until peritoneal fluid is obtained
- Aspirate 10–15 mL fluid for culture, biochemistry (protein, sugar), other investigations (amylase, lactate dehydrogenase, adenosine deaminase), cell count and gram stain.
- Replace the needle with a catheter by Seldinger method if paracentesis is done for decompression.
- Allow the patient to rest in lateral position with the puncture site up (to prevent fluid leak) for 2 hours after paracentesis.

COMPLICATIONS

- Hemorrhage
- Fluid leak
- Bowel/bladder perforation
- Hypotension (if large volume of fluid is removed)
- Infection at the puncture area or peritoneum.

CONCLUSION

Ascitic fluid tap is occasionally a procedure needed for diagnostic and therapeutic purposes in the pediatric intensive care unit.

Chapter 123

Suprapubic Urine Aspiration

S Sushamabai

ABSTRACT

The main indication is to collect noncontaminated urine for culture purpose in small children. Use 22/23G needle with 5 mL syringe attached to it. The baby should not have passed urine for 2 hours. Percuss the suprapubic area to assess the bladder distension. Palpate the symphysis pubis, plunge the needle in the midline just above the symphysis pubis and insert downward perpendicular applying continuous and gentle pressure to obtain urine.

INDICATIONS

- Diagnostic—to collect sterile urine for culture purpose.
- Therapeutic—for the evacuation of paralyzed and/or distended bladder.

EQUIPMENT AND MATERIALS

- Povidone iodine and alcohol for cleaning the puncture area
- No 22 or 23G needle
- 5 mL syringe.

PROCEDURE

- Assure that the child has not voided for 2 hours.
- Percuss the suprapubic area and ascertain dullness of the distended bladder.
- Ultrasonography-guided aspiration is of superior efficacy.
- Wash your hands and wear sterile gloves.
- Clean the suprapubic area of the patient (Chapter 116).
- Attach the needle to the syringe.
- Palpate the symphysis pubis; plunge the needle just above the symphysis pubis in the midline, insert downward perpendicularly applying continuous and gentle negative pressure to the syringe (Fig. 123.1).

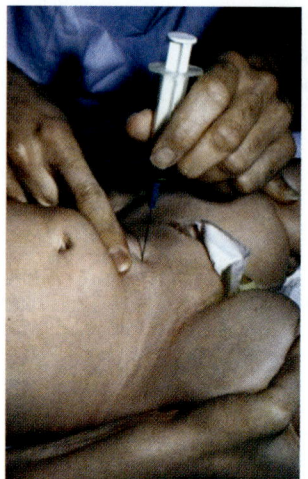

Fig. 123.1: Suprapubic aspiration.

- As the bladder is penetrated, urine enters into the syringe.
- Remove the needle and transfer the urine into a sterile container; send immediately for culture and sensitivity.

COMPLICATIONS

- Hematuria
- Perforation of bowel.

CONCLUSION

Suprapubic urine aspiration is a common procedure needed in small children to collect uncontaminated urine so that all pediatricians should master the technique.

Chapter **124**

Liver Biopsy

S Sushamabai

ABSTRACT

The indications for liver biopsy are to diagnose the etiology and to assess the progression of liver diseases. The absolute contraindication for the procedure is INR >1.5 or coagulation abnormality. Blood for transfusion should be kept ready for all patients undergoing liver biopsy irrespective of the coagulation status. Ultrasonography (USG) guided liver biopsy is ideal and better in specimen collection. The methods are Menghini 1 second liver biopsy (safer, small bit of tissue, better expertise needed) and Vim–Silverman needle biopsy (larger bit, less expertise needed but bleeding tendency more). Pathologist should be available during the procedure for observing specimen collection. Fasting for 4 hours is a must, start IV maintenance solution prior to the procedure and sedate the child. The needle is introduced at 10th intercostal space in the right midaxillary line. After the procedure, the patient should be monitored for 12 hours; the earliest evidence of bleeding is unaccountable tachycardia.

INDICATIONS

- To diagnose the etiology of asymptomatic hepatomegaly/suspected liver disease (clinically/by imaging studies/persistently abnormal liver function tests).
- To assess the progression of a known liver disease/response to therapy in chronic liver disease/drug toxicity.

CONTRAINDICATIONS

Absolute

Overt bleeding, international normalized ratio more than 1.5, low platelet count (<50,000), and bleeding diathesis.

Relative

Tense ascites, deep jaundice, peritonitis, and subphrenic or pleural effusion or infection.

PRECAUTIONS

- Blood grouping, typing, crossmatching; keep blood ready for transfusion since hemorrhage and shock can occur unexpectedly.
- In hemophiliacs, bring up factor VIII/IX level 50% for 48 hours prior to the procedure.
- Give vitamin K 5 mg intravenous daily for 3 days to prior to the biopsy.
- Ultrasonography-guided liver biopsy is safer and yields better result.
- Inform the pathologist regarding the provisional diagnosis and biopsy specimen preservation.
- Monitor and document, pulse, blood pressure (BP) and abdominal girth at the umbilicus prior to the procedure.

EQUIPMENT NEEDED

- Menghini/Vim–Silverman biopsy needles are commonly used
- For local anesthesia—23/24G needles, 2/5 mL syringes, and 1% lignocaine
- 5 or 10 mL syringe with normal saline for Menghini needle biopsy, and petri dish with saline for specimen collection
- Materials and chemicals for sterile procedure (Chapter 116)
- Specimen collection bottles with preservatives (formalin/alcohol) for specimen transport to the laboratory.

PROCEDURE

Menghini 1 Second Liver Biopsy

Menghini's 1-s liver biopsy—less traumatic, but small bit of liver tissue yield.
- Child should be fasting for 4 hours. Start intravenous maintenance solution prior to the procedure.
- Locate the site of needle introduction—10th intercostal space in the mild axillary line/subcostal or epigastric if large hepatomegaly (Fig. 124.1); clean and drape the area.
- Sedate the child with ketamine or midazolam.
- Administer local anesthesia up to the liver capsule.
- Make a stab wound of the skin with a surgical blade.
- Using the lancet make a track to the liver capsule (since the Menghini needle is blunt).

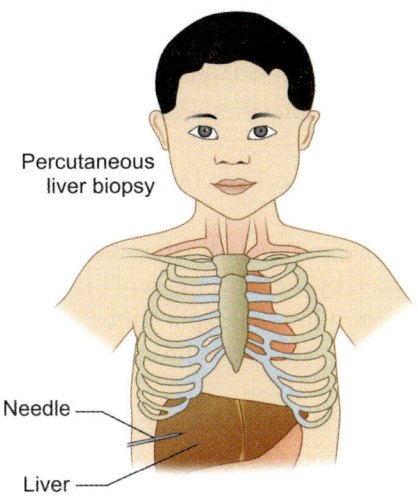

Fig. 124.1: Liver biopsy site.

- The assistant should fix the liver by firm upward pressure from the right hypochondrium.
- Assemble the inner nail inside the biopsy needle with the flat end of the inner nail at the hub of the Menghini needle.
- Attach the needle to the saline containing syringe (3 mL saline); push out the air collected through the needle.
- Through the track made by the lancet, introduce the needle, to pass through the intercostal muscle.
- As the needle pierces the liver (as evidenced by the movement of the needle with respiration), push out some saline to remove the debris in the needle.
- While applying negative pressure in the syringe by pulling the piston with your dominant hand, plunge the barrel of the piston with the needle to a distance up to 3 cm with the other hand and immediately withdraw the syringe and the needle (in 1 s). The biopsy material is obtained by the negative pressure created inside the syringe.
- Push out the saline through the needle into the petri dish. The biopsy tissue will be observed floating on saline.
- Withdraw the saline from the dish with syringe. Transfer the tissue into the preservative containing bottle using a fine needle.
- Correct labeling of the specimen bottle is needed.
- Monitor, pulse, BP, and abdominal girth of the patient every 30 minutes for 12 hours.
- Early evidence of hemorrhage is increasing tachycardia.
- The Menghini needle parts (lancet, needle, inner nail) should be carefully replaced.

Vim–Silverman Needle Biopsy

In this technique, biopsy sample is larger but hemorrhagic complication is more. Procedure up to local anesthesia administration is as for Menghini needle biopsy.

- The assistant should fix the liver by firm upward pressure from the hypochondrium.
- Introduce the outer needle along with the stylet till the capsule of the liver is pierced as evidenced by the movement of the needle with respiration.
- Remove the stylet; introduce the split inner needle through the outer needle. Advance the short outer needle up to the length of the split inner needle.
- Rotate the whole needle assembled to 90° to obtain the biopsy bit.
- Withdraw the needles together. Gently separate the large bit of liver tissue entangled between the blades of the split inner needle.
- Apply firm pressure over the puncture area for 10 minutes; seal the area.
- Place the biopsy material in the preservative fluid and label.
- Monitor the patient for 12 hours every 30 minutes as described for Menghini needle procedure.

COMPLICATIONS

- Hemorrhage and shock
- Injury to the biliary system
- Visceral perforation
- Infection.

CONCLUSION

Liver biopsy is an important procedure to diagnose the disease process and the prognosis and should be done carefully with arrangements for blood transfusion.

Section 16

PEDIATRIC DRUG FORMULARY

Chapter 125

Pediatric Drug Formulary

S Sushamabai

Drug	Dose and Route
N-acetyl cysteine	Infant: 2–4 mL q 6–8 hr; child: 6 mL q 6–8 hr,[1] Given as nebulization up to 10 mL as 10% solution (IV, PO—see Chapter 93 paracetamol poisoning)
Acetazolamide	Prevention of acute mountain sickness: 2.5 mg/kg PO q 12 hr, ceiling dose 125 mg/dose[2]
Acetylsalicylic acid	Pain, inflammation, fever: 10–15 mg/kg/dose q 4–6 hr Kawasaki's disease, acute phase: 80–100 mg/kg/24 hr div q 6 hr Rheumatic fever: 60–100 mg/kg/24 hr div q 6 hr, all PO
Adrenocorticotropic hormone	Infantile spasms: 150 U/kg/24 hr IM div q 12 hr for 2 weeks, followed by tapering in 2 weeks
Activated charcoal	Single dose: 1 g/kg, add 8 mL water/1 g or sorbitol (10%) 1 g/kg as sweetening agent; multiple dose: 0.5 g/kg q 4–6 hr for ≤24 hr PO
Acyclovir	HSV: Perinatal infections: 60 mg/kg/24 hr IV div q 8 hr × 21 days,[3] followed by oral suppressive therapy 300 mg/m² per dose × 6 months; children with HSV encephalitis and immunocompromised: 10 mg/kg IV q 8 hr as 1 hr infusion till resolution; oral dosing for HSV recurrent infections: 800 mg q 8 hr × 2 days; long-term suppressive therapy: 400 mg bid PO;[4] VZV infections: severe illness and in immunocompromised patients—500 mg/m² q 8 hr × 7–10 days or until no new lesions appear × 48 hr[5]
Adenosine	SVT: See Chapter 26
Albumin, human	Neonates 0.5–1 g/kg/dose IV, max: 1 g/kg/24 hr
Albendazole	1–2 year: 200 mg, >2 years 400 mg single dose, PO
Amlodipine	See Chapter 32
Amikacin sulfate (IV/IM)	Newborn age ≤7 days; weight: 1.2–2 kg—7.5 mg/kg q 12–18 hr; >2 kg—10 mg/kg q 12 hr; age >7 days, weight: 1.2–2 kg—7.5 mg/kg q 8–12 hr; >2 kg—10 mg/kg q 8 hr; children: 15–25 mg/kg/24 hr q 8–12 hr[3,6]

Contd...

Contd...

Drug	Dose and Route
Ammonium chloride	75 mg/kg/day div q 6 hr IV; max 6 g/day
Amoxicillin	20–50 mg/kg/24 hr div q 8–12 hour PO/IV; higher dose 80–90 mg/kg/24 hr div q 12 hr for otitis media[3,6]
Amoxicillin-clavulanate	Babies ≤28 days age: 30 mg/kg/24 hr div q 12 hour PO; children 20–45 mg/kg/24hr q 8–12 hr PO; higher dose 80–90 mg/kg/24 hr PO for otitis media or high-risk cases;[3,6] IV 30 mg/kg/dose q 8 hr[1]
Amphotericin B deoxycholate	1 mg/kg IV q 24 hr[7]
Lipid amphotericin B formulations	5 mg/kg/day IV[7]
Ampicillin (IM, IV, PO)	Newborn age ≤7days, weight ≤2 kg: 50 mg/kg/24 hr div q 12 hr (meningitis: 100 mg/kg/24 hr div q 12 hr IV); weight >2 kg: 75 mg/kg/24 hr div q 8 hr (meningitis: 150 mg/kg/24 hr IV div q 8 hr); age >7 days, weight >2 kg: 100 mg/kg/24 hr div q 6 hr (meningitis: 200 mg/kg/24 hr div q 6 hr IV or IM); children: 100–200 mg/kg/24 hr div q 6 hr (meningitis: 200–400 mg/kg/24hr div q 4–6 hr IV[3,6]
Ampicillin-sulbactam	100–200 mg/kg/24 hr div q 4–8 hr IV/IM[6]
Artesunate	2.4 mg/kg/ dose IV × 3 days at 0, 12, 24, 48 and 72 hr.[8] Should be followed by single dose of mefloquine 25 mg/kg in malaria (*see* Chapter 72).
Atropine sulfate	Bradycardia: 0.02 mg/kg (minimum 0.1 mg): IV or intratracheal (max 0.5 mg): may be repeated 5 min later;[9] Organophosphate poisoning: *See* Chapter 93A.
Atenolol	0.8–1.5 mg/kg/24 hr, max: 2 mg/kg/24 hr PO[10]
Azithromycin	First day10 mg/kg PO, then 5 mg/kg PO q 24 hr for 4 days; Group A *Streptococcus* pharyngitis—12 mg/kg/24 hr PO for 5 days.[3] *Naegleria* encephalitis: 20 mg/kg IV once daily[8]
Baclofen	0.2–2 mg/kg/24 hr div q 8 12 hr PO[11]
Betamethasone	Topical application to affected area: 2–4 times daily
Biotin	Treatment of primary biotin deficiency: 5–20 mg/day PO
Bisacodyl	5–10 mg given 6 hr before the desired effect PO
Budesonide aerosol	Inhalation 2 puffs (200 µg/puff) twice daily
British anti-Lewisite (BAL)/dimercaprol	For arsenic poisoning: 2.5–3 mg/kg/dose IM q 6 hr for 2 days, then q 12 hr on day 3 and q 24 hr for 10 days; inorganic mercury poisoning: 5 mg/kg load then 2.5 mg/kg/dose q 12–24 hr × 10 days; lead poisoning: 300–500 mg/m^2/day IM div q 4 hr × 3–5 days
Caffeine citrate	Neonate: loading dose 20 mg/kg; maintenance dose 5 mg/kg/24 hr PO/IV[12]

Contd...

Contd...

Drug	Dose and Route
Calcium gluconate	1–2 mL/kg (10% solution) IV infusion slowly under cardiac monitoring (elemental Ca 9%)
Captopril	0.3–0.5 mg/kg/dose, titrate up to maximum 6 mg/kg/24 hr div q 6–12 hr PO[12]
Carbamazepine	<6 years: 5 mg/kg/24 hr initially div q 12 hr; may increase q 5–7 days by 5 mg/kg based on effect or toxicity and serum concentration; 6–12 years: 10 mg/kg/24 hr q 12 hr initially then increase by 100 mg, or 5 mg/kg/24 hr weekly PO
Cefaclor	20–40 mg/kg/24 hr div q 8–12 hr PO (max dose 2 g)[6,12]
Cefadroxil	30 mg/kg/24 hr div q 12 hr PO (max dose 2 g)[6]
Cefoperazone	Newborns: 100 mg/kg/24 hr div q 12 hr; children: 100–150 mg/kg/24 hr div q 12 hr[3,6]
Cefpodoxime proxetil	10 mg/kg/24 hr div q 12 hr PO[13]
Cefotaxime sodium (IV/IM)	Newborns age ≤7 days: 100 mg/kg/24 hr div q 12 hr; >7 days, weight <1.2 kg: 100 mg/kg/24 hr div q 12 hr; >1.2 kg: 150 mg/kg/24 hr div q 8 hr; children: 150 mg/kg/24 hr div q 8 hr (meningitis: 200 mg/kg/24 hr div q 6 hr IV)[6,13]
Cefixime	8 mg/kg/24 hr div q 12–24 hr PO[3,6]
Cefuroxime	Neonates: 40–100 mg/kg/24 hr div q 12 hr IV or IM; children: 200–240 mg/kg/24 hr div q 8 hr IV or IM; 20–30 mg/kg/24 hr div 8 q hr PO[3,6]
Ceftazidime (IV/IM)	Babies age ≤7 days: 100 mg/kg/24 hr div q 12 hr; >7 days age, weight ≤1.2 kg: 100 mg/kg/24 hr div q 12 hr; weight >1.2 kg: 150 mg/kg/24 hr div q 8 hr; children: 150 mg/kg/24 hr div q 8 hr[6,13]
Ceftriaxone (IV/IM)	Newborns: 50–75 mg/kg q 24 hr; children: 50–75 mg/kg/24 hr; (Meningitis: 75 mg/kg as 1st dose, followed by 80–100 mg/kg/24 hr div q 12–24 hr IV or IM)[3,6]
Cefepime	100–150 mg/kg/24 hr div q 8–12 hr IV or IM[6]
Cephalexin	25–100 mg/kg/24 hr div q 6–8 hr PO[3,6]
Chloramphenicol	Newborn: 20 mg/kg OD followed 12 hr later by-postnatal age ≤7 days: 25 mg/kg/24 hr q 24 hr IV; >7 days age, ≤2 kg: 25 mg/kg/24 hr q 24 hr IV; >2 kg: 50 mg/kg/24 hr div q 12 hr IV.[6,13] children: 50–75 mg/kg/24 hr div q 6–8 hr IV or PO (meningitis: 75–100 mg/kg/24 hr div q 6 hr)[6,13]
Chloral hydrate	Neonate: 25 mg/kg/dose. Infants and children: 25–100 mg/kg/dose PO
Chloroquine	Malaria:10 mg/kg base PO (max 600 mg); then 5 mg/kg base 6 hr later; then 5 mg/kg base at 24 hr and 48 hr;[8,14] IM: 5 mg/kg initial dose, 5 mg/kg 6 hr later (max IM dose 10 mg/kg/24 hr)[8,15,16]
Chlorthiazide	10–40 mg/kg/24hr div q 12 hr PO; 4 mg/kg/24 hr IV[12]

Contd...

Contd...

Drug	Dose and Route
Chlorpheniramine maleate	2–6 years: 1 mg q 4–6 hr 6–12 years: 2 mg q 4–6 hr >12 years: 4 mg q 4–6 hr PO, IM, IV
Chlorpromazine	>6 months: 0.5–1 mg/kg/dose q 6–8 hr PO[1]
Ciprofloxacin	Neonate: 10 mg/kg q 12 hr PO or IV;[3] children: 15–30 mg/kg/24 hr div q 12 hr PO or IV; cystic fibrosis: 20–40 mg/kg/24 hr div q 8–12 hr PO, IV[6]
Citrate solution	3 mEq/kg/24 hr div q 8 hr diluted in water PO[12]
Clarithromycin	15 mg/kg/24 hr div q 12 hr[16]
Clindamycin (Neonates IM/IV)	Neonates: age ≤7 days, weight < 2 kg: 10 mg/kg/24 hr div q 12 hr; weight >2 kg: 15 mg/kg/24 hr div q 8 hr; age >7 days, weight < 1.2 kg: 10 mg/kg/24 hr div q 12 hr; 1.2–2 kg: 15 mg/kg/24 hr div q 8 hr; >2 kg: 20 mg/kg/24 hr div q 8 hr;[3,6] children: 10–40 mg/kg/24 hr div q 6–8 hr IV/IM/PO[3,6]
Clonazepam	< 10 year or < 30 kg: 0.01–0.03 mg/kg/24 hr div q 8–12 hr; >10 years or >30 kg: Initial dose up to 2.5 mg PO q 8 hr; may increase by 0.5–1 mg/day every 3 days; maintenance dose: 0.05–0.2 mg/kg/day up to 20 mg/day[17]
Clonidine	Hypertension: 5–10 µg/kg/24 hr in 2–4 div doses; max: 0.9 mg/24 hr.[18] Clonidine tolerance test for GH release: 4 µg/kg × 1 dose PO
Cromolyn sodium	Asthma: 1–2 puff (MDI) or 2 mL (Nebulizer solution) 3–4 times daily; rhinitis: 1 spray each nostril q 6–8 hr; conjunctivitis: 1–2 drops q 4–6 times/day
Cyproheptadine	2–6 years: 2 mg/dose PO q 8–12 hr; 7 years: 4 mg/dose q 8–12 hr[19]
Cloxacillin	50–100 mg/kg/24 hr PO div q 6 hr[3]
Cotrimoxazole	Trimethoprim + sulfamethoxazole (TMP–SMZ): 6 mg SMZ 20 mg TMP/kg/24 hr div q 12 hr IV/PO[3]
Deferoxamine mesylate	Acute iron intoxication: 90 mg/kg/dose IM q 8 hr; 15 mg/kg/hr IV (max 6 g/24 hr);[15] chronic iron overload: 15 mg/kg/hr (max 12 g/24 hr). IV; 40 mg/kg/24 hr SC over 8 hr[16]
Desipramine Hcl	1–3 mg/kg/24 hr PO[16]
Desmopressin (DDAVP) acetate	Nocturnal enuresis: >6 years: 0.2–0.6 mg at bed time PO
Dexamethasone	Before extubation to prevent rebound airway edema: Neonate: 0.25 mg/kg IV q 12 hr 3–4 doses (start 4 hr before extubation); children: 0.5–2 mg/kg/24 hr IV, IM, PO div q 6 hr. start 24 hr before extubation.[13] In bacterial meningitis as anti-inflammatory: 0.6 mg/kg/24 hr IV div q 6 hr on first 4 days of antibiotic therapy; start 30 minutes prior to the antibiotics.[3] Cerebral edema: loading dose 1–2 mg/kg then 1–1.5 mg/kg/24 hr;[1] IV, IM, PO div q 4–6 hr, taper over 1–6 weeks

Contd...

Contd...

Drug	Dose and Route
Dextran 40	Plasma volume expander: 20 mL/kg D1, 10 mL/kg D2–D5 IV in 20–60 min
Diazepam	Immediate control in status epilepticus: infants and children: 0.05–0.3 mg/kg/dose IV given over 2–3 min, may repeat q 30 min; maximum total dose 5–10 mg; rectal: 0.5 mg/kg, then 0.25 mg/kg in 10 min, if needed; sedation: 0.04–0.3 mg/kg IV (max 30 mg/8 hr)[20]
Diazoxide	Hyperinsulinemic hypoglycemia: Newborns and infants: 15 mg/kg/24 hr PO div q 8–12 hr;[3] children: 3–8 mg/kg/24 hr PO div q 8–12 hr;[3] hypertension: 1–3 mg/kg PO; may repeat after 5 min and then every 4 hr
Digoxin (PO)	Neonates: Loading dose 10–30 µg/kg IV, maintenance 5–10 µg/kg;[21] 1 month to 2 years: Loading dose 30 µg/kg, maintenance 10–15 µg/kg/24 hr; 2–10 years: 30 µg/kg load, 5–10 µg/kg/24 hr maintenance; >10 years: 10 µg/kg load, 2–5 µg/kg/24 hr maintenance (maintenance dose to be given div q 12 hr)[22]
Dicyclomine	Infants >6 months: 5 mg/dose PO q 6–8 hr
Diphenhydramine	5 mg/kg/24 hr div q 6 hr as needed IM, IV, PO (max 300 mg/24 hr)[3]
Dobutamine	See Chapter 25
Domperidone	0.3–0.6 mg/kg/24 hr PO div q 8 hr[3]
Dopamine	Hypotension and shock: neonates, children: 1–20 µg/kg/min IV (see Chapter 25).
Doxycycline	2–5 mg/kg/24 hr PO, IV q 12–24 hr; max: 200 mg/24 hr[6]
Enalapril	See Chapter 32
Epinephrine	Cardiac arrest, bronchospasm, anaphylactic reaction: neonate: IV, intratracheal 0.01–0.03 mg/kg (0.1–0.3 mL/kg of 1:10,000 solution) q 3–5 min; infants and children: SC 0.01 mg/kg (0.01 mL/kg/dose of 1:1,000 solution); IV—0.01 mg/kg (0.1 mL/kg of 1:1000 solution);[21] IT 0.1 mg/kg/dose (0.1 mL/kg of 1:1,000 solution);[21] continuous infusion—0.1–1 µg/kg/min as per response; nebulization: 0.25–0.5 mL of 2.25% racemic epinephrine in 3 mL NS
Erythromycin	30–50 mg/kg/24 hr PO div q 6–8 hr[6,16]
Ethambutol	20 mg/kg/24 hr PO once daily[16]
Fluconazole	See Chapter 75
Fentanyl	Narcotic analgesic for pain relief, sedation: neonates and infants: 1–4 µg/kg/dose IV, repeat q 2–4 hr or as infusion 0.5–5 µg/kg/hr; children: 1–3 µg/kg/dose IV, IM, repeat q 30–60 min or as infusion 1–5 µg/kg/hr[17]
Fludrocortisone acetate	Adrenocortical insufficiency: Infants and children: 0.05–0.2 mg/24 hr[16]
Flumazenil	Loading dose of 0.005–0.01 mg/kg IV, then continuous infusion of 0.005–0.01 mg/kg/hr (max cumulative dose 1 mg)[16]

Contd...

Contd...

Drug	Dose and Route
Folic acid	Treatment of folic acid anemia: PO Neonates—6 months: 25–35 μg/24 hr; 6 months to 3 years: 50 μg/24 hr; 4–6 years: 75 μg/24 hr; 7–10 years: 100 μg/24 hr;[12] 11–14 years: 150 μg/24 hr;[12] >15 years: 200 μg/24 hr; folic acid deficiency: 1 mg/24 hr
Fosphenytoin	See Chapter 35
Furosemide	Premature infants: 0.5–2 mg/kg IV or 4 mg/kg PO q 12–48 hr (dose to response);[1] infants and children: 1–2 mg/kg IV or 1–4 mg/kg PO q 6–24 hr or continuous infusion (start at 0.05 mg/kg/hr and adjust dose to response)[16]
Gabapentin	2–12 years: 15–35 mg/kg/24 hr PO div q 8 hr, max 50 mg/kg/24 hr;[3] >12 years: start 300 mg daily, then increase by 300 mg daily,[1] max: 3,600 mg/24 hr div q 8 hr
Gentamicin	Neonates: ≤7 days, 1,200–2,000 g: 2.5 mg/kg IV/IM q 12–18 hr; >2,000 g: 2.5 mg/kg q 12 hr; children: 7.5 mg/kg/24 hr div q 8–12 hr; may administer 5–7.5 mg/kg/24 hr IV/IM once daily[6]
Glucagon	Hypoglycemia: neonates: 0.3 mg/kg/dose (max 1 mg) IV, IM, SC; children: 0.025–0.1 mg/kg/dose (max 1 mg), repeat in 20 min[22]
Glycopyrrolate	Anticholinergic, inhibits salivation; 40–100 μg/kg/dose PO q 6–8 hr;[1] 4–10 μg/kg/dose IM/IV q 3–4 hr
Haloperidol	3–12 years: start 0.25–0.5 mg/24 hr div q 8–12 hr, increase weekly by 0.25–0.5 mg daily based on response to max 0.15 mg/kg/24 hr[12]
Heparin	See Chapter 87
Homatropine hydrobromide	2% solution 1 drop for mydriasis, repeat q 10 min as needed
Hydralazine	Neonates: 0.1–0.5 mg/kg/dose IV q 6–8 hr; 0.25–1 mg/kg/dose PO q 6–8 hr; infants and children: start 0.1–0.2 mg/kg/dose IV/IM q 4–6 hr;[19] titrate to effect to maximum dose of 3.5 mg/kg/24 hr; 0.75–1 mg/kg/24 hr PO div q 6–12 hr, max 7.5 mg/kg/24 hr[22]
Hydrocortisone	Neonates, infants and young children: acute adrenal insufficiency: see Chapter 49; maintenance therapy: give doses as ¼ at am, ¼ at noon and ½ at night; anti-inflammatory: 1–5 mg/kg/24 hr IV/IM in 1–2 doses;[3] 2.5–10 mg/kg/24 hr PO div q 6–8 hr; Shock: 50 mg/kg/dose IV q 4 hr: See Chapter 25
Hydrochlorothiazide	Neonates and infants: 2–4 mg/kg/24 hr PO div q 12 hr; infants >6 months and children: 2 mg/kg/24 hr div q 12 hr[3]
Hydroxyzine	0.6 mg/kg/dose IM/PO q 6 hr[22]
Hyoscyamine hydrobromide	0.1 mL/kg/dose PO q 4 hr max 5 mL or 1 tab q 8 hr[22]
Ibuprofen	Pain, fever: 5–10 mg/kg/dose PO q 6–8 hr;[12] JIA: 50 mg/kg/24 hr div q 6 hr[3]

Contd...

Contd...

Drug	Dose and Route
Immunoglobulin IV	Neonate: 500–750 mg/kg one dose; children: immunodeficiency syndromes: 100–400 mg/kg/dose q 2–4 weeks;[19] ITP: 1 g/kg/dose for 2–5 consecutive days, then q 3–6 weeks;[22] Kawasaki disease: 2 g/kg/single dose;[22] severe systemic infection: 500–1,000 mg/kg/week;[22] cytomegalovirus infection: 500 mg/kg/dose q on alternate day for 7 doses;[22] chronic lymphocytic leukemia: 400 mg/kg/dose q 3 weeks;[22] polyneuropathy: 1 g/kg/24 hr for 2 consecutive days monthly[22]
Indomethacin	PDA: neonates: 0.10–0.25 mg/kg/dose IV q 12 hr for 3–6 doses.[22] Rheumatoid diseases: 1–2 mg/kg/24 hr PO div q 6–12 hr (max 4 mg/kg/24 hr)[16,22]
Insulin	Neonates: regular insulin 0.01 U/kg/hr by continuous IV infusion or SC 0.1–0.2 U/kg q 6 hr;[20] children and adults: 0.5–1 U/kg/24 hr; adjust dose to blood glucose and HbA1C value;[12] adolescents: 0.8–1.2 U/kg/24 hr [DKA: continuous infusion 0.1 U/kg/hr adjusted to serum glucose value (Chapter 48); hyperkalemia: give calcium gluconate and $NaHCO_3$ first, then dextrose 50% 0.5–1 mL/kg and regular insulin 1 U/5g dextrose (Chapter 53)]
Ipratropium bromide	Neonates: nebulization 100 µg/dose or MDI 1–2 puffs tid-qid; infants and children: nebulization 125–250 µg or MDI 1–2 puffs 3–6 times daily; >5 years: 500 µg q 6 hr[22]
Iron (elemental)	For prevention of anemia: 1–2 mg/kg/24 hr PO;[12] deficiency: 3–6 mg/kg/24 hr PO div q 8–12 hr[22]
Isoniazid	5–10 mg/kg/24 hr PO as q d. max: 300 mg[13]
Ivermectin	Choice drug for strongyloidiasis: 200 µg/kg /day PO × 2 days[8]
Ketorolac	For analgesia: 2–16 years: IV, IM 0.4–1 mg/kg/dose; PO 1 mg/kg/dose q 6 hr as needed.[22]
Labetalol	Children: Start 4 mg/kg/24 hr PO div q 12 hr, then gradually increase (max 40 mg/kg/24 hr);[12,18] IV start 0.2–1 mg/kg/dose (max 20 mg/dose); continuous infusion of 0.4–1 mg/kg/hr (max 2 mg/kg/hr)
Lactulose	Hepatic encephalopathy, constipation: to yield 2–3 loose stools/day; infants: 2.5–10 mL/24 hr PO in 3–4 doses; children: 40–90 mL/24 hr in 3–4 doses[10]
Lamotrigine (PO)	2–12 years: 0.6 mg/kg/24 hr in 1–2 doses for 2 weeks; increase to 1.2 mg/kg/24 hr div q 12 hr for 2 weeks;[10] depending on response can increase the dose up to 5–15 mg /kg/24 hr div q 12 hr (max dose 400 mg/24 hr).[3,22] For patients on valproate: 0.15 mg/kg/24 hr in 1–2 doses for 2 weeks, increase to 0.3 mg/kg/24 hr in 2 doses for 2 weeks, up to 1–5 mg/kg/24 hr in 2 doses[22,23]
L-carnitine	Premature infants: 8–16 mg/kg/24 hr IV infusion;[12] children: 50–100 mg/kg/24 hr in 2–3 div doses PO, 50 mg/kg/dose q 4–6 hr IV[22]
Lansoprazole	15–30 mg/day administered early morning PO[22]

Contd...

Contd...

Drug	Dose and Route
Levamisole	Immunopotentiation: 2 mg/kg/day PO × 3 days/week for 4–6 weeks[20,22]
Levothyroxine	Thyroid replacement therapy: PO 0–6 months: 8–10 µg/kg/24 hr; 6–12 months: 6–8 µg/kg/24 hr; 1–5 years: 5–6 µg/kg/24 hr; 6–12 years: 4–5 µg/kg/24hr; >12 years: 2–3 µg/kg/24 hr;[22] IV, IM 50–75% of PO dose. Myxedema coma: 200–500 µg for 1 dose Thyroid suppression therapy: 2–6 µg/kg/24 hr × 7–10 days[12]
Linezolid	10 mg/kg q 12 hr IV, PO[3]
Lidocaine	Arrhythmias: children: loading dose of 1 mg/kg (may repeat q 5–10 min, max 3 mg/kg);[22] IV continuous infusion: 20–50 µg/kg/min;[12] ET route: 2–2.5 × IV dose[22]
Loratadine	< 3 years < 30 kg: 5 mg/24 hr, >30 kg: 10 mg/24 hr (0.2 mg/kg/day OD)[22]
Lorazepam	Status epilepticus: See Chapter 35 Neonates: 0.05–0.2 mg/kg/dose IV over 2–5 min, repeat in 10–15 min; infants and children: loading dose of 0.1 mg/kg IV over 2–5 min; give additional 0.05 mg/kg bolus in 10–15 min if needed[12]
Magnesium hydroxide	Constipation: given once daily PO < 2 years: 0.5 mL/kg/dose;[12] 2–5 years: 5–15 mL; 6–12 years: 15–30 mL; >12 years: 30–60 mL[22]
Magnesium sulfate	Hypomagnesemia: Neonates: 25–50 mg/kg/dose IV q 8 hr for 2–3 doses;[1] children: 100–200 mg/kg/dose PO q 6 hr; 25–50 mg/kg/dose IV/IM q 6 hr × 3–4 doses;[20] daily maintenance: neonates, infants and children: IV 30–60 mg/kg/24 hr; Seizure, hypertension: children: 20–100 mg/kg/dose IV/ IM q 4–6 hr as needed;[1] acute asthma: (as third-line drug): 30–50 mg/kg in 30 mL NS as IV infusion in 30 min[10]
Mannitol	Raised ICP, promotion of diuresis: IV test dose 200 mg/kg, initial 0.5–1 g/kg, maintenance 0.25–0.5 g/kg q 4–6 hr;[12] (or 20% solution 2.5–5 mL/kg in 10–15 min)
Mebendazole	Pinworm: 100 mg PO once, repeat after 2 weeks; roundworm, hookworm, whipworm—100 mg PO q 12 hr for 3 consecutive days;[1] 2nd course, if needed, after 3–4 weeks
Methadone	Newborns (abstinence syndrome): 0.05–0.2 mg/kg/dose q 12 hr, adjust or taper as per response;[24] children: analgesia: IV, IM, PO: 0.1 mg/kg/dose q 4 hr 2–3 doses, followed by q 6–12 hr as needed[22]
Metolazone	0.2–0.4 mg/kg/24 hr PO as single or 2 div doses[12]
Metoprolol	1–5 mg/kg/24 hr PO[16]
Meropenem	Children: 60 mg/kg/24 hr IV div q 8 hr (meningitis: 120 mg/kg/24 hr div q 8 hr, max: 6 g/24 hr)[6]

Contd...

Contd...

Drug	Dose and Route
Metronidazole	35–50 mg/kg/24 hr PO/IV div q 6–8 hr[8]
Methotrexate	JIA: 5–15 mg/m2/week PO/IM as a single dose[25]
Methylene blue	Cyanide poisoning, drug-induced methemoglobinemia: 1–2 mg/kg IV over 5–10 min; may repeat after 1 hr if needed[22]
Methylphenidate	Attention deficit disorder: >5 years: 0.3–0.6 mg/kg/dose PO (max 2 mg/kg/24 hr)[22]
Methylprednisolone	Anti-inflammatory and immune suppression: 0.5–2 mg/kg/24 hr IV/IM/PO div q 6–12 hr; pulse dose: 30 mg/kg in 30 mL NS as infusion in 30 min daily; acute spinal cord injury: pulse dose infusion in 15 min followed in 45 min by continuous infusion of 5.4 mg/kg/hr for 23 hr[22]
Midazolam	Status epilepticus: See Chapter 35 Intranasal: 2.5 mg (0.5 mL) in each naris for seizure prevention[22]
Montelukast	Asthma long-term therapy: 2–5 years: 4 mg OD, 6–14 years: 5 mg OD, >15 years: 10 mg OD; PO, evening[22]
Morphine sulfate	Newborns: for pain relief: 0.05 mg/kg/dose IV q 2–4 hr;[16] continuous infusion 0.025–0.5 mg/kg/hr; infants and children: 0.1–0.2 mg/kg/dose IV/IM/SC q 2–4 hr; 0.2–0.5 mg/kg/dose PO q 4–6 hr[22]
Mefloquine	Malaria treatment: PO 15 mg/kg (max 750 mg) followed by 10 mg/kg 12 hr later;[8] prophylaxis: 5 mg/kg (max 250 mg) weekly once
Naloxone	Newborns, infants and children: 0.1 mg/kg IV (max dose 2 mg); can repeat the dose q 2–3 min until desired effect is observed; continuous infusion in severe painful situations[22]
Naproxen	5–7 mg/kg PO q 8–12 hr[1]
Nalidixic acid	50–55 mg/kg/24 hr PO div q 6 hr; suppressive therapy: 25–33 mg/kg/24 hr div q 6–8 hr[3]
Neomycin sulfate	Infants: 50 mg/kg/24 hr PO div q 6 hr; children: 50–100 mg/kg/24 hr div q 6–8 hr[3,6]
Niclosamide	As an alternative drug: beef and fish tapeworm: 50 mg/kg, PO once;[8] dwarf tapeworm: 11–34 kg: 1 g D1 then 500 mg/day × 6 days; >34 kg:1.5 g D1, then 1 g/day × 6 days, all PO[8]
Nifedipine	See Chapter 32 Hypertrophic cardiomyopathy: 0.2–0.3 mg/kg PO q 8 hr[22]
Nitrofurantoin	PO 5–7 mg/kg/24 hr div q 6 hr max: 400 mg/24 hr; suppressive therapy: 1–2.5 mg/kg/24 hr q 12–24 hr; max: 100 mg/day[22]
Neostigmine methylsulfate	See Chapter 41

Contd...

Contd...

Drug	Dose and Route
Nitroprusside sodium	See Chapter 32
Norepinephrine bitartrate	See Chapter 25
Ofloxacin	15 mg/kg/day PO div q 12 hr[14]
Ondansetron	0.15 mg/kg/dose PO/IV q 8 hr;[16] 0.45 mg/kg/24 hr as IV infusion[22]
Oxcarbazepine	8–10 mg/kg/day PO div q 12 hr;[22] increase over 2 weeks to 30–40 mg/kg/24 hr[12]
Pancreatin	Dose titrated to desirable stool frequency and consistency
Paracetamol or acetaminophen	10–15 mg/kg/dose q 4–6 hr PO, PR, IM[22]
Pentazocine	>14 years: 50 mg q 3–4 hr max dose 600 mg/day; for IV / IM reduce oral dose by 1/3;[22]
Phenylephrine	Nasal decongestant:[22] Infants: 1–2 drops per nare q 3–4 hr 0.16% solution; children: 1–6 year: 1–2 drops/spray per nare q 3–4 hr 0.125% solution; 6–12 years: 1–2 drops/spray per nare q 3–4 hr 0.25% solution; >12 years: 1–2 drops/spray per nare q 3–4 hr 0.25–0.5% solution
Phytonadione (vitamin K1)	1–2 mg/dose IM/IV/SC; PO 2.5 mg[10]
Penicillin G	1–2.5 lakhs U/kg/24 hr div q 4–6 hr IV/IM (max: 4 lakhs units/kg/24 hr)[6]
Penicillin G benzathine (IM)	Newborns weight >1.2 kg: 50,000 U/kg single dose; children: 3 lakhs to 1.2 million Units/kg q 3–4 weeks, max: 1.2–2.4 million Units/dose[3,5,12]
Penicillin G procaine (IM)	Newborns weight <1.2 kg: 50,000 U/kg/24 hr; children: 25,000–50,000 U /kg/24 hr (max dose: 4.8 million U/dose); gonorrhea: 100,000 U/kg (max: dose 4.8 million U/24 hr) single dose with probenecid 25 mg/kg (max dose: 1 g)[6]
Penicillin V	25–50 mg/kg /24/hr div q 4–6 hr PO[6]
Phenazopyridine	12 mg/kg/24 hr PO div q 8 hr[16,22]
Permethrin	Scabies: apply and leave on for 8–16 hr followed by wash with water
Pethidine	1–2 mg/kg/dose IM or IV[10]
Pralidoxime	Children: 20–50 mg/kg/dose IV/IM; repeat dose after 1–2 hr if muscle weakness is persisting.[15] Continue dose q 12 hr till muscle weakness recovers: See Chapter 93A
Prazosin	See Chapter 94(2) 0.1 mg/kg/24 hr PO div q 6 hr titrating dose to desired blood pressure;[12] max dose: 0.4 mg/kg/24 hr or 15 mg total dose[22]
Prednisolone	Asthma: Children: 0.5–4 mg/kg/24 hr PO, IV div q 6–12 hr;[3,22] Anti-inflammatory: 0.1–2 mg/kg/24 hr PO, IV div q 6–24 hr[3]

Contd...

Contd...

Drug	Dose and Route
Piperacillin	Neonates ≤7 days: 150 mg/kg/24 hr IV div q 8–12 hr;[6] >7 days: 200 mg/kg/24 hr div q 6–8 hr IV;[6] children 200–300 mg/kg/24 hr IV div q 4–6 hr[3] (cystic fibrosis: 350–500 mg/kg/24 hr IV)
Piperacillin-tazobactum	Children 300–400 mg/kg/24 hr IV/IM div q 6–8 hr[3,6]
D-Penicillamine	Wilson disease: dose titrated to maintain >1 mg/24 hr of urinary Cu excretion;[22] infants and children: 20 mg/kg/24 hr PO q 6–12 (max dose: 1 g/24 hr);[22] lead intoxication: infants and children: 30–40 mg/kg/24 hr PO div q 8–12 hr (max 1.5 g/24 hr)[3]
Phenobarbital	Seizure loading dose: refer Chapter 35, 104; maintenance dose: neonates: 3–4 mg/kg/24 hr PO/IV div q 12–24 hr; children and adults: 5–6 mg/kg/24 hr PO/IV div q 12–24 hr[3] Sedation: children: 2 mg/kg/dose PO, IV[22]
Phenoxybenzamine	Pheochromocytoma: Children: 3–8 mg/kg/24 hr, titrate to desired effect on BP[12]
Primaquine–malaria	Therapy: 0.5 mg base/kg/24hr PO once daily for 14 days; Prevention: 0.6 mg/kg base daily[8]
Promethazine	Motion sickness: 0.5 mg/kg/dose PO 30–60 min before departure, then q 8–12 hr as needed[1,22]
Propoxyphene	2–3 mg/kg/24 hr PO div q 4–6 hr[3,22]
Propranolol	Cardiac arrhythmias: See Chapter 26 Migraine prophylaxis: children: 0.6–2 mg/kg/24 hr PO div q 6–8 hr (max 4 mg/kg/24 hr)[14]
Prostaglandin E1	For keeping the ductus arteriosus patent in the newborn and as afterload reducer in shock: 0.01–0.2 μg/kg/min IV infusion; maintenance 0.01 μg/kg/min[15]
Pyridostigmine	Myasthenia gravis: See Chapter 41
Pyridoxine	Dependent seizures: 100–200 mg IV/IM/PO; maintenance dose 100–200 mg/day PO; drug-induced neuritis: 1 mg/kg/24 hr q 24 hr; dietary deficiency: 5 mg/24 hr for 3–4 weeks[16]
Quinine sulfate	30 mg/kg/24hr PO q 8 hr 3–7 days with another antimalarial agent[8]
Quinupristin/dalfopristin	For vancomycin resistant *Enterococcus faecium* (VRE) and MRSA: 7.5 mg/kg dose IV q 8 hr[1,6]
Ranitidine	1–5 mg/kg/dose PO, IM, IV q 8 hr; may be given as continuous infusion[1]
Rifampicin	10 mg/kg/24 hr single dose on empty stomach PO (max: 600 mg)
Risperidone	0.25 mg q 12 hr PO, increase per response to 3 mg q 8 hr[22]
Salbutamol	0.1 mg/kg/dose PO q 8 hr;[16] inhalation: 1–6 puffs of 100 μg q 2–6 hr; 4–6 μg/kg/dose SC, IM, IV q 6–8 hr
Sodium polystyrene sulfonate	4 mg/kg/24 hrs PO div q 4–8 hr[22]

Contd...

Contd...

Drug	Dose and Route
Sodium thiosulfate	1 g thiosulfate for every 100 mg nitroprusside IV, infuse in same IV line[22]
Spironolactone	1–3 mg/kg/24 hr PO div q 8–24 hr
Streptokinase	*See* Chapter 22 for intrapleural instillation
Streptomycin	15–20 mg/kg/24 hr IM div q 12 hr[3]
Sucralfate	40–80 mg/kg/24 hr PO div q 6–8 hr[3,22]
Terbutaline sulfate	< 12 years: 0.01 mg/kg/dose SC/IV, max 0.5 mg, can repeat in 15–20 min; 0.05 mg/kg/dose PO q 8 hr, max 5 mg; >12 years: 0.25 mg/dose SC, can repeat in 15 min; 2.5 mg/dose PO q 6–8 hr[1]
Terfenadine	3–6 years: 15 mg bid PO; 6–12 years: 30 mg bid; >12 years: 60 mg bid[22]
Tetanus antitoxin	Prophylaxis: 3,000–5,000 units IM after skin test; treatment: 50,000–100,000 units ½ IM and ½ IV
Tetanus immunoglobulin	Treatment: 500–6000 units IM. Prophylaxis: 4 U/kg IM
Theophylline	Neonatal apnea: *See* Chapter 109 As a bronchodilator: PO 6 weeks to 6 months: 10 mg/kg/24 hr div q 6–8 hr;[5] 6 months to 1 year: 12–18 mg/kg/24 hr div q 6–8 hr;[5] 1–9 years: 20–24 mg/kg/24 hr div q 6–8 hr;[12] >9 years: 13–16 mg/kg/24 hr div q 6–8 hr[22]
Thiamine	10–25 mg/24 hr IM/IV div q 6–8 hr
Thiopental sodium	Sedation: 5–10 mg/kg/dose IV; seizures: 2–3 mg/kg/dose IV, repeat as needed; raised ICP: 1.5–5 mg/kg/dose IV[22,23]
Tiagabine	>2 years: PO 0.5–2 mg/kg/day div q 6–12 hr; adolescents: starting dose 4 mg daily, increase by 4–8 mg q week until response (max: 56 mg/week)[15]
Topiramate	2–16 years: start 1–3 mg/kg/24 hr PO for 1 week;[12] increase 1–2 week by 1–3 mg/kg/24 hr;[10] administer q 12 hr up to 5–10 mg/kg/24 hr div q 12 hr[22,23]
Tropicamide	0.5% instill 1–2 drops for mydriasis; may repeat in 5 min
Urokinase	*See* Chapter 22 for intrapleural administration
Ursodeoxycholic acid	Neonate: 10–18 mg/kg/24 hr PO div q 8–24 hr; infants: 30 mg/kg/24 hr PO div q 8–12 hr[13,22]
Vancomycin IV	Neonates ≤7 days, < 1,200 g: 15 mg/kg/24 hr q 24 hr; 1,200–2,000 g: 15 mg/kg/24 hr div q 12–18 hr; >2000 g: 30 mg/kg/24 hr div q 12 hr; >7 days < 1,200 g: 15 mg/kg/24 hr div q 24 hr; 1,200–2,000 g: 15 mg/kg/24 hr div q 8–12 hr; >2,000 g: 45 mg/kg/24 hr div q 8 hr; children: 45–60 mg/kg/24 hr div q 6–8 hr[3,6,13]

Contd...

Contd...

Drug	Dose and Route
Valproic acid	Neonates: refractory seizures: loading dose 20 mg/kg PO, then 10 mg/kg/dose q 12 hr. Children: seizures: 10–15 mg/kg/24 hr div q 8–12 hr; may need up to 100 mg/kg/day div q 6–8 hr especially when used with concurrent enzyme inducers (phenytoin)[24]
Varicella zoster immunoglobulin	125 units (1 vial) for each 10 kg body weight IM (≤2 kg ½ vial) as early as possible after exposure to varicella, may be effective up to 10 days[5]
Vasopressin	Diabetes insipidus: 2.5–10 U/dose IM, SC 2–4 times/24 hr Gastrointestinal (GI) hemorrhage— (*See* Chapter 66)
Vecuronium	*See* Chapter 8
Vigabatrin	Infantile spasm, partial seizure: 50–150 mg/kg/24 hr PO div q 12–24 hour[3]
Xylometazoline	2–12 years: instill 2–3 drops 0.05% solution in each nostril q 8–10 hr (nasal drops 0.05%, 0.1%) >12 years: instill 2–3 drops 0.1% solution in each nostril q 8–10 hr[14]
Zinc	Zinc deficiency: infants and children: 0.5–1 mg/kg/24 hr PO in 1–3 doses. TPN supplement: preterm: 400 µg/kg/24 hr; infants < 3 months: 250 µg/kg/24 hr; >3 months: 100 µg/kg/24 hr; children: 50 µg/kg/24 hr[22]

REFERENCES

1. Deglin JH, Vallerand AH. Drug monographs in alphabetical order by generic name. Davis's Drug Guide for Nurses, 11th edition. Philadelphia: F.A. Davis Company; 2008.
2. Neirmeyer.S, Yaron M. Altitude associated illness in children. Nelson Textbook of Pediatrics. Philadelphia: Elsevier; 2016.
3. https://archive.org/stream/nelson20/1102_djvu.txt. [Accessed September, 2018].
4. Stanberry LR. Herpes Simplex Virus. In: Stanton Bonita F, Kleigman Robert M, Joseph G (Eds). Nelson Textbook of Pediatrics; 2016. pp. 1572-9.
5. La Russa PS, Marin M. Varicella Zoster Virus. Nelson Textbook of Pediatrics, 19th edition. Philadelphia: Elsevier; 2016.
6. Schleiss MR. Principles of Antibacterial Therapy. In: Kleigman RM, Behrman RE, Jenson HB (Eds). Nelson Textbook of Pediatrics, 18th edition. Philadelphia, PA: WB Saunders; 2016.
7. Steinbach WJ, Cohen-Wolkowiez, Benjamin Jr DK. Principles of Antifungal Therapy. Nelson Textbook of Pediatrics, 19th edition. Philadelphia: Elsevier; 2016.
8. Schleiss MR. Principles of Antiparasitic Therapy. Nelson Textbook of Pediatrics. Philadelphia: Elsevier; 2016.
9. http://www.beyazhastane.com/Print.aspx?Ctrl=HTML&HTMLID=40. [Accessed September, 2018].
10. http://www.alhadapedia.com/hospen/Edu/PDFbks/pedoncall.pdf. [Accessed September, 2018].
11. Johnston MV. Cerebral Palsy. Nelson Textbook of Pediatrics; 2016.

12. Lee Carlton KK, Megan M, Krishnan M, et al. Drug Doses. The Harriet Lane Handbook; 2012.
13. Mark RS. Principles of Antibacterial Therapy. Nelson Textbook of Pediatrics, 2011.
14. http://dokumen.tips/documents/daftar-indonesiapdf.htm. [Accessed September, 2018].
15. http://www.onestopnursing.org/wp-content/uploads/2015/06/Saunders-Nursing-Drug-handbook-2014.pdf. [Accessed September, 2018].
16. http://documents.mx/science/harriet-lane-20-ed.html. [Accessed September, 2018].
17. UIIrich.C, Duncan J, Joselow M, et al. Pediatric Palliative Care. In: R Kleigman, B Stanson, J St. Geme (Eds). Nelson Textbook of Pediatrics, 20th edition. Philadelphia: Elsevier; 2016. pp. 256-67.
18. Lande MB. Systemic Hypertension. In: RM Kleigman, BF Stanton, JW St. Geme, (Eds). Nelson Textbook of Pediatrics. Philadelphia: WB Saunders; 2016.
19. Kishore D Phadke, Paul Goodyer, Martin Bitzan, et al. Manual of Pediatric Nephrology. Berlin: Springer; 2014.
20. http://www.docstoc.com/docs/417843/Pediatric_ Drug_ Reference. [Accessed September, 2018].
21. http://necipfazildh.saglik.gov.tr/index.php/kaliteyonetim/dokumanlar/send/52-Is/530-pediatrik-dozlari-olari-listesi.html. [Accessed September, 2018].
22. Gal P, Reed MD. Medications. Nelson Textbook of Pediatrics, 18th edition. Saunders: Elsevier; 2007.
23. http://www.federaljack.com/ebooks/My%20collection%20off%medical%20books.%2028%20books%20%28part%202%20off%203%29/clinician%27s%20Pocket%20Reference_0838515525.pdf (Internet from 21-Apr-2016). [Accessed September, 2018].
24. LSU Health. Pediatrics Residency. [Online] Available from http://www.medschool.lsuhsc.edu/pediatrics/residents/docs/HemeOncGuidelinesWebsiteversion.doc. [Accessed September, 2018].
25. Robinson NE. Table of Common Drugs and Approximate Dosages. Amsterdam: Elsevier; 2015.

Index

Page numbers followed by *b* refer to box, *f* refer to figure,
fc refer to flowchart, and *t* refer to table

A

AACI *See* Acute adrenocortical insufficiency
ABC *See* Airway, breathing and circulation
Abdominal injuries, blunt 328
Abdominal pain 227, 298
ABG *See* Arterial blood gas
Abscess, epidural 192
Accidents 421
ACE *See* Angiotensin-converting enzyme
ACEI *See* Angiotensin-converting enzyme inhibitor
Acetaminophen 217, 447, 564
 poisoning 308
Acetazolamide 555
Acetylsalicylic acid 418, 555
ACHD *See* Acyanotic congenital heart diseases
Acid 447
Acid-base
 disurbances, interpretation of 77*fc*
 gases 72
Acidosis
 causes of 291
 correction of 294
Acinetobacter 371
Acquired immunodeficiency syndrome 273
Acute adrenocortical insufficiency 232, 234
 differential diagnosis 233
 etiology 232
 management, algorithm of 234*fc*
Acute laryngotracheobronchitis 95, 99
Acute respiratory distress syndrome 89, 124, 339, 356, 423, 427, 434
 causes 124
 chest skiagram 125
 clinical presentation 125
 clinical stages 125
 CT scan chest 126
 investigations 125
 management 126
 pathophysiology 125
Acyanotic congenital heart diseases 146
Acyclovir 555
Addison disease 131, 232, 248, 250, 292
Adenosine 38, 47, 555
Adherent labia 300
Adrenal hyperplasia, congenital 251, 252, 292
Adrenal insufficiency 246
Adrenaline 47, 56, 106
Adrenergic stimulation, late phase of 458
Adrenocorticotropic hormone 555
Advanced life support 24, 31
 pediatric 31
 steps in 31
AED *See* Automated external defibrillator
AEP *See* Asthma education program
Airway 32, 178
 breathing, circulation 234, 327, 443, 445
 disease 91
 laryngeal mask 32
 nasopharyngeal 32
 obstruction, treatment of 97
 oropharyngeal 32
 positioning of 45
 protection of 44
Albendazole 555
Albumin 555
Alkalis 448

ALS *See* Advanced life support
ALTB *See* Acute laryngotracheobronchitis
Aluminum phosphide rat poison 451
Amanita poisoning 308
Ambu bag 61, 61*f*
Amikacin 118
    sulfate 555
Amino acidopathy 262
Aminomethane 74
Amiodarone 38, 47, 432
Amitriptyline 218
Amlodipine 164, 555
Ammonium chloride 556
Amoxicillin 154, 556
    clavulanate 556
Amphotericin B deoxycholate 556
Ampicillin 111, 505, 556
    sulbactam 556
Anaphylaxis 54, 57, 397
    differential diagnosis 55
    etiology 54
    investigations 55
    manifestations 54
    onset 55
    patient approach 55
    treatment, algorithm for 56*fc*
Anemia 289, 413 414, 514
    in newborns 514
        clinical presentation 515
        common causes 514
        treatment 515
    mild 237
    moderate 237
    severe 236, 237, 276, 393
Anesthesia 434
    bags 62
Angioedema 95, 96
Angiotensin-converting enzyme 150, 152
    inhibitor 143, 146
Anion gap metabolic acidosis
    increased 76
    normal 76
Antibiotic 47
    Acute Illness Observation Scale
Anticoagulant protein 389
Anticoagulant therapy 416

Anticonvulsants 47
Antifungal agents 372
Antiganglioside antibodies 193
Antihistamines 448
Antimicrobial prophylaxis 300
Antinuclear antibody 198
Antituberculosis 306
Aorta, coarctation of 143
Aplastic crisis 406
Apnea 222, 496
    in newborns 509
        common causes 509
        management 510
    of prematurity, treatment of recurrent 511*fc*
    test 222
Apneic neonate, clinical approach to 510*fc*
ARDS *See* Acute respiratory distress syndrome
Areflexia 191
Arsenic 450
Artemether 354
Artemisinin combination therapy 352, 355, 357
Arterial blood gas 32, 51, 74, 121, 126, 132, 143, 425, 444, 487, 536
    analysis 63, 74
        indications for 74
Artesunate 354, 556
Arthritis 368, 464
Ascites 332
    abdominal distension 333
    clinical presentation 333
    common causes of 332*b*
    fluid examination 334
    subsequent treatment 334
Ascitic fluid tap 545, 546*f*
    complications 546
    diagnostic 545
    indications 545
    procedure 545
    requirements 545
    therapeutic 545
Aseptic meningitis 358
Aspergillosis 364, 366
Aspiration 118

Aspirin 217, 416, 418
Assist-control mode 86, 86*f*
Asthma 341
   acute 100
      life-threatening 100, 103
      pathophysiology 100
      patient approach 101
   education program 104
   exacerbation 101
   management, algorithm for acute
      104*fc*
   triad of 100
Asystole 36*f*
   management of 37*fc*
Atenolol 556
Atracurium 432
Atrial fibrillation, treatment of 141
Atrial flutter, treatment of 141
Atropine 37, 43, 432
   sulfate 47, 556
Autoimmune
   disease 232, 305, 328
      encephalitis 195
      hepatitis 308
Automated external defibrillator 23, 24
Azathioprine 328
Azithromycin 109, 154, 360, 361, 556

B

Baby inside oxygen hood 61*f*
Back blows, method of 27, 28*f*, 29*f*
Baclofen 556
Bacterial dysentery 317
Bacterial infection, antibiotic for 158
Bacterial meningitis 185, 187
   acute 185
      differential diagnosis 186
      empirical antibiotic therapy 187
      pathophysiology 185
Bacterial peritonitis, spontaneous 332
Bacterial pneumonia, antibiotic therapy
   of 116
Bacterial tracheitis, acute 95, 96
Bag and mask ventilation 32-34
Barbiturates 448
Barium study 121

Bartter and Gitelman syndrome 253
Basic life support 23, 24, 31
Bee and wasp stinging 461
Belladona alkaloids 448
Benzathine penicillin IM 157
Benzoate therapy 260
Benzodiazepines 178
Benzyl benzoate 448
Benzylpenicillin 114
Beta blockers 145, 448
Betamethasone 556
Bicarbonate 294
Biliary system, injury to 552
Biopsy bit 552
Biotin 267, 556
Birth asphyxia 482
Bisacodyl 556
Bleeding
   disorders 205
   severity of 296
   time 236
   types of 411
Blood
   and blood
      component therapy 387, 404
      products 344
   gas 72, 211
      abnormality 487
      derangement, therapy in 78
   glucose 211, 425
   loss 286
   oxygen saturation 106
   pressure 252
   sample, collection of 75
   sugar, random 132, 233, 323, 425
   transfusion 207
   urea 425
BLS *See* Basic life support
Body ammonia, elimination of 263, 263*t*
Body mass index 236
Body surface area 428
Bone marrow suppression 414
   causes 414
   manifestations 414
Botulism 197, 198

Bowel infarction 332
Bowel sterilization 313
BP *See* Blood pressure
Bradyarrhythmias 138, 141
Bradycardia 168
Brain
　abscess 167, 183
　death 221
　edema, development of 260
　functions of entire 221
　herniation 173*b*
　injury, severe acute 222
　insults, prevention of secondary 214
　ischemia 423
　parenchyma 182
　　inflammation of 184
　tumors 167, 205
Brainstem 195
　auditory evoked response 522
　reflexes 172
　　absence of 222
Breastfeeding 471
Breath holding spells 147
Breathing 68, 162, 178
　irregular 168
　trial, spontaneous 92
British anti-Lewisite 556
Bronchiolitis 106
　grading of severity in 107*t*
Bronchiolitis, acute 106, 144
　clinical presentation 106
　complications 109
　differential diagnosis 107
　indications for hospitalization 108
　investigations 108
　monitoring 109
　pathogenesis 106
　patient approach 107
　treatment 108
Bronchopneumonia 144
Budd-Chiari syndrome 332, 334
Budesonide aerosol 556
Bulging fontanel 260
Burn injuries 427
　investigations 429
　management 428, 430
　pathophysiology 428
　prevention 430

C

Caffeine citrate 509, 556
CAH *See* Congenital adrenal hyperplasia
Calcium 291
　channel blockers 448
　gluconate 47, 557
Camphor 448
Campylobacter 315
Candida 365
　glabrata 365
　krusei 365
Candidiasis 364
　clinical presentation 365
　diagnosis 365
　specific treatment 365
Capillary refill time 68, 135
Captopril 557
Carbamate 448
　poisoning 446
Carbamazepine 557
Cardiac arrest 427
Cardiac arrhythmia 137, 142, 150, 244, 268, 270, 382, 427, 544
　clinical presentation 138
　etiology 137
　investigations 138
　types 138
Cardiac failure 161, 243
　evidence of 488
Cardiac irregularities 426
Cardiomyopathy 159
Cardiopulmonary resuscitation 23, 24, 27, 31, 37, 38, 222, 423, 438
　steps in 24*fc*
Cardiovascular system 51, 127
Carnitine 263, 267
Catch-up growth 277
Catecholamines, dose and administration of 133*t*
Cathartics 443
Catheter ablation 139
CBC *See* Complete blood count
CCHD *See* Cyanotic congenital heart diseases
Cefaclor 557
Cefadroxil 557

Cefepime 557
Cefixime 557
Cefoperazone 557
Cefotaxime 360
   sodium 557
Cefpodoxime proxetil 557
Ceftazidime 557
Ceftriaxone 114, 118, 187, 348, 405, 557
Cefuroxime 557
Celecoxib 218
Central nervous system 240, 367, 378, 381, 457
   aspergillosis 367
Central venous access 532
   catheter care 535
   complications 535
   equipment 532
   indications 532
   procedure in general 533
   technique 533
Central venous pressure 135
Cephalexin 154, 557
Cephalosporins, third-generation 347
Cerebellar ataxia, acute 195
Cerebellar tumors 195
Cerebral blood flow 221
Cerebral edema 230
   treatment of 313
Cerebral malaria 171
Cerebrospinal fluid 183, 188, 189, 191, 262, 359, 529
Cervical
   spinal cord 434
   spine, protecting 213
Cetirizine 56
Chaotic breathing 168
Charcoal, activated 555
Chemistry tests 72
Chest
   retraction 106
   skiagram 106, 108
      indications for 113
Child
   choking 27
   on ventilator, care of 89
Childhood pneumonia
   classification of 113*t*
   treatment of 113*t*
Chloral hydrate 557

Chloramphenicol 557
Chloromycetin 347, 361
Chloroquine 557
   resistant *Plasmodium falciparum* malaria 354
   sensitive
      group, therapy in 354*t*
      malaria 353
Chlorpheniramine maleate 456, 558
Chlorpromazine 218, 558
Chlorthiazide 557
Cholecystitis 407
Cholelithiasis 405, 407
Cholera 318
Choline magnesium salicylate 218
Cholinergic crisis 200
Cholinergic stimulation 458
Cholinesterase 445
Ciprofloxacin 347, 558
Circulatory dysfunction 129
Citrate solution 558
Clarithromycin 361, 558
Clindamycin 558
Clinical brain death, components of 221
Clinical scoring systems 70
Clonazepam 558
Clonidine 558
Clostridium 371
Clotting time 236
Cloxacillin 118, 558
Coagulase-negative staphylococci 370
Coagulation profile 211
Cold injuries 438
   clinical presentation 439
   pathophysiology 438
Cold stress 439
Coma 161, 171, 182, 244
   common causes of 173
   grading of 171
   irreversible 221
Comatose child 171
   algorithm for management of 175*fc*
   continuing treatment 175
   monitoring 175
Compartmental syndrome 270, 455*fc*
Complete blood count 32, 118, 132, 168, 183, 206, 211, 214, 223, 235, 425
Compression syndromes 415

Congestive cardiac failure 137, 288, 378
Congestive heart failure 143, 150, 273
   cardiac 143
   chronic 146
   critically ill 146
   diagnosis of 144
   differential diagnosis 144
   disease-specific drug therapy in 146*t*
   drug therapy for 145
   etiology 143
   investigations 144
   noncardiac 143
   recovering 146
   signs 144
   therapy in 146*t*
   treatment 144
Connective tissue disorders 375
Conscious child 27
Constipation 300
Continuous positive airway pressure 87*f*, 106, 110, 478, 479, 482, 483, 511
   complications of 485
   contraindications to 483
   protocol for 484*t*
   types of ventilators for 483
Convulsions 161
Copper sulfate 448
Coronary artery disease 377
Corticosteroid 47, 188, 190
Cotrimoxazole 558
Cough 161
Counseling family 53
Cow's milk protein 325
Coxiella burnetii 361
CPR *See* Cardiopulmonary resuscitation
Cranial computed tomography 214
C-reactive protein 132
Creatine phosphokinase 193
CRFT *See* Capillary refill time
Cricoid pressure 44*f*
Critically ill children 150
Crohn's disease 326
Cromolyn sodium 558
Cryoprecipitate 387, 390
   indications 390

Cryptococcosis 364, 365
   clinical presentation 365
   diagnosis 365
   specific treatment 366
Cryptococcus neoformans 365
Cryptosporidium parvum 315
Cushing's syndrome 162, 251
Cushing's triad 168
Cutaneous reaction 462, 463
CVP *See* Central venous pressure
Cyanosis 496
Cyanotic congenital heart diseases 146
Cyproheptadine 558
Cytomegalovirus 494

D

Dalfopristin 565
Damp cold, exposure to 441
Dapsone 449
Datura 449
Decompressive craniotomy 215
Deferoxamine mesylate 558
Deficit therapy 280
Dehydration 227, 272, 274, 286, 314, 316
   assessment of 316*t*
   correction of 294
   signs of 299
Delirium 243, 268
Delivery room, care in 471
Demyelination 194
   acute 205
Dengue 352, 359
   illness 340*f*
   severe 342
   shock 131
   shock syndrome 130, 278, 339, 345, 389, 393
     severity classification 339
   with fluid overload 344
   with organ dysfunction 344
   with warning signs, fluid therapy in 342*fc*
Dermatological disorders 395
Dermatomyositis 192
Desipramine 218, 558
Dexamethasone 47, 185, 187, 558

Dextran 40 559
Dextrose 47, 178
  normal saline 234
  ringer lactate 427
  water 480
Diabetes 341
  insipidus 239
    acute central 241
    diagnostic criteria 239
    diagnostic features of 240
    differential diagnosis of 239*b*
    management 241
    nephrogenic 241
    permanent central 241
  mellitus 240, 273
Diabetic ketoacidosis 227, 252
  clinical presentation 227
  diagnostic criteria 227
  in children, severity grading of 228*t*
  treatment 230
Dialysis
  indications for 289
  types of 289
Diaphoresis 268
Diarrhea 286, 298, 314, 399
  acute 314
  chronic 314
  drug therapy in 317
  persistent 318
    clinical presentation 318
    etiopathogenesis 318
    indications for hospitalization 319
Diarrheal disease, acute 314
  clinical presentation 315
  etiology 314
  pathophysiology 315
Diazepam 47, 178, 559
Diazoxide 559
DIC *See* Disseminated intravascular coagulation
Dicyclomine 559
Digoxin 145, 559
Dimercaprol 556
Dimercaptosuccinic acid 300
Dimorphic fungus 367
Dinitrophenylhydrazine 262
Diphenhydramine 47, 56, 559
Direct Coombs test 400

Discharge protocol 520
Disseminated intravascular coagulation 402, 413, 415, 501, 512
  clinical presentation 403
  common causes of 402
  investigations 404
  pathogenesis 403
  treatment 404
Diuretics 286
Dizziness 161
DKA *See* Diabetic ketoacidosis
DNS *See* Dextrose normal saline
Dobutamine 47, 133, 145, 559
  administration, early 268
Domperidone 559
Dopamine 47, 133, 145, 287, 559
  infusion 459
Down syndrome 217
Downe's score 97*t*
Doxapram 509
Doxycycline 360, 465, 559
D-penicillamine 565
Drowning 423
Drowsiness 182
Drugs
  first-line 178
  rashes 346
  second-line 178
  third-line 179
Dry cold, exposure to 441
Dural sinus thrombosis 167
DW *See* Dextrose water
Dyselectrolytemia 244, 272, 275, 413, 425
Dysentery 314
Dyspnea 161

E

Ear-nose-throat 434
ECG *See* Electrocardiograph
Echocardiography 143
ECMO *See* Extracorporeal membrane oxygenation
Edema 161, 287, 288
Edrophonium test 199
EEG *See* Electroencephalography
Electrocardiography 143, 158, 234

Electrocution and lightning 429
Electroencephalography 170
Electrolyte
   disorders 391
   management 288
   metabolism, disorders of 244
Emergency department 423
   care at 428
Emergency room 47, 56
   assessment in 67
   primary assessment 67
   secondary assessment 69
   tertiary assessment 69
Empirical antibiotic therapy 118, 347
   in neonatal sepsis 507*t*
Empyema 116, 119
   chest skiagram 117
   drainage of 118
   etiology 116
   investigations 117
   prognosis 119
   signs 117
   symptoms 117
   treatment 118
Enalapril 164, 559
Enalaprilat 164
Encephalitic syndrome, acute 171
Encephalitis 167, 182, 205, 239, 358
   differential diagnosis 183
   pathophysiology 183
   specific therapy 184
Encephalomyelitis
   acute disseminated 183, 194
      differential diagnosis 195
      etiopathogenesis 194
Encephalopathy 161, 461
   severity of 307
Enclosure systems 60
End-expiratory pressure, positive 485
Endocrine emergencies 225
Endotracheal tube 42, 51, 62, 83, 222, 480
   placement 45
Entamoeba histolytica 315
Enteroviral infection 308
   diarrhea in 182
Envenomation 421

Enzyme-linked immunosorbent assay 361
Epiglottitis, acute 95, 96
Epileptic syndrome 494
Epinephrine 37, 133, 559
Episodic viral wheeze 144
Epistaxis 411
Equipment 6
   diagnostic 6
   miscellaneous 7
   monitoring 6
   procedural 6
Erythema palms 377
Erythrocyte sedimentation rate 381
Erythromycin 154, 559
Escherichia coli 298, 315, 399
   pathogen 299
Esmolol 164
Ethambutol 559
Ethylene glycol 449
Etomidate 43, 48
ETT *See* Endotracheal tube
Euglycemia, maintain 214
Extracorporeal membrane oxygenation 150, 152
Extubation, procedure for 92
Eye
   opening 172
   response 172

F

Fanconi syndrome 258
Fatal disease 188
FB *See* Foreign body
Febrile neutropenia 414
Febrile seizures 298
Femoral vein 534
Fenoldopam 164
Fentanyl 43, 48, 432, 559
Fever 182
   high 269
FFP *See* Fresh frozen plasma
Flaccid paralysis, acute 191-193
   causes of 192
Flow-inflating bags 62
Fluconazole 368, 559

Fludrocortisone acetate 559
Fluid
   and electrolyte balance 459
   composition 280
   loss 286
   maintenance 56, 489
   management 48
   resuscitation, start 316
   therapy 316*t*
   type of 229
Flu-like illness 358
Flumazenil 559
Fluoxetine 218
Focal neurologic
   deficits 182
      stage of 189
      signs, stage of 188
Folic acid 275, 317, 560
Foreign body 99
   aspiration 93, 95, 96
   obstruction 94, 144
   of airway 93
Fosphenytoin 47, 426, 560
Fractional inspired oxygen 84
Fresh frozen plasma 343, 387, 427, 480
Fresh whole blood transfusion 343
Fulminant hepatic failure 305
   common causes 306
   differential diagnosis 306
   pathophysiology 306
   signs 306
   symptoms 306
Fulminant meningococcemia 346
   clinical presentation 346
   differential diagnosis 346
   prevention 348
   subsequent management 347
Furosemide 328, 560
FWBT *See* Fresh whole blood transfusion

G

Gabapentin 218, 560
Galactosemia 262
Ganglioside-disialic acid 193
Gastric lavage 443
Gastroesophageal reflux 159
Gastrointestinal absorption, prevent 443
Gastrointestinal bleeding 321
   common causes of 321
   lower 321, 324
      clinical presentation 325
      common causes of 325
      diagnostic workup 326
      patient approach 325
      physical examination 326
      subsequent management 326
   upper 321
      clinical presentation 322
      patient approach 322
Gastrointestinal system 52, 303
Gastrointestinal tract 378
GCS *See* Glasgow coma scale
Genetic disease 265
Genitourinary system 378
Gentamicin 111, 118, 560
Gestational age, small for 501
Giardia lamblia 315
Gitelman and Bartter syndromes 256
Glasgow coma scale 168, 170, 172*b*, 210, 424
Glomerular diseases 296
Glomerulonephritis 285
Glucagon 560
Glucose administration 229
Glycopyrrolate 560
Graft-versus-host disease 391, 413, 415
Gram stain 203, 544
Gram-negative bacteria 370
Grand mal seizures, early 182
Granulocyte 387
   transfusion 389
      dose 389
      indications 389
Granulomatous disease 253
Guillain-Barre syndrome 162, 191, 192, 198, 395, 396, 529
   clinical features 191
   differential diagnosis 192
   investigations 193
   pathogenesis 192
   treatment 193

H

Haemophilus influenzae B 96, 116, 158, 185, 406
   infection 201

Haloperidol 218, 560
Hand-foot-mouth disease 182
Handwashing
    prevention 469
    steps for effective 469
    steps in 470*f*
Hanging 434
    complete 434
    detailed evaluation 436
    incomplete 434
    investigations 436
    management 435
    pathophysiology 435
Head injury 167, 212
    goals of therapy 213
    types of 212, 213
Headache 161, 205, 464
Healthcare providers, guidelines for 23
Hearing
    impaired 523
    impairment, high-risk newborns for 523
Heart
    block, complete 141, 142*f*
    disease, congenital 273, 475
    failure 152
    rate 478
Heartbeats, irregular 138
Heat stroke 268
    clinical presentation 268
    complications 270
    differential diagnosis 269
    exertional 268
    investigations 270
    monitoring 270
    nonexertional 269
    prevention 271
    subsequent management 270
Hemarthrosis 411
Hematologic system 52
Hematology
    oncology 385
    tests 73
Hematuria 161, 295
    assess degree of 295
    causes of 295
    common causes of gross 295

Hemodialysis, intermittent 289
Hemoglobin 236, 405, 501
Hemolytic anemia 352
Hemolytic reactions 391
    management 391
Hemolytic uremic syndrome 210, 359, 389, 399
    clinical presentation 400
    diarrhea-associated 401
    etiology 399
    prognosis 401
    subsequent management 401
Hemophilia 210, 409
    A 390
        and B, treatment of 411*t*
    subsequent management 412
    types of 409
Hemorrhage 552
    epidural 209*f*
Hemorrhagic disease 512
Hemorrhagic fevers 295, 296, 346, 352
Henoch-Schönlein vasculitis 346
Heparin 560
    flushing 417
Hepatic encephalopathy 260, 305
    clinical staging of 308*t*
Hepatic failure 270, 360
    chronic 389
Hepatic sickle cell crisis 407
Hepatitis 358
    A 372
    B virus chronic infection 308
Hepatomegaly 260
Herald severe disease 329
Herpes infections 494
Herpes simplex 194
    virus infection 308
Hirschsprung disease 325
Histoplasma capsulatum 367
Histoplasmosis 364, 367
    clinical presentation 368
    diagnosis 368
    treatment 368
HMD *See* Hyaline membrane disease
Homatropine hydrobromide 560
Hormone therapy, avoid 237

Hospital-acquired infections 370
  clinical presentation 372
  organisms 371
  predisposing factors 370
    environmental factors 371
    host factors 370
  prevention 373
  source of 371
  types of 371
Hospital-acquired pneumonias 115
Hudson mask 59, 60*f*
Human immunodeficiency virus 273, 366
Hungry bone syndrome 258
Hurst disease 195
Hyaline membrane disease 510
Hydralazine 164, 560
Hydrocarbons 444
Hydrochlorothiazide 560
Hydrocortisone 47, 56, 560
Hydroxymethyl 74
Hydroxyzine 560
Hyoscyamine hydrobromide 560
Hyperammonemia 260, 264
  causes 260
  clinical presentation 261
  diagnosis 262
  differential diagnosis 262
  laboratory evaluation 261
  laboratory interpretation in 262*t*
  pathophysiology 261
  treatment 263
    of unconjugated 502
Hypercalcemia 253
  causes 253
  clinical presentation 253
  investigations 254
  treatment 254
Hypercalciuria nephrocalcinosis 256
Hypercarbia 74
Hypercatabolic disease 273
Hypercyanotic attacks 147
  differential diagnosis 147
  etiopathogenesis 147
  investigations 148
  treatment 148

Hypercyanotic spells, algorithm for management of 148*fc*
Hyperglycemia 205, 240, 425, 426
Hyperkalemia 233, 249
  causes 249
  clinical presentation 249
  correction of 250
  ECG changes in 250*t*
  management of 251*fc*
  true 249
Hyperleukocytosis 413, 415
Hypermagnesemia 255
  causes 255
  clinical presentation 255
  diagnosis 256
  investigations 256
  pathophysiology 255
  treatment 256
Hypernatremia 244
  causes 244
  clinical presentation 244
  complications 245
  management of 246*fc*
  pathophysiology 245
Hyperornithinemia-hyperammonemia-homocitrullinuria syndrome 260
Hyperphosphatemia 257
  causes 257
  chronic 258
  clinical features 257
  laboratory evaluation 258
  treatment 258
Hypertension 161, 168, 205, 216, 288
  cause for 163
Hypertensive crisis 161, 164
  classification 161
  diagnosis 162
  drug therapy in 164*t*
  etiology 162
  primary 162
  secondary 162
Hypertensive urgency, drugs for 164*t*
Hyperthermia 268
Hypertriglyceridemia 328
Hyperuricemia 413
Hyperventilation 215

Hypervolemia 287
Hypoaldosteronism 291
Hypocalcemia 254, 494
    causes 254
    clinical presentation 254
    symptomatic 255
Hypoglycemia 233, 272, 274, 494
    asymptomatic 496
    correction of 147
Hypokalemia 192, 251, 275
    causes 251
    clinical presentation 252
    correction of 229, 253, 294
    diagnostic approach to 252*fc*
    suspect 252
    treatment 252
Hypomagnesemia 256, 275
    causes 256
    clinical presentation 256
    investigations 257
    severe 257
    treatment 257
Hyponatremia 233, 246
    asymptomatic 248
    chronic 248
    clinical presentation 247
    etiology 246
    hypervolemic 248
    mild 247
    monitoring 248
    pathophysiology 247
    severe 247
Hypophosphatemia 192, 258
    causes 258
    clinical features 258
    diagnosis 259
    investigations 259
    treatment 259
Hypotension 223, 546
Hypothermia 215, 223, 272, 274, 439, 475, 477
    correct 519
    differential diagnosis 439
    investigations 440
    mild 169, 439
        and moderate 476
    moderate 439
    monitoring 440
    oxygen, severe 475
    profound 439
    severe 476
Hypotonia 191
Hypovolemia 286, 288
Hypoxemia 216
Hypoxia 223
    hypercarbia 213

I

Ibuprofen 218, 560
ICP *See* Intracranial pressure
Idiopathic thrombocytopenic purpura 454
Iliopsoas hemorrhage 411
Illness observation scale, acute 70
Immune
    deficiency disorders
        primary 396
        secondary 396
    modulation 396
    thrombocytopenia 346
    thrombocytopenic purpura 210, 395, 396
Immunoglobulin IV 561
Indomethacin 561
Infant 27
    chest thrusts in 28*f*
Infection 205, 272, 275, 289, 295, 402, 552
    severe 402
    source of 371
    types of 371
Infectious diseases 337
Infectious laryngitis, acute 95, 96
Infective endocarditis 155
Inflammatory bowel disease 325, 326
Inflammatory disease 106
    chronic 100
Influenza 194
    A virus 95
Infusion, rate of 279
Inhaler, metered dose 100
Initiate breastfeeding 472
Innocent cardiac murmurs 155
Insulin 561

infusion 229
    preparation of 229
Intensive bronchodilator therapy 103
Intensive care
    concept of 1
    unit 210, 373
Intermittent mandatory ventilation, ventilator controls in 485
Intra-arterial blood pressure 536
Intra-arterial injection 432*t*
    inadvertent 431
Intracranial hemorrhage 167, 208, 211
    classification 208
    clinical presentation 210
    etiology 210
    outside brain 208
    pathophysiology 210
    within brain 208
Intracranial pressure 43, 170
    increased 261
    management of raised 170*fc*
    raised 167, 415
    signs of 173*b*
Intraosseous access 539, 540*f*
    complications 540
    infusion sites 539
    procedure 540
    requirements 539
Intrauterine infections 522
Intravenous 74
    ampicillin 299
    calcium gluconate 255
    cefotaxime 299
    ceftriaxone 299
    dexamethasone 169
    edrophonium chloride 199
    furosemide 169
    mannitol 169
    methylprednisolone 102
    quinine combination therapy 355
Intravenous fluid 48, 102, 342
    therapy 278
        complications of 281
        components of 279
        indications 278
        maintenance 279
        replacement 280
        routes of administration 279

Intravenous immunoglobulin 146, 152, 191, 194, 349, 395
    administration of 377
    therapy 395
        indications 396
        mode of action 395
Intubation equipment 480
Invasive aspergillosis 366
    clinical presentation 366
    diagnosis 367
    treatment 367
Invasive fungal infections 364, 369
Ipratropium 102
    bromide 561
Iron 275, 561
    elemental 561
    salts 449
Irritability 182
Isoniazid 188, 328, 449, 561
Itchy rash 392
ITP *See* Idiopathic thrombocytopenic purpura
Ivermectin 561
IVIG *See* Intravenous immunoglobulin

J

Jatropha curcas 449
Jaundice 260, 298
    severity of 500
Jerky movements, short-lived 494
Jitteriness 496
Jugular vein
    external 534
    internal 533
Juvenile idiopathic arthritis 155, 395

K

Kadallavanakku 449
Kawasaki disease 155, 186, 377, 395, 397, 416
    atypical 378, 380
    clinical presentation 377
    complicated 380
    IVIg-resistant 379
    treatment 379
    uncomplicated 379, 380
Kernicterus 494

Kerosene 444
    lethal dose of 444
Ketamine 43, 48, 432
Ketoacid correction 229
Ketone body 261
Kidney injury
    acute 285, 290, 358
        common causes 286
        complications 289
        diagnostic criteria 285
        fluid management 288
        investigations 287
        management 287
        network 285
    cause of acute 399
    staging of acute 286*t*
Klebsiella 298, 371, 505

L

Labetalol 164, 561
Lactate dehydrogenase 400
Lactic dehydrogenase 287
Lactulose 561
Lamotrigine 561
Lansoprazole 561
L-asparaginase 328
Lay rescuers, guidelines for 23
L-carnitine 561
Lead 450
Leptospira antibody 307
Leptospirosis 352, 358
    anicteric 358
    clinical presentation 358
    differential diagnosis 359
    icteric 359
    pathogenesis 358
    specific therapy 360
    subsequent management 360
    supportive therapy 360
    suspect 359
Lethal illness 265
Leukemia 158, 205, 239
Leukopenia 506
Levamisole 562
Levetiracetam 328
Levosimendan 134
Levothyroxine 562

LFT *See* Liver function test
LGIB *See* Lower gastrointestinal bleeding
Liddle syndrome 253
Lidocaine 43, 48, 562
    cream 219
    infiltration 219
Life support, withholding and withdrawing 19
Life-threatening reaction 393
Linezolid 372, 562
Lipid amphotericin B formulations 556
Listeria monocytogenes 185
Liver biopsy 549, 552
    complications 552
    contraindications 549
    equipment needed 550
    indications for 549
    menghini 1 second 550
    precautions 550
    procedure 550
    site 551*f*
    ultrasonography-guided 550
Liver cell
    failure, acute 305
    necrosis 305
Liver disease 255, 260, 269, 549
    acute 310
    chronic 236, 305
    suspected 549
Liver failure 268
    acute 260, 305, 313
    chronic 260
Liver function test 126, 132, 168, 206, 211, 238, 299, 307, 323, 400
Local tissue damage 441
Loratadine 562
Lorazepam 47, 178, 562
Lower gastrointestinal bleeding 323
    diagnostic workup of 323*b*
Low-molecular-weight heparin 416, 417
Lumbar cerebrospinal fluid 215
Lumbar puncture 202, 230, 529, 530*f*
    complications 531
    contraindications 529
    indications 529
    procedure 530

Lung
  crackles 287, 444
  disease, chronic 273
  parenchyma, inflammation of 111
Lymphoma 158, 205, 239

M

Macrolides 109
Macrophage activation syndrome 381
  clinical presentation 381
  diagnostic criteria 382
  differential diagnosis 382
  subsequent management 382
Magnesium
  hydroxide 562
  sulfate 562
Malabsorption syndrome 273
Malaria 352, 359, 565
  clinical presentation 352
  differential diagnosis 352
  late treatment failure 357
  monitoring 356
  peripheral smear for 132
  response to therapy 356
  severe complicated 352, 355
  subsequent management 353
  supportive therapy in severe 355
Malarial parasite 173
Mallory-Weiss tears 321
Malnutrition
  severe 332
  severe acute 272
    causes 272
    clinical presentation 273
    differential diagnosis 273
    investigations 273
Mannitol 240, 562
MAO *See* Monoamine oxidase
MAP *See* Mean arterial pressure
Maple syrup urine disease 267
MAS *See* Meconium aspiration syndrome
Massive hematemesis 323
Mastoiditis 206
Mean airway pressure 85
Mean arterial pressure 135, 167

Mebendazole 562
Mechanical ventilation 83, 103, 109, 208
  controlled 85*f*
  expiratory phase characteristics 87
  extubation 91
  indications for 84
  inspiratory phase characteristics 87
  laboratory investigations 89
  normal versus 83
  phases of 85
  preparation and monitoring 88
  radiological 89
  starting of 88
  termination of inspiration 87
  terminologies used 84
  ventilator assessment 89
  weaning 91
Meckel's diverticulum 325
Meconium aspiration syndrome 486
Mediastinal disease, severe 368
Mediastinal tumors 159
Mefloquine 563
Megavitamin therapy 260
Menghini needle biopsy 550
Meningeal irritation
  signs of 182
  stage of 188
Meningitis 167, 183, 205, 206, 239, 352, 359, 494
Meningococcal vaccine 401
Meningococcemia 352
Mental status 434
Meropenem 347, 562
Metabolic abnormalities 413
Metabolic acidosis 77, 78, 233, 294
Metabolic alkalosis 77, 78
  causes 78
  clinical features 79
  treatment 79
Metabolic complications, management of 268
Metabolic emergencies 225
Metabolic problems 52
Metabolism 509
  inborn errors of 205, 260, 265
Metabolites, deficient 267

Methadone 562
Methanol 449
Methicillin-resistant *Staphylococcus aureus* 370
Methotrexate 563
Methylene blue 563
Methylphenidate 563
Methylprednisolone 47, 56, 104, 194, 382, 563
Metolazone 562
Metoprolol 562
Metronidazole 328, 563
Micronutrient deficiency 272, 275
Microorganisms causing pneumonia 112*t*
Midazolam 43, 47, 83, 178, 432, 563
Migraine 205
Miller-Fisher syndrome 192
Milrinone 134
Mitral valve prolapse 155
Monoamine oxidase 43
Montelukast 563
Morphine 83, 432
    sulfate 563
Mortality, pediatric risk of 71
Multidrug-resistant *Plasmodium falciparum* 354
Multiorgan
    dysfunction syndrome 131, 461
    failure 452
Multisystem disease, acute 349
Myalgia 464
    in influenza 182
Myasthenia gravis 192
Myasthenia, mild 199
Myasthenic crisis 200
Myasthenic paralysis 197, 200, 452
    confirmatory tests 199
    differential diagnosis 198
    investigations 198
    pathogenesis 197
    treatment 199
Mycobacterium tuberculosis 158
Mycoplasma pneumoniae 106, 194
Myocardial hypoxia 423
Myocarditis 150
    causes of 151

N

N-acetyl cysteine 308, 555
Nalidixic acid 563
Naloxone 48, 563
Naphthalene 450
Naproxen 218, 563
Nasal cannula, high flow 108
Nasal prongs 59, 59*f*
Nasogastric aspiration 323
Nebulization 104, 106
Nebulized adrenaline 57
Nebulized ipratropium 102
Nebulized salbutamol 57, 102
NEC *See* Necrotizing enterocolitis
Neck stiffness 161
Necrotizing enterocolitis 510, 513
Needle thoracocentesis 541
    complications 542
    contraindications 541
    indications 541
Neisseria meningitides 185, 406
Neomycin sulfate 563
Neonatal anemia, diagnostic approach to 516*fc*
Neonatal convulsions 493
    causes 493
    clinical presentation 493
    investigations 494
Neonatal hypocalcemia 498
    causes 498
    clinical presentation 499
    investigations 499
    management of 499*fc*
Neonatal hypoglycemia 496
    clinical presentation 496
    management of 497*fc*
    risk factors 496
Neonatal hypothermia 475
    clinical presentation 476
    differential diagnosis 476
    grading 475
    management 476
    pathophysiology 475
    prevention 477
    supportive measures 477
Neonatal intensive care unit 491
    admission to 491

Index   585

Neonatal jaundice 500
    diagnostic approach to 501*fc*
    physical examination 500
Neonatal resuscitation 478
    algorithm 479*fc*
    equipment checklist 479
Neonatal seizures, anticonvulsant
        therapy in 495*fc*
Neonatal sepsis 395, 505
    approach to 507*fc*
    clinical features 506
    differential diagnosis 506
    etiology 506
    risk factors for 505
Neonatal transport 518
Neonatal ventilation 482
    mechanical 485
    normal 485
Neonate
    audiology screening in 522
    bleeding 512
Neonatology 467
Neostigmine methylsulfate 563
Neostigmine test 199
Nephrogenic diabetes insipidus 240
Nephrotic syndrome 130, 205, 273, 332,
        334, 389, 390, 461, 463
Nephrotoxic drug 285
Nervous system 51, 165
    examination 174
Neuritis 461
Neurologic vital signs 71
Neurological function 493
Neurometabolic screening 261, 262
Neuroprotective therapy 206
Neutral head position 26*f*, 214
Neutropenia 413
Newborn
    care of normal 471
    danger signs in 474
    fluid therapy in 488
    visual screening in 524
        indications 524
    with anemia, transfusion protocol for
        516*t*
    with bloody stools, approach to 513*fc*
    with generalized bleeding, approach
        to 512*fc*

Niacin 275
Nicardipine 164
Niclosamide 563
Nifedipine 164, 563
Nitrofurantoin 563
Nitroglycerine 134
Nitroprusside 134
    sodium 564
NMS *See* Neurometabolic screening
Nonconvulsive seizures, treatment for
        169
Nonhemolytic reactions 392, 393
    febrile reaction 392
Non-rebreathing masks 60
Nonshockable rhythm 36, 37*fc*
Nonsteroidal anti-inflammatory drugs
        158
Norepinephrine 133
    bitartrate 564
Normal newborn, care of 471
    basic principles 471
    care of cord 472
    examine 472
    eye care 472
    postnatal care 472
    prevention of infection 473
    skin care 472
Normothermia 214
Normovolemia 169
Nortriptyline 218
Nutrition 289

O

Obstructive airway disease 510
OCS *See* Oral corticosteroids
Odollam 450
Ofloxacin 564
Oleander
    white 450
    yellow 450
Oliguria 161
Ondansetron 564
OPA *See* Oropharyngeal airway
Opioids 450
Oral contraceptive pills, combined 235
Oral corticosteroids 104
Oral itraconazole 368

Oral medroxyprogesterone acetate 237
Oral rehydration solution 246
Organ donation 223
Organic acidemias 262
Organization and staffing 7
   ancillary staff 8
   doctor-in-charge 7
   medical staff 8
   nursing staff 8
Organochlorines 450
Organophosphate poisoning 192, 198, 328, 445
   management of 445, 445*fc*
   specific therapy 446
   symptoms 445
Organophosphorus poisoning 197
Oropharyngeal airway 31, 33*f*
   advancing 33*f*
   method of insertion of 32, 33*f*
   position 33*f*
   rotating 33*f*
ORS *See* Oral rehydration solution
Oseltamivir therapy 109
Osmotherapy 169
Otoacoustic emission 522
Oxcarbazepine 564
Oxygen 56
   delivery systems 59
      high-flow 60
      low-flow 59
   therapy 58
      adverse effects of 63
      indications 58
      monitoring of 63

P

Packed cell volume 132
Pain management
   and sedation 216
   drug therapy for 217*t*
Pancreatin 564
Pancreatitis 332
Pancreatitis, acute 327, 331
   classification 327
   clinical presentation 328
   differential diagnosis 329
   etiology 328
   mild 327
   pathogenesis 328
   severe 328
   subsequent management 330
Pancuronium 48, 432
Papilledema 161, 205, 260
Paracetamol 306, 456, 564
   for fever 214
Paralysis 44, 161, 244
Paralytic agents 43
Paralytic poliomyelitis 191, 192
Parenteral fluid therapy 488
Parenteral therapy 488
Patent ductus arteriosus 143
PBS *See* Peripheral blood smear
PEA *See* Pulseless electrical activity
Peak inspiratory pressure 84, 89, 486, 487
Pediatric bradycardia 37
   algorithm 38*fc*
   drug dosages 37
Pediatric chain of survival 25*f*
Pediatric Drug Formulary 553
Pediatric intensive care unit 3, 9, 54, 83, 147, 148, 150, 154, 167, 192, 199, 206, 233, 234, 243, 245, 425, 438
   admission
      indications for 333
      notes 13
   care 342
      levels of 8
   communication in 16
   critically ill children in 18
   daily routine in 9
   discharge summary 15
   documentation in 11
   equipment, essential 6*b*
   ethics in 18, 19
      autonomy 18
      beneficence 18
      justice 18
      nonmaleficence 18
   general guidelines 13
   prescriptions 14
   procedure notes 14
   progress notes 13
   rounds 11

systematic approach for examination 12
transfer notes 14
Pediatric pain 216
Pediatric tachycardia 38
   algorithm 39*fc*
   drug dosages 38
Pediatrician's responsibilities in brain death 222
PEEP *See* Positive end-expiratory pressure
PEM *See* Protein-energy malnutrition
Penicillin
   G 360, 465, 564
      benzathine 564
      procaine 564
   V 154, 564
Pentagon, assessment 68*f*
Pentazocine 564
Pentobarbital infusion 169, 215
Pericardial cyst 159
Pericardial effusion 158, 160*f*
   common causes 158
   differential diagnosis 159
   pathophysiology 159
Pericardiocentesis 543
   complications 544
   equipment 543
   indications 543
   preambles 543
   procedure 544
Peripheral arterial cannulation 536
   arteries used 536
   complications 538
   contraindications 536
   equipment 537
   indications 536
   procedure 537
Peripheral blood smear 238, 323, 379, 506
Peritoneal dialysis 289
Permanent pacemaker 141
Permethrin 564
Persistent diarrhea 314, 318
Persistent pulmonary hypertension of newborn 146
Pethidine 564
Peutz-Jeghers syndrome 326

Phenazopyridine 564
Pheniramine 56
Phenobarb 426
Phenobarbitone 47
Phenol 450
Phenothiazines 450
Phenoxybenzamine 565
Phenylephrine 564
Phenytoin 432, 451
Phototherapy 502
   unit, quality assessment of 503
Phytonadione 564
PICU *See* Pediatric intensive care unit
Pinworm infestation 300
PIP *See* Peak inspiratory pressure
Piperacillin 372, 565
Piperacillin-tazobactum 565
Plasma
   ammonia 173, 260, 307
   phosphorus 257
   transfusion 389
      dose and administration 390
      indications 389
Plasmodium falciparum 352
Platelet 387
   count 132, 339
   transfusion 388
      indications 388
   type of 389
Pleural effusion 340*f*
Pleural fluid
   needle aspiration of 542
   study 118
Pleurodynia 159
Pneumocystis jiroveci 414
Pneumomediastinum 120, 122
   clinical features 122
   common causes 122
   diagnosis 123
   pathogenesis 122
   treatment 123
   with pneumopericardium, chest X-ray 123*f*
Pneumonia 111, 358, 399
   adjuncts to treatment 118
   clinical presentation 112
   complications of 115

etiology 111
management 112
Pneumothorax 120, 121*f*, 544
   aspiration pneumonia 51
   clinical presentation 121
   investigations 121
   pathogenesis 120
   physical examination 121
   treatment 122
Poison
   and drugs, clues for 442
   promote excretion of 443
Poisoning 171, 421, 447
   common 444
   in children 442
   management 447
   symptomatology 447
   to hydrocarbons, management of 444*fc*
Polydipsia, primary 240
Polymorphonuclear cell 203
Polymorphonuclear leukocytosis 186
Polyuria 280, 286
Poor urine stream 286
Portal hypertension 332
Positive airway pressure 132
Positive end-expiratory pressure 59, 84, 89, 487
Positive pressure ventilation 478, 479
   intermittent 106, 110
Postdiphtheritic paralysis 192
Post-intubation care 45
Post-resuscitation care 50
   approach 50
   system-wise approach 51
Postresuscitation management 480*fc*
Poststreptococcal glomerulonephritis 295
Post-transfusion care 504
Potassium chloride 48
PPHN *See* Persistent pulmonary hypertension of newborn
PPV *See* Positive pressure ventilation
Pralidoxime 564
Prazosin 564
Prednisolone 102, 564
Pre-existing disease, chronic 269

Prematurity
   recurrent apnea of 511
   retinopathy of 524
Primaquine 565
Promethazine 565
Prophylactic anticoagulant therapy 416
Propofol 43, 48, 432
Propoxyphene 565
Propranolol 565
Prostaglandin E1 134, 565
Protein-energy malnutrition 252
Proteus groups 298
Prothrombin time 236
Proton pump inhibitor 513
Pseudohyperkalemia 249
Pseudomonas 371
   aeruginosa 185
Pseudotumor cerebri 167
Puberty menorrhagia 235
   etiology 235
Pulmonary aspergillosis 367
Pulmonary blood flow 147
Pulmonary disease, moderate 387
Pulmonary edema 459
Pulmonary histoplasmosis
   acute 368
   chronic 368
Pulmonary score 100, 102
Pulseless
   cardiac arrest, management of 35, 35*fc*
   electrical activity 36*f*, 37, 37*fc*
   ventricular tachycardia 36, 37*fc*
Pyelonephritis, acute 298
   subsequent management 300
Pyogenic meningitis, complication of 201
Pyrazinamide 188
Pyridostigmine 565
Pyridoxine 178, 565

Q

Q fever 361
QT syndrome, long 140, 141*f*
Quetiapine 218
Quinine 355
   sulfate 565
Quinupristin 565

R

Radial artery 537
    puncture, stabilizing wrist for 537*f*
Ranitidine 48, 565
Rapid digitalization, digoxin for 145*t*
Rapid sequence intubation 41, 42, 46, 180, 206, 213
    algorithm 46*fc*
    contraindications for 42
    indications for 41
    medications in 43*t*
    preparation 42*t*
    procedure 42
    sedatives for 44*t*
Rat-bite fever 464
    differential diagnosis 465
    pathophysiology 464
    treatment 465
RBC *See* Red blood cell
RBS *See* Random blood sugar
RDS *See* Respiratory distress syndrome
Rebreathing mask, partial 59
Red blood cell 235, 323, 387, 404, 405
    transfusion 387, 409
        indications 387
        precautions 388
    types of 388
Refeeding syndrome 258
Refractory status epilepticus 179, 180
Rehabilitation, subsequent 277
Renal angle tenderness 298
Renal disease 245, 255, 269, 333
Renal failure 161, 268, 270, 397
    acute 285
    chronic 273
    intrinsic 288
Renal function
    normal 258
    test 126, 132, 168, 206, 211, 234, 238, 245, 299, 307, 323, 339, 392, 400
Renal replacement therapy, continuous 289
Renal system 52, 283
Renal tubular acidosis 252, 273, 291, 294
    clinical presentation 293
    clinical types 292
    differential diagnosis 293
    hyperkalemic 292
    pathophysiology 292
    proximal 292
    subsequent management 294
    type of 293
Replacement therapy 396
Respiration 172
Respiratory acidosis 77, 78
    causes 78
    clinical features 78
    treatment 78
Respiratory alkalosis 77, 79
    bag for 74
    causes 79
    clinical features 79
    treatment 79
Respiratory depression 178
Respiratory distress 287, 491
Respiratory distress syndrome 483, 486
    causes of acute 124*t*
Respiratory infection, upper 106
Respiratory rate 106, 491
Respiratory sound, abnormal 95
Respiratory syncytial virus 106
    infection 109
Respiratory system 51, 81
Restlessness 243
Resuscitation 21
    equipment and drugs 47
Retinopathy 161
    of prematurity 524
        clinical manifestations 525
        diagnosis 525
        pathogenesis 524
        screening 525*fc*
        treatment 525
Retropharyngeal abscess 95, 96, 99
Revised National Tuberculosis Control Program 188
Reye syndrome 217, 261, 266, 306, 311, 313
    clinical features 312
    clinical staging of 312*t*
    differential diagnosis 312
    etiology 311
    investigations 312

pathogenesis 311
subsequent management 313
treatment 313
RFT *See* Renal function test
Rheumatic carditis 154, 157
    antibiotic therapy 156
    anti-inflammatory therapy 156
    differential diagnosis 155
    rest in 156*t*
    subsequent management 156
    supportive therapy 156
Rheumatic fever 157*t*
Rheumatoid disease 219
Rheumatological disorders 195
Ribavirin 109
Riboflavin 267, 275
Rickets, development of 291
Rickettsia conorii 361
Rickettsia tsutsugamushi 361
Rickettsial disease 186
Rickettsial fever 347
Rickettsial infections 361, 363
    clinical presentation 361
    differential diagnosis 362
    management 362
    pathogenesis 361
    specific therapy 363
    subsequent management 362
    supportive therapy 363
Rifampicin 187, 188, 348, 361, 565
Ringer's lactate 435
Risperidone 218, 565
Rocuronium 43, 48, 432
Rotavirus 314
RPA *See* Retropharyngeal abscess
RSE *See* Refractory status epilepticus
RSI *See* Rapid sequence intubation
RTA *See* Renal tubular acidosis
Rubella 494
Rule of palm 428

S

SABA *See* Short-acting beta agonists
Salbutamol 101, 106, 565
    nebulization 48, 102
Salicylates 451
Saline, normal 148, 278, 339

Salmonella 185, 315, 371, 372, 406
Sarcoid-like disease 368
SBP *See* Systolic blood pressure
SBR *See* Serum bilirubin
SCH *See* Succinylcholine
Sclerosis, multiple 195
Scorpion envenomation 457, 460
    clinical presentation 458
    differential diagnosis 458
    management 459
    monitoring 460
    pathophysiology 457
    poor prognostic indicators 460
    systemic symptoms 458
Scrub typhus 361
Seizure 147, 205, 244, 260, 270, 288, 493, 496
    continuing 179
    control 268
Self-inflating bags 61
Sellick maneuver 44
Sensorium 260, 452
    altered 177
Sensory stimulation 277
Sensory symptoms, mild 191
Sepsis 206
    prevention 469
    syndrome 347
Septic arthritis 346
Septic shock 352
Serum 400
    ascites albumin gradient, interpretation of 334*t*
    bilirubin 501
    electrolytes 126, 132, 143, 206, 211, 296, 299, 307, 339, 392, 400, 425
    glutamic oxaloacetic transaminase 311
    glutamic pyruvic transaminase 311
    osmolality 240
    sickness 461
Severe dengue
    with compensated shock, fluid therapy in 343*fc*
    with hypotensive shock, fluid therapy in 343*fc*
    with organ failure, fluid therapy in 343*fc*

Sexual maturity rating 236
Shigella 315
  dysentery 399
Shock 129, 137, 150, 213, 270, 356, 426, 552
  additional therapies 135
  cardiogenic 130
  catecholamine-resistant 133
  cold 131
  distributive 130
  fluid refractory 133
  hemodynamic management of 135*fc*
  hypovolemic 130
  management 131
  monitoring 135
  obstructive 130
  patient approach 131
  poor prognostic factors 136
  refractory 135
  septic 131
  severe dehydration with 274
  signs of recovery from 133*b*
  therapy 132
  vasoactive drugs in 134*t*
  warm 131
Shockable rhythm 23, 36
Short-acting beta agonists 100, 104
Sick child 240
  ethical issues in treating 18
Sick neonates, transporting 518
Sickle cell
  anemia 205, 207
  crisis 405
    diagnosis 407
    infectious 405
    management 407
    noninfectious 406
    nonspecific fever 405
  disease 296, 405
Simple oxygen mask 59
Snake envenomation 197, 198, 452, 454, 454*fc*
  complications 455
  in hospital, management of 455*fc*
  pathophysiology 453
  prehospital management 454
  supportive therapy 455
  with complications, management of 456*fc*

Sodium
  bicarbonate 48, 294
  nitroprusside 164, 459
  polystyrene sulfonate 565
  thiosulfate 566
  valproate 47
Soft-tissue neck radiographs 436
Solitary rectal ulcer syndrome 325
Spasmodic croup 95, 96
Spinal cord compression 415
Spine, arthritis of 155
Spirillum minus 464
  infection 465
Spironolactone 566
Splenic sequestration, acute 406
Spontaneous mode 86
Spotted fever 361
Stabilize airway 162
Staphylococcus 406
  aureus 96, 116, 185, 349, 371, 505
  pneumonia 111, 117
    chest X-ray in 117*f*
Starvation 286
Status epilepticus 171, 176
  algorithm for management of 180*t*
  clinical presentation 177
  common causes 176
  mechanism of 177
  prevention of complications 179
  prognostic factors in 177*t*
  treatment 179
Steroid 328
  therapy 187
Streptobacillus moniliformis 464
Streptococcus
  pneumoniae 96, 116, 185, 406
  pyogenes 96
Streptokinase 566
Streptomycin 188, 566
Stridor 95
  child with acute 99*fc*
Stridor, acute 95
  common causes 95
  investigations 98
  monitoring 98
  prognosis 98
  salient features 95
Stroke in children, acute 204
  classification 204

clinical presentation 205
differential diagnosis 205
management of 204
patient approach 206
Subclavian vein access 534
Subdural empyema 201
clinical features 201
diagnostic investigations 201
differential diagnosis 202
procedure 202
treatment 202
Subdural fluid tap 202
Subdural hemorrhage 209*f*
Submersion duration 426
Submersion injuries 423
Succinylcholine 43, 48, 432
dose of 44
Sucralfate 566
Sulphonyl ureas 451
Superior vena cava syndrome 415
Suprapubic aspiration 548*f*
Suprapubic urine aspiration 547
complications 548
equipment 547
materials 547
procedure 547
Supraventricular tachycardia 138
algorithm for treatment of 139*fc*
ECG in 139*f*
Sweating 496
erythema and pain 428
Synchronized cardioversion 38
Synchronized intermittent mandatory
ventilation 86, 86*f*
Syndrome of inappropriate antidiuretic
hormone 248
Systemic analgesia 219
Systemic diseases 236
chronic 273
Systemic infections 317
Systemic reactions 462
Systolic blood pressure 343

T

Tachyarrhythmias 138
Tachycardia 216, 243, 296, 496

Tachypnea 216, 269, 405, 444, 491, 496
Tardieu spots 436
Temperature homeostasis 52
Tension pneumothorax, needle
decompression for 541
Terbutaline sulfate 566
Terfenadine 566
Tet spells 147
Tetanus
antitoxin 566
immunoglobulin 566
toxoid 459
TFT *See* Thyroid function test
Theophylline 509, 566
Therapeutic food 276
ready to use 276
Thiamine 267, 275, 566
Thiopental 43, 432
sodium 566
Thrombocytopenia 383, 413, 414
Thromboembolic diseases 416
Thrombolytic therapy 416, 418
Thromboplastin time, partial 409
Thrombotic disorders 205
Thyroid
crisis 242
differential diagnosis 243
management 243
pathogenesis 242
function test 238
hormones 242
stimulating hormone, low 242
storm 242
Thyroxine 242
Tiagabine 566
Tibia, upper end of 540*f*
Tick
paralysis 197, 198
typhus 361
Tidal volume 84, 486
Tincture iodine 451
Tissue injury 403
Topiramate 566
Toxic liver damage 305
Toxic reactions 462
Toxic shock syndrome 349
clinical presentation 349
diagnostic criteria 350

etiology 349
exclusion criteria 350
treatment 351
Toxins 403
Toxoplasmosis 494
Tracheal compression 415
Transfusion
exchange 503
indications 503
requirements 503
reactions 391
Transverse myelitis, acute 192
Traumatic acute cord compression 192
Traumatic brain injury 208, 210, 212
causes of 212
Tricuspid atresia 143
Tricyclic antidepressants 451
Triiodothyronine 242
Tropicamide 566
Tuberculin skin test 189
Tuberculosis disease 188
Tuberculous meningitis 183, 188-190, 195
radiology 189
specific treatment 190
Tumor lysis syndrome 249, 254, 257, 413
Typhoid 359
fever 352
Tyrosine kinase, muscle-specific 198

U

Umbilical vein 488
Unfractionated heparin 417
Unit design 3
central station 4
clean and dirty utility rooms 5
communication area 5
crash cart 4
entry doors 4
ICU beds 4
power supply and temperature control 4
resuscitation trolley 4
room layout and bed area 3
storage 5
waste disposal 5
United Nations International Children's Emergency Fund 272

Upper airway obstruction 97*t*
Urea cycle disorder 262
Urinary tract hematuria, lower 295
Urine output, normal 489
Urokinase 566
Urolithiasis 295, 296
Ursodeoxycholic acid 566
Uterine bleeding
abnormal 235
algorithm of management of abnormal 238*fc*
dysfunctional 235
Uterine problems 236
Utero-ovarian mass 235

V

VAD *See* Ventricular assist devices
Valproic acid 328, 567
Valvular heart disease, chronic 154
Vancomycin 187, 370, 372
Varicella 194
Vasculitis 195, 461
syndrome 205
Vaso-occlusive
complications 405
incidents, acute 407
Vasopressin 567
deficiency 241
Vecuronium 43, 48, 567
Veins 533
Venomous snakes of Kerala 452
Venoms and toxins 402
Venous blood gas 233, 307
Ventilation bags 61
Ventilator dyssynchrony 216
Ventilator parameters, disease-based 89*t*
Ventilator problems encountered 90
Ventilator settings, initial 486*t*
Ventilatory support
for hypoxia 74
types of 482
Ventricular assist devices 152
Ventricular fibrillation 23, 36*f*, 140
Ventricular tachycardia 36*f*, 140, 140*f*
management of 37*fc*
Venturi masks 60

Verbal output 172
Vessel wall defects 210
Vibrio cholerae 315
Vigabatrin 567
Vim-Silverman needle biopsy 549, 550, 552
Vincristine 192
Viral hepatitis 352, 359
Viral markers 307
Viral myocarditis 150, 155
   common organisms 150
   diagnosis of 151
   differential diagnosis 151
   investigations 151
   management of 152, 152*fc*
Viral pericarditis 155
Visceral perforation 552
Vision, blurring of 161
Visual screening in newborns 524
Vitamin
   A 275, 317
   B_{12} 267
   B_6 267
   D 275, 291
   K 275, 305, 471
      antagonists 416, 418
      injection 475
   K_1 564

Vomiting 227, 286, 464
von Willebrand disease 236, 390, 410

W

Warfarin 416, 451
Warm transport 519
WBCT *See* Whole blood clotting time
WBT *See* Whole blood transfusion
Weil syndrome 359
Wheeze 444
Whole blood transfusion 343, 387
Wilson's disease 306, 307
Wiskott-Aldrich syndrome 396
Wong-Baker faces pain 217*f*
World Health Organization 216, 272

X

Xylometazoline 567

Y

Yersinia 315

Z

Zinc 275, 451, 567
Zoonotic infection 358